Multidisciplinary Approach to Cancer Care

Guest Editors

Kimberly M. Brown, MD
Margo Shoup, MD, FACS

SURGICAL CLINICS OF NORTH AMERICA

www.surgical.theclinics.com

Consulting Editor
RONALD F. MARTIN, MD

February 2009 • Volume 89 • Number 1

SAUNDERS an imprint of ELSEVIER, Inc.

W.B. SAUNDERS COMPANY
A Division of Elsevier Inc.
1600 John F. Kennedy Blvd., Suite 1800, Philadelphia, PA 19103-2899
http://www.theclinics.com
SURGICAL CLINICS OF NORTH AMERICA Volume 89, Number 1
February 2009 ISSN 0039–6109, ISBN-10: 1-4377-0545-6, ISBN-13: 978-1-4377-0545-4
Editor: Catherine Bewick

This journal and the individual contributions contained in it are protected under copyright by Elsevier, and the following terms and conditions apply to their use:

Photocopying

Single photocopies of single articles may be made for personal use as allowed by national copyright laws. Permission of the Publisher and payment of a fee is required for all other photocopying, including multiple or systematic copying, copying for advertising or promotional purposes, resale, and all forms of document delivery. Special rates are available for educational institutions that wish to make photocopies for non-profit educational classroom use. For information on how to seek permission visit www.elsevier.com/permissions or call: (+44) 1865 843830 (UK)/(+1) 215 239 3804 (USA).

Derivative Works

Subscribers may reproduce tables of contents or prepare lists of articles including abstracts for internal circulation within their institutions. Permission of the Publisher is required for resale or distribution outside the institution. Permission of the Publisher is required for all other derivative works, including compilations and translations (please consult www.elsevier.com/permissions).

Electronic Storage or Usage

Permission of the Publisher is required to store or use electronically any material contained in this journal, including any article or part of an article (please consult www.elsevier.com/permissions). Except as outlined above, no part of this publication may be reproduced, stored in a retrieval system or transmitted in any form or by any means, electronic, mechanical, photocopying, recording or otherwise, without prior written permission of the Publisher.

Notice

No responsibility is assumed by the Publisher for any injury and/or damage to persons or property as a matter of products liability, negligence or otherwise, or from any use or operation of any methods, products, instructions or ideas contained in the material herein. Because of rapid advances in the medical sciences, in particular, independent verification of diagnoses and drug dosages should be made.

Although all advertising material is expected to conform to ethical (medical) standards, inclusion in this publication does not constitute a guarantee or endorsement of the quality or value of such product or of the claims made of it by its manufacturer.

Surgical Clinics of North America (ISSN 0039–6109) is published bimonthly by Elsevier Inc., 360 Park Avenue South, New York, NY 10010-1710. Months of publication are February, April, June, August, October, and December. Business and Editorial Offices: 1600 John F. Kennedy Blvd., Suite 1800, Philadelphia, PA 19103-2899. Customer Service Office: 6277 Sea Harbor Drive, Orlando, FL 32887-4800. Periodicals postage paid at New York, NY and additional mailing offices. Subscription prices are $269.00 per year for US individuals, $432.00 per year for US institutions, $134.00 per year for US students and residents, $330.00 per year for Canadian individuals, $537.00 per year for Canadian institutions, $371.00 for international individuals, $537.00 per year for international institutions and $185.00 per year for Canadian and foreign students/residents. To receive student/resident rate, orders must be accompanied by name of affiliated institution, date of term, and the *signature* of program/residency coordinator on institution letterhead. Orders will be billed at individual rate until proof of status is received. Foreign air speed delivery is included in all *Clinics* subscription prices. All prices are subject to change without notice. POSTMASTER: Send address changes to *Surgical Clinics*, Elsevier Periodicals Customer Service, 11830 Westline Industrial Drive, St. Louis, MO 63146. **Customer Service: 1-800-654-2452 (US). From outside of the United States, call 1-314-453-7041. Fax: 1-314-453-5170. E-mail: JournalsCustomerService-usa@elsevier.com (for print support), journalsonlinesupport-usa@elsevier.com (for online support).**

Reprints. For copies of 100 or more, of articles in this publication, please contact the Commercial Reprints Department, Elsevier Inc., 360 Park Avenue South, New York, New York 10010-1710. Tel. (212) 633-3812, Fax: (212) 462-1935, e-mail: reprints@elsevier.com.

The Surgical Clinics of North America is also published in Spanish by McGraw-Hill Interamericana Editores S.A., P.O. Box 5-237 06500 Mexico D.F. Mexico; and in Portuguese by Interlivros Edicoes Ltda., Rua Comandante Coelho 1085, CEP 21250, Rio de Janeiro, Brazil; and in Greek by Paschalidis Medical Publications, Athens Greece.

The Surgical Clinics of North America is covered in *MEDLINE/PubMed (Index Medicus)*, *EMBASE/Excerpta Medica*, *Current Contents/Clinical Medicine*, *Current Contents/Life Sciences*, *Science Citation Index*, and *ISI/BIOMED*.

Printed and bound by CPI Group (UK) Ltd, Croydon, CR0 4YY

Transferred to Digital Print 2011

Contributors

CONSULTING EDITOR

RONALD F. MARTIN, MD
Staff Surgeon, Marshfield Clinic, Marshfield; and Clinical Associate Professor, University of Wisconsin School of Medicine and Public Health, Madison, Wisconsin; Lieutenant Colonel, Medical Corps, United States Army Reserve

GUEST EDITORS

KIMBERLY M. BROWN, MD
Assistant Professor, University of Missouri-Kansas City; Section of Surgical Oncology, Saint Luke's Hospital, Kansas City, Missouri

MARGO SHOUP, MD, FACS
Associate Professor of Surgery, Loyola University Medical Center; Chief, Division of Surgical Oncology, Loyola University Medical Center, Maywood, Illinois

AUTHORS

GERARD J. ABOOD, MD, MS
Resident, Department of General Surgery, Loyola University Medical Center, Maywood, Illinois

GLEN BALCH, MD
Assistant Professor of Surgery, Department of Surgery, Northwestern University Feinberg School of Medicine, NorthShore University HealthSystem, Evanston, Illinois

KIMBERLY M. BROWN, MD
Assistant Professor of Surgery, University of Missouri-Kansas City; Section of Surgical Oncology, Saint Luke's Hospital, Kansas City, Missouri

COURTNEY L. BUI, MD
Radiation Oncology, Cancer Care Associates, St. Luke's Hospital & Health Network, Bethlehem, Pennsylvania

RICHARD CHENEY, MD
Professor of Oncology, Department of Pathology and Laboratory Medicine, Roswell Park Cancer Institute, Buffalo, New York

MARK S. CHOH, MD
Resident, Department of General Surgery, Rush University Medical Center; and Fellow, Department of Minimally Invasive and Robotic Surgery, University of Illinois-Chicago, Chicago, Illinois

RONALD P. DEMATTEO, MD
Vice Chair, Department of Surgery, Memorial Sloan-Kettering Cancer Center, New York, New York

DARIUS C. DESAI, MD
Division of Surgical Oncology, St. Luke's Hospital and Health Network, Bethlehem, Pennsylvania

AILEEN GO, MD
Fellow, Division of Hematology and Oncology, Loyola University Medical Center, Cardinal Bernardin Cancer Center, Maywood, Illinois

CAPRICE C. GREENBERG, MD, MPH
Instructor in Surgery, Department of Surgery, Brigham and Women's Hospital; Center for Surgery and Public Health, Brigham and Women's Hospital; and Center for Outcomes and Policy Research, Dana-Farber Cancer Institute, Boston, Massachusetts

NORA M. HANSEN, MD
Department of Surgery, Northwestern University Feinberg School of Medicine; Lynn Sage Comprehensive Breast Center; and Robert H. Lurie Comprehensive Cancer Center, Chicago, Illinois

SARAH E. HOFFE, MD
Assistant Professor of Radiation Oncology, Department of Radiation Oncology, Moffitt Cancer Center and Research Institute, Tampa, Florida

MELISSA C. HULVAT, MD
Department of Surgery, Northwestern University Feinberg School of Medicine; Lynn Sage Comprehensive Breast Center; and Robert H. Lurie Comprehensive Cancer Center, Chicago, Illinois

DAVID P. JAQUES, MD
Professor of Surgery, Department of Surgery, Washington University School of Medicine; and Vice-President, Barnes-Jewish Hospital, St. Louis, Missouri

JACQUELINE S. JERUSS, MD, PhD
Department of Surgery, Northwestern University Feinberg School of Medicine; Lynn Sage Comprehensive Breast Center; and Robert H. Lurie Comprehensive Cancer Center, Chicago, Illinois

ROBERT J. KENNEY, DO
Resident, Department of Surgery, University of Missouri, Kansas City, Kansas City, Missouri

T. PETER KINGHAM, MD
Fellow, Department of Surgery, Memorial Sloan-Kettering Cancer Center, New York, New York

WILLIAM KRAYBILL, MD
Professor of Surgery, Department of Surgery, University of Missouri, Kansas City, Kansas City, Missouri

MIRIAM N. LANGO, MD
Associate Member, Department of Surgical Oncology, Head and Neck Section Fox Chase Cancer Center; and Assistant Professor, Department of Otolaryngology, Temple University Hospital, Philadelphia, Pennsylvania

JAMES A. MADURA II, MD
Attending Surgeon, Department of Surgery, John H. Stroger Hospital of Cook County; and Associate Professor of Surgery, Department of General Surgery, Rush University Medical Center, Chicago, Illinois

DEEPAK MALHOTRA, MD
Assistant Professor, Division of Hematology and Oncology, Loyola University Medical Center, Cardinal Bernardin Cancer Center, Maywood, Illinois

KENNETH L. MEREDITH, MD
Assistant Professor of Surgery, Department of Gastrointestinal Oncology, Moffitt Cancer Center and Research Institute, Tampa, Florida

THOMAS J. MINER, MD
Assistant Professor, Associate Program Director, Director, Surgical Oncology, Department of Surgery, The Alpert Medical School of Brown University, Rhode Island Hospital, Providence, Rhode Island

AUNDREA OLIVER, MD
Surgical Resident, Department of Surgery, Brigham and Women's Hospital, Boston, Massachusetts

LEE B. RILEY, MD, PhD
Medical Director, Oncology Service Line, Section Chief of Surgical Oncology, St. Luke's Hospital and Health Network, Bethlehem, Pennsylvania

RODERICK M. QUIROS, MD
Surgical Oncology, Cancer Care Associates, St. Luke's Hospital & Health Network, Bethlehem, Pennsylvania

DAVID SHIBATA, MD, FACS
Associate Professor of Surgery, Head, Section of Colorectal Oncology, Department of Gastrointestinal Oncology, Moffitt Cancer Center and Research Institute, Tampa, Florida

MARGO SHOUP, MD, FACS
Associate Professor of Surgery, Loyola University Medical Center; Chief, Division of Surgical Oncology, Loyola University Medical Center, Maywood, Illinois

MARGARET A. STULL, MD
Director of Musculoskeletal Imaging, Department of Diagnostic Radiology, St. Luke's Hospital of Kansas City; and Clinical Associate Professor of Radiology, University of Missouri – Kansas City School of Medicine, Kansas City, Missouri

ALAN A. THOMAY, MD
Surgical Resident, Department of Surgery, The Alpert Medical School of Brown University, Rhode Island Hospital, Providence, Rhode Island

SHARON WEBER, MD
University of Wisconsin Department of Surgery, Clinical Science Center, Madison, Wisconsin

DAVID J. WINCHESTER, MD
Professor of Surgery and Chief, Division of Surgical Oncology and General Surgery, Department of Surgery, Northwestern University Feinberg School of Medicine, NorthShore University HealthSystem, Evanston, Illinois

BRETT YAMANE, MD
Department of Surgery, University of Wisconsin, Clinical Science Center, Madison, Wisconsin

KATHARINE YAO, MD
Assistant Professor of Surgery, Department of Surgery, Northwestern University Feinberg School of Medicine, NorthShore University HealthSystem, Evanston, Illinois

Contents

> The sequencing of the human genome and the ability to rapidly identify genes and proteins, both normal and mutant, that are involved in tumorigenesis and malignant phenotypes, have changed the ability to understand malignant cells. Understanding and applying this information to the diagnosis and treatment of cancer are facilitated best with a multidisciplinary team. The cancer surgeon plays a pivotal role in this team. This article briefly summarizes: (1) the clinically relevant applications of molecular biology to the cancer surgeon, (2) the current understanding of the molecular basis for cancer, and (3) the current targeted agents and their clinical applications.

> An important component of quality healthcare is that it be patient-centered with a focus on the patient, including his or her preferences, values, and beliefs. The goal of this article is to provide a broad overview of patient-centered outcomes in oncologic research. It starts with an introduction to the different types of patient-centered measures including patient satisfaction, decision regret, patient preference, and health-related quality of life. It then offers an overview of survey instrument design and selection. Finally, it provides examples of existing approaches to measurement and previously validated instruments for each type of patient-centered outcome.

> This article provides an overview of the approach to patients who may benefit from palliative care. While the article's details lend themselves

to the treatment of complications secondary to advanced malignancies, the data herein can also be extrapolated to other chronic, terminal diseases. Guidelines for patient selection are discussed, using currently available outcomes data as a platform for the critical decision making process. Suggestions for a multidisciplinary team approach are offered, using the palliative triangle as the ideal model of communication and cooperation. Finally, methods for measuring success are detailed, along with proposals for how to better equip the surgeons of tomorrow with the knowledge and experience needed to tackle these difficult and intimate problems.

Head and neck cancers are relatively less common tumors, but with complex anatomic and physiologic relationships to the structures from which they arise. Multimodal management is required for advanced stage disease, while single modality treatment is usually sufficient for early lesions. Treatment paradigms have shifted toward more functional preservation of speech and swallowing, when possible. Increased use of radiation, systemic/targeted therapies and function-preserving surgical approaches have allowed for organ preservation without compromising oncologic outcomes in properly selected patients.

This article reviews the use of minimally invasive surgical and endoscopic techniques in the field of surgical oncology. It reviews the indications and techniques of the use of minimally invasive surgery for several oncologic indications in general surgery. In particular, it reviews the currently published literature discussing the oncologic outcomes of these techniques.

The incidence of esophageal and gastric malignancies has increased over the last decade. Historically, surgery has been considered the best treatment for these cancers. However, long-term survival after surgery is fair at best, because of the tendency of disease to recur locally and distantly. Presently, the management of these cancers involves surgery, chemotherapy, and radiation therapy. This article discusses various treatment strategies that employ these modalities either alone or in combination, in an attempt to improve survival rates for patients who have gastroesophageal malignancies.

Colorectal cancer liver metastases and hepatocellular carcinoma remain significant health problems in the United States and worldwide. Although surgical resection is often the treatment of choice, patient comorbidities or disease extent may preclude this option. Alternative approaches to primary and secondary hepatic malignancies have been developed, and their impact on disease control has been the subject of much recent study. These therapies can be administered alone but can also be effective when used in combination, or with other chemotherapeutic regimens. This article reviews the different techniques of liver-directed therapy and the available literature on short- and long-term outcomes.

Tumors of the pancreas and biliary tree remain formidable challenges to patients and clinicians. These tumors elude early detection, rapidly spread locally and systemically, and frequently recur despite apparently complete resection. Cystic tumors of the pancreas, however, may represent a subset of patients who do not uniformly require aggressive resection, and a thoughtful, evidence-based approach to work-up allows for the rational application of surgical therapy. Increasing evidence supports treating patients who have pancreaticobiliary disease in a multidisciplinary setting.

The care of patients with breast cancer has become increasingly complex with advancements in diagnostic modalities, surgical approaches, and adjuvant treatments. A multidisciplinary approach to breast cancer care is essential to the successful integration of available therapies. This article addresses the key components of multidisciplinary breast cancer care, with a special emphasis on new and emerging approaches over the past 10 years in the fields of diagnostics, surgery, radiation, medical oncology, and plastic surgery.

Advancements have been made in multiple aspects of diagnostic and therapeutic approaches to rectal cancer. These advances include clinical staging such as endorectal ultrasound and pelvic MRI, surgical approaches such as transanal excision, and adjuvant treatments such as new chemotherapeutic agents and refined radiotherapy techniques. Optimal patient outcomes depend on multidisciplinary involvement for tailored therapy. The successful management of rectal cancer requires a multidisciplinary approach, with treatment decisions based on precise patient evaluations by a group of clinicians, including surgeons, gastroenterologists, medical and radiation oncologists, radiologists, and pathologists. The accurate identification of patients who are candidates for combined modality treatment is particularly essential to optimize outcomes. Technical and technologic advances have led to the availability of a wide range of surgical approaches for managing rectal cancer. Concomitantly, similar critical developments and refinements have also occurred in the administration of radiation and chemotherapeutic agents. This article provides an overview of the multimodal treatment of patients who have rectal cancer, with a focus on staging, surgical techniques, and the application of chemotherapy or radiation in the adjuvant and neoadjuvant settings.

Gastrointestinal stromal tumor (GIST) has been recognized as a unique tumor only in the last decade. Although rare as a clinical entity, there is much interest in the pathology and treatment because the *KIT* protooncogene mutation common to most GISTs can be inhibited by imatinib mesylate. Diagnosing and treating GIST requires a multidisciplinary approach, given the combination of pathologic and radiographic evaluation, surgical treatment, and oncologic care required to successfully treat patients with GIST.

This article reviews the current state of diagnosis and treatment of soft tissue sarcomas. Etiology, staging, imaging, tissue sampling, and current treatment are all reviewed using updated references. Current standards for surgical treatment are emphasized and the future directions of treatment addressed.

Neuroendocrine tumors of the pancreas comprise a class of rare tumors that can be associated with symptoms of hormone overproduction. Five distinct clinical endocrinopathies are associated with neuroendocrine tumors; however, most of these tumors remain asymptomatic and follow an indolent course. Complete surgical resection offers the only hope for cure, but understanding the basic biology of the tumors has advanced the medical management in metastatic disease. Surgical resection of hepatic metastases offers survival advantage and should be performed when feasible. Although hepatic artery embolization is currently the preferred mode of nonsurgical palliation for pain and hormonal symptoms, other modalities may play a role in metastatic disease.

This article covers the multidisciplinary treatment of primary melanoma. Excision margins and the need for sentinel lymphadenectomy are mainly dictated by the Breslow thickness although exceptions to this dictum do exist. Interferon is the only FDA approved adjuvant therapy for high risk melanoma although its overall survival benefit is minimal. Trials examining different doses or duration of interferon therapy have not demonstrated any promising survival data so far. There have been several randomized vaccine trials for melanoma but none have shown an overall survival benefit. Research into T-cell regulation continues and will hopefully bring promise for the future of melanoma treatment.

THE CLINICS ARE NOW AVAILABLE ONLINE!

Access your subscription at:
www.theclinics.com

Foreword

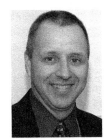

Ronald F. Martin, MD
Consulting Editor

"Biology is the king, case selection is the queen, and the technical maneuvers undertaken are the princes and princesses of the realm."
—*Blake Cady, MD Presidential Address to the Society of Surgical Oncology, 1988*

Several years ago, Blake Cady, Ricardo Rossi, and I co-edited an issue of the *Surgical Clinics of North America* entitled "Multidisciplinary Approach to Cancer." It was an extremely valuable and rewarding experience for me for many reasons, but chief among them was being able to work with two phenomenal surgeons whom I respect enormously as we tried to outline how we surgeons fit into the "big picture" of patient care. Since that time, there have been such sufficient developments and changes in our approach as a team that we felt it necessary to revisit this topic—not only for the freshness of the information but also because of the overwhelming relevance of the topic on so many levels.

Much of the history of surgery is attributed to the efforts of great individuals (some of that credit is justly deserved, while in some cases it may belong to another unnamed individual or, more likely, other groups of people). Yet, despite that, history seems to over-attribute credit and blame to specific individuals. I cite, for example, sports, war, economics, and politics as matters in which credit and blame are distributed in a nonproportional manner to worthiness. But, if anything distinguishes the current era of health care delivery from the past, it would be that the successes of exceptional people who deliver excellent care are due to the coordinated efforts of groups, instead of the heroic efforts of isolated individuals. Please do not mistake me; I do not want to diminish the impact of the highly motivated individual (especially to a collection of surgeons). But if we truly check our egos at the door, then we will realize how dependent we have become on the efforts of others to achieve our own needs.

It was not so long ago that it was considered a surgical dictum that when dealing with cancer, the surgeon was the "captain of the ship." I am not sure that all of our

Surg Clin N Am 89 (2009) xiii–xiv
doi:10.1016/j.suc.2009.01.003
0039-6109/09/$ – see front matter © 2009 Elsevier Inc. All rights reserved.

surgical.theclinics.com

nonsurgical colleagues always agreed with that sentiment, but I was certainly taught that philosophy. Today, it comes as no surprise that such a comparison is no longer sensible when the captain is "off the ship" most nights, and the ship is staffed largely by other captains. The days of surgeons "always" being on call for "their" patients have long since passed and have evolved into group coverage and shared responsibility. Also, one would be hard pressed to find a non-surgeon physician who thinks that he or she works "for" a surgeon. And, since the division of labor is a time-honored tenet of advancing civilizations, it would also stand to reason that combining our expertise might benefit us as well. However, accepting the notion that we no longer live in the "one riot, one ranger" era of surgery should not cause us to abdicate our responsibility to be valued members, or often leaders, of the team.

Effective leadership and team membership in the care of patients who have cancer requires both an excellent knowledge of one's own skill set as well as a good fundamental knowledge of the skills of the other team members. We might not strive to be an expert in our colleagues' matters, but we cannot abandon our need to speak their languages fluently and with understanding (for those of you who may be considering certifying board exams, you may rest assured that an understanding of theses ideas is not considered frivolous by most examiners).

As the treatment of other life-ending diseases becomes more effective (such as atherosclerotic coronary artery disease), the likelihood is that the incidence and prevalence of neoplastic diseases will increase along with other "chronic" illnesses. This, of course, will be a matter of increasing national economic significance. The advances in therapeutic intervention will need to be measured not only on their efficacy but also on their relative cost-effectiveness and trade-off value against other disease treatments and social priorities.

When a patient who has cancer comes to us, he or she is often terrified. This can lead us in two directions: to care for the patient as well as treat the disease, or to treat the disease and lose sight of what the patient really wants or needs. People who are terrified can be easily convinced of many things; we must be as certain as possible that we are putting the needs of the patient first and be honest with them as well as with ourselves of what we can and cannot accomplish. While we must maintain our proud history of avoiding nihilism and shrinking from difficult challenges when confronting such devastating illness, we must also remember to care for patients—as least as much as we hate cancer, but preferably more.

As always, the path to good decision making begins with good information and knowledgeable analysis. Drs. Brown and Shoup have assembled an excellent collection of articles for your consideration. It is an excellent place to begin but we must never forget—biology is king.

Ronald F. Martin, MD
Department of Surgery
Marshfield Clinic
1000 North Oak Avenue
Marshfield, WI 54449, USA

E-mail address:
martin.ronald@marshfieldclinic.org

Preface

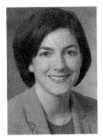 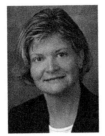

Kimberly M. Brown, MD   Margo Shoup, MD, FACS
Guest Editors

Since the last issue of *Surgical Clinics of North America* on the multidisciplinary approach to cancer care was published in April of 2000, the field of oncology has continued to evolve in the understanding of the biology of cancer and how biology impacts the treatment strategy in a given patient. The dynamics of this relationship are described in this issue's article by Drs. Riley and Desai. Advancements in surgery, radiation, and chemotherapy have occurred across the spectrum of malignancies, and, as a result, cancer care is more frequently delivered in the setting of a multidisciplinary team of physicians. More and more evidence accumulates that suggests patients may be better served when cared for under a multidisciplinary paradigm. Furthermore, for certain complex tumor types such as pancreas and esophagus, patient outcomes may be improved when they receive care in higher-volume referral centers.

The concept of outcomes for cancer patients has expanded beyond the traditional endpoints of overall survival and disease-free survival, as discussed in the article by Drs. Oliver and Greenberg. Organ preservation, quality of life, pain control, and other patient-centered outcomes are now used in the comprehensive assessment of the quality of cancer care. Newer tools to reproducibly measure these outcomes have been developed and continue to be tailored and improved. In addition, palliation may be a treatment goal for those patients in whom a cure is not a realistic outcome. The field of palliative care is a relatively new one, and Dr. Thomay and colleagues discuss the approach to palliative care within the framework of the palliative triangle.

Surgeons maintain a central role in the treatment of many types of cancer, often assuming a leadership position in the decision-making team. Therefore, it is critical for surgeons to have a comprehensive knowledge of the treatment modalities employed in the multidisciplinary approach to cancer care. Well-designed studies have shown that less invasive treatments can yield comparable oncologic outcomes to more radical treatments, allowing for organ preservation. One example includes treating certain early-stage squamous cell cancers of the upper aerodigestive tract with radiation instead of surgery, as discussed by Dr. Lango in this issue. Minimally invasive treatment may extend to local therapies, such as radiofrequency ablation in the liver or trans-anal local excision for early-stage rectal cancer, sparing patients larger surgeries or allowing for sphincter preservation.

Surg Clin N Am 89 (2009) xv–xvi
doi:10.1016/j.suc.2009.01.002
0039-6109/09/$ – see front matter

Another impact of tumor biology on treatment strategy is the alteration of the order in which treatments are traditionally delivered. Chemotherapy or chemoradiotherapy prior to surgery may be employed in cancers of the esophagus, stomach, breast, liver, pancreas, or rectum, with the goals of decreasing the risk of positive margins, allowing for less radical surgery, serving as an "in vivo assay" of the effectiveness of the treatment (alternatively the behavior of the tumor), or realizing a benefit in overall or disease-specific survival.

The ultimate application of our increasing understanding of tumor biology is seen in the development and tailoring of targeted agents to patient- or tumor-specific factors. Targeted agents, such as imatinib for the treatment of gastrointestinal stromal tumors (GIST), represent an entirely new era in the delivery of optimally effective therapy with fewer side effects. Assessing tumor characteristics for particular gene expression such as Her2/Neu or mutations such as exon-11 mutation in GIST that render the tumor most susceptible to imatinib also allows for more specific selection of therapies most likely to be effective in a given patient.

As surgeons and other providers for cancer patients move forward, it is clear that tumor biology will play an increasing role in cancer-related research and clinical decision making. Surgery remains a cornerstone in the treatment of many cancer types, but the application of this therapy and the anticipated outcomes may be influenced by the underlying tumor biology, and an understanding of this can contribute to appropriate patient selection for surgery. The selection of patients for clinical trials may include stratification for underlying tumor characteristics, which may affect decisions such as whether to obtain a preoperative tissue diagnosis. Finally, with more widespread use of an ever-expanding array of preoperative therapies, it is important for surgeons to understand the impact these agents have on perioperative decisions. For example, operative timing may be influenced by the administration of bevacizumab, which has been associated with increased bleeding complications in certain situations.

Oncology is evolving as a multi-disciplinary field, and it is more important than ever that surgeons have a familiarity with other disciplines involved in cancer care. The articles presented in this issue of *Surgical Clinics of North America* serve to update the practicing surgeon on the recent changes in the multidisciplinary approach to cancer care.

Kimberly M. Brown, MD
Department of Surgery
University of Missouri—Kansas City
Saint Luke's Hospital
4401 Wornall Road
Suite 420
Kansas City, MO 64108, USA

Margo Shoup, MD, FACS
Department of Surgery
Loyola University
2160 South First Avenue
Building 110
Maywood, IL 60153, USA

E-mail addresses:
kbrown4@saint-lukes.org (K.M. Brown)
mshoup@lumc.edu (M. Shoup)

The Molecular Basis of Cancer and the Development of Targeted Therapy

Lee B. Riley, MD, PhD[a],*, Darius C. Desai, MD[b]

KEYWORDS

- Targeted • Molecular • Genomic oncogenes
- Epigenetic • Breast tumor suppressor

The Human Genome Project started in 1990 as a 15-year program to sequence an estimated 3 billion base pairs and identify all human genes. Because of rapid technological advances, the project was completed 2 years ahead of schedule and was published in 2003.[1,2] The genetic information provided by the project, the advanced technologies, and the creation of advanced bioinformatic systems forever changed the field of medical research. In addition to elucidating the origins and mechanisms of cancer development, the ability to screen, diagnose, image, and treat cancer have changed substantially. To appropriately manage cancer today, not only do surgeons, radiation oncologists, and medical oncologists need to understand cancer at the molecular level, but so do radiologists, pathologists, genetics counselors, and others. This article briefly summarizes three areas of interest to the surgeon: (1) clinically relevant applications of molecular biology to cancer screening, imaging, pathology, and treatment; (2) the current understanding of the molecular basis for cancer; and (3) a brief summary of the agents and uses of current targeted therapies.

THE SURGEON'S ROLE IN MOLECULAR ONCOLOGY

The surgeon always has played a cardinal role in coordinating the multidisciplinary management of most solid cancers. Additionally, because of anatomic considerations, the discipline of surgery formed disease-specific subspecialties (eg, neurologic, thoracic, urologic, gynecologic, colorectal) that facilitate the surgeon's ability to acquire a detailed understanding of a disease process and coordinate the care of specific cancer patients. This pivotal position heightens the need for the surgeon to

[a] St. Luke's Hospital and Health Network, 801 Ostrum Street, Bethlehem, PA 18015, USA
[b] Division of Surgical Oncology, St. Luke's Hospital and Health Network, 801 Ostrum Street, Bethlehem, PA 18015, USA
* Corresponding author.
E-mail address: rileyl@slhn.org (L.B. Riley).

Surg Clin N Am 89 (2009) 1–15
doi:10.1016/j.suc.2008.09.016
0039-6109/08/$ – see front matter © 2009 Elsevier Inc. All rights reserved.
surgical.theclinics.com

understand the molecular discoveries as they relate to screening, diagnosis, and the pre-, intra-, and postoperative management of cancer.

Molecular and Genetic Screening

There are several known genetic defects that are associated with elevated risks of cancer. Genetic tests to evaluate patients and their families are commercially available for several genes, including:

BRCA1 and BRCA2, which are associated with breast and ovarian cancer[3]

MLH1, MSH2, and MSH6, which are responsible for most hereditary forms of hereditary nonpolyposis colon cancer (HNPCC) and are associated with up to a 70% chance of endometrial cancer[4]

The APC and MYH genes, which cause the adenomatous polyposis syndromes[5]

The RET oncogene, which is responsible for medullary thyroid cancer in patients who have the multiple endocrine neoplasia type 2 syndrome[6]

Although these and other tests are used to direct prophylactic surgery, additional tests are being developed that will impact the surgical management of patients who have cancer and their family members.

MOLECULAR DIAGNOSIS AND PATHOLOGY

The radiologic detection of cancer based on anatomy (eg, CT) or physiology (positron emission tomography, PET) is known to the practicing physician; however, molecular imaging using various probes to detect tumor-specific molecules is finding its way into the clinical realm. Historically, radiolabeled antibodies have been used with some success to localize, image, and treat tumors. Molecular engineering has provided small antibody structures with improved pharmacokinetics that maintain the specificity of the original antibody. These radiolabeled minibodies have shown promise in preclinical models for both human epidermal growth factor (HER)-2neu and carcinoembryonic antigen localization.[7–9] Similarly, ^{18}F-labeled ligands like estradiol or dihydrotestosterone can detect estrogen or androgen receptors in patients who have breast or prostate cancer, respectively.[10,11] Other targets for molecular imaging include oncogenes, surface receptors, and angiogenic and apoptotic pathways. Akin to anatomic imaging, which measures responses to therapy, molecular imaging ultimately may be used to evaluate responses to chemotherapy or other treatments.

Perhaps more germane to the multidisciplinary cancer team is the field of molecular pathology. Traditionally, tumors have been characterized by their microscopic appearance. Additional immunohistochemical analysis has provided molecular characteristics of the tumor; the composite evaluation yields a global phenotype of the tumor. Recent advances in genomic technologies have allowed a more precise characterization of human cancers. One of the most useful approaches uses DNA microarray analysis to evaluate the entirety of gene expression within a tumor.[12] The application of microarrays to cancer has enhanced the understanding of the molecular architecture and heterogeneity of human cancers greatly and is improving how physicians diagnose, treat, and predict clinical outcomes.

Gene expression analysis using microarrays initially was shown to have clinical utility in patients with hematologic malignancies.[13] Subsequently, significant differences in gene expression patterns were shown between solid tumors from different primary sites. Focusing this technology on a single histology has allowed investigators to divide tumors into various subclasses with prognostic and therapeutic implications.[14] This perhaps is demonstrated best in breast tumors, which now classified into five subtypes (luminal A, luminal B, HER-2+/ER−, basal-like, and normal breast-like) that predict overall patient survival.[15,16] Similar analyses have identified gene expression patterns that are associated with prognosis in prostate cancer and lung cancer.[17,18] For example, patients who have stage 1A nonsmall cell lung cancer have up to a 25% chance of recurrence; gene expression profiles can reclassify these patients into those at low risk (with an estimated 5-year survival of 90%) and those at high risk (less than 20% 5-year survival).[18] Although this expression profile has not been validated in large trials, it offers considerable benefit, and similar profiles in breast cancer have been incorporated into clinical practice.[15,19] For an increasing number of cancers, appropriate management depends on a thorough understanding of the molecular basis of the disease, its diagnosis, and treatment. Participating in multidisciplinary teams to coordinate and provide this care will continue to be a benefit to surgeons and their patients.

MOLECULAR BASIS OF CANCER

The evolution from a normal cell to a metastatic cancer cell requires multiple genetic and epigenetic changes. Overall, there are at least three mechanisms that allow these changes to be transferred to the progeny of a cell undergoing malignant transformation: an inherited mutation, a somatic mutation, and methylation of the cell's DNA (**Fig. 1**, green arrows). These genetic events typically affect at least four pathways; however,

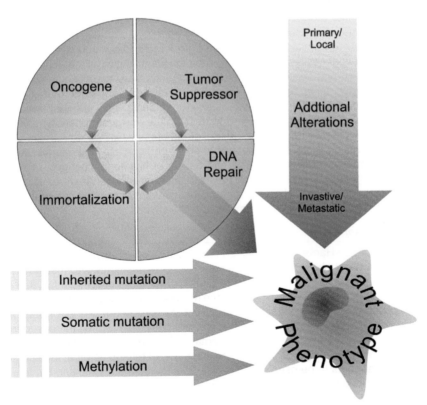

Fig. 1. Multistep evolution of the malignant phenotype (see text for description).

the order in which the genes are affected is not critical. For example, a mutation in a tumor suppressor gene may occur before a mutation in either an oncogene, or a gene involved in DNA repair (see **Fig. 1**, blue region). Although the changes represented in the blue and green regions of **Fig. 1** may result in a malignant cell, the biologic behavior of that cell can vary dramatically. Various additional alterations that involve interactions between the malignant cell and the surrounding stromal elements are needed for a cell to transition from well differentiated to poorly differentiated, or locally recurrent to aggressively metastatic. Conceptualizing a patient's tumor in the context of these categories may help the physician direct individualized diagnostic and therapeutic interventions for the patient and his or her family members.

Oncogenes

In the 1970's it was clear that there were several viruses closely associated with human cancers, including human papilloma virus associated with cervical carcinoma, Epstein-Barr virus associated with both Burkitt's lymphoma and nasopharyngeal carcinomas, and hepatitis B and C viruses closely associated with hepatocellular carcinomas (HCCs).[20] Although these viruses could account for as many as 20% of the tumors worldwide, most human cancers had no obvious associations with viruses, and it became accepted that mutant cellular genes were responsible for most cancers. In the 1970's, however, the experimental technologies for directly testing this hypothesis were not available. Shortly thereafter, Varmus and Bishop demonstrated that the oncogenic gene v-src and the Rous sarcoma virus originated from a normal cellular gene, the c-src gene.[21] This gene, termed a proto-oncogene, has the ability to become activated into a cancer-causing gene. Shortly after this discovery, several tumorigenic viruses were shown to have cellular oncogene correlates.[21] In the early 1980s, the ability to transfer DNA extracted from tumors to nontransformed cells to identify these oncogenes became feasible. After the identification of the Rous and sarcoma oncogenes, numerous other cellular oncogenes were identified.[22] As further transfection experiments ensued, it became increasingly apparent that a single gene seldom could transform normal cells into tumorigenic cells, and that frequently two or more genes seem to be required to develop the malignant phenotype.[23] This led to the development of a multistep model of tumorigenesis.[24]

This theory was consistent with that observed by pathologists who had discovered that tumor formation begins through a succession of histologic changes ultimately leading to malignancy. Over the ensuing years, numerous oncogenes were described, and investigators sought to characterize additional mutant genes that appeared to be involved with the progression of the malignant phenotype.

Tumor Suppressor Genes

Pioneering work by Harris first suggested the presence of genetic material that could suppress the tumor phenotype.[25] Using cell hybridization studies and fusing normal cells with malignant cells, he was able to demonstrate more often than not that the genes present in the normal cell suppress the malignant phenotype and subsequently hypothesized that cancer cells seemed to have lost the presence of these genes with tumor suppressive capability. These genes subsequently were termed tumor suppressor genes. Knudson, studying retinoblastoma, demonstrated the clinical impact of these tumor suppressor genes.[26] There are two forms of retinoblastoma, the sporadic form, which appears to be caused exclusively by somatic mutations, and the familial form, which appears to be caused by transmission of a mutated gene in the germ line. The retinoblastoma gene ultimately paved the way for the identification of various tumor suppressor genes that are distributed throughout the cellular genome and have a spectrum of physiologic functions united by their ability to impact cellular proliferation in a negative way. In contrast to the identification of oncogenes, the identification of tumor suppressor genes has been more difficult; however, based on experiments in loss of heterozygosity, it is anticipated that several dozen additional tumor suppressor genes ultimately will be identified.[27]

Genomic Instability

Pathologic observations suggest that the transformation to a full-blown malignancy requires multiple steps, presumably each associated with a mutational event.[24] These random mutational events occur with an estimated frequency of approximately one per-million divisions. The infrequent nature of these random events and the need to have mutations in several specific genes within the same cell suggest that people rarely should develop cancers. This is inconsistent with published incidences. The high incidence is easy to explain in families with inherited mutations of tumor suppressor genes; however, this does not explain the observed incidence in nonfamilial cancers. The observation that the rate of mutations increases throughout a tumor's pathogenesis suggests that other mechanisms promote cancer development. Phenotypically, this genomic instability appears to be a characteristic of many human malignancies.[28] There are at least six pathways of DNA repair that can be disrupted to account for the observed genomic instability.[29] These pathways differ in their ability to repair specific DNA bases and DNA cross-links. Different histologies depend on different repair mechanisms. Patients who have xeroderma pigmentosum (XP), for example, are unable to repair ultraviolet radiation induced pyrimidine dimers. These mutations subsequently are transmitted to the daughter cells, and this ultimately leads to a high rate of skin tumors, including squamous cell carcinomas and melanomas.[30] There are several different defects in the mismatch repair system in patients who have HNPCC, and each defect appears to be associated with a unique histologic subtype.[31] Other defects in DNA repair are found in patients who have ataxia telangiectasia, and more recent evidence suggests that BRCA-1 and BRCA-2, originally thought to be tumor suppressor genes, are involved in repair of double-stranded DNA breaks.[32] Investigators continue to unravel the implications of DNA repair defects. Although it remains unclear why defects in HNPCC only affect intestinal histologies or why BRCA-1/BRCA-2 mutations result in tumors restricted to breast and ovarian histologies, it is becoming clear that DNA repair defects participate in most human tumors.

Cellular Immortality

Normal cellular populations have a finite ability to replicate. A control system limits the number of cell divisions, starting in the embryonic stage and continuing through differentiation and senescence. This effect is achieved through the specialized ends of the DNA (telomeres), which shorten with each division. Once the telomeric DNA is gone, the unprotected chromosomal ends fuse to one another, leading to cell death.[33] Cancer cells overcome this regulatory system by activating or increasing the expression of a telomerase enzyme, which maintains the telomeric length. This telomeric activity is present in approximately 90% of human tumors and virtually absent in normal tissues.[34] Specifically, the telomerase gene, hTERT, is not itself mutated, but its expression is increased by several mechanisms, including activated oncogenes like MYC.[35] Consequently, increased activation of the hTERT gene is one more common step leading to a malignant phenotype.

Loss of Gene Function

Clearly, there are several genes that need to be inactivated or altered for a cell to ultimately undergo malignant transformation. These alterations can occur through several mechanisms. Direct somatic mutation occurs with many oncogenes and is one such mechanism, whereas deletion of a tumor suppressor gene is another. Both of these mutations can be passed on to cellular progeny. Another mechanism that regulates the genetic function of cellular progeny, but does not involve a somatic mutation, is DNA methylation. This regulatory system adds methyl groups to cytidine residues within the promoters of various genes. When a segment of DNA containing a methylated cytidine residue is replicated, the new DNA strand also is methylated rapidly by a series of enzymes. In this way, genes can be inactivated in a heritable fashion without any change to the actual nucleotide sequence. DNA methylation plays a substantial role in the development of cancer; several studies have demonstrated that tumor suppressor genes and DNA repair genes are more frequently inactivated through DNA methylation than mutation.[36]

Nongenetic Mechanisms that Accelerate Tumor Progression

The progressive alteration of normal cellular genomes through oncogenic activation, inactivation of tumor suppressor genes, increased expression of hTERT, and loss of DNA repair mechanisms all lead to an increased capacity for unregulated proliferation (see Fig. 1). It is the ability of cancer cells to invade neighboring tissues and metastasize throughout the body, which results in most cancer-related mortalities. The complexity and number of mutations needed to create a successful metastatic cell that can survive in histologically different tissues are thought to require additional diverse mutations. Although considerable evidence suggests this, other research indicates an alternative or complimentary mechanism. This alternative process, referred to as "epithelial–mesenchymal transition" (EMT), is a normal embryologic process, whereby epithelial cells undergo rapid differentiation and acquire a mesenchymal phenotype, including the properties of motility and invasion.[37] Several transcription factors activated in embryogenesis, including Snail, Slug, and Twist, are capable of facilitating this normal invasive activity. Recent evidence indicates that cancer cells use these embryonic pathways to affect most steps needed to acquire the invasive metastatic phenotype.[37,38] Additional work suggests that the signals that induce the EMT are derived from activated stromal elements present in the primary tumor. Consequently, the numerous mutations required for metastatic potential can, for some tumors, occur rapidly, through these normal embryologic pathways.

Invasive and Metastatic Phenotypes

The use EMT pathways by neoplastic cells can expedite the metastatic phenotype but does not necessarily impart the ability of these cells to colonize and expand in different histologic sites. This requires additional properties, including the ability to successfully interact with surrounding stromal elements and stimulate the development of new blood vessels. Without neovascularization, tumor growth is limited to an area of approximately 1 mm in diameter. Angiogenesis depends on a complex coordination of cytokines and cells, including existing endothelial cells, macrophages, myofibroblasts, neutrophils, and recruited pericytes and angioblasts.[39] Some of these processes can be induced by the local disturbance of surrounding elements; however, some tumor cells can facilitate these processes by secreting various cytokines themselves. Many of these pathways and those described previously have been characterized sufficiently well so that targeted agents exist or can be developed to specifically abrogate the malignant cell.

TARGETED MOLECULAR AGENTS

Agents used in targeted cancer therapy interfere with specific receptors and signaling pathways that promote tumor cell growth. These agents include monoclonal antibodies and small molecule tyrosine kinase inhibitors (TKIs). The receptor tyrosine kinase family includes: epidermal growth factor (EGF), epidermal growth factor receptor (EGFR), vascular endothelial growth factor receptor (VEGFR), and platelet-derived growth factor receptor (PDGFR) families. The therapeutic agents inhibit receptor tyrosine kinase signaling by binding to the extracellular component of the growth receptors. They can bind the ligand that triggers the receptor or bind intracellular sites that interfere with downstream signaling events. The toxicity profiles of targeted agents differ substantially from those of standard chemotherapy, because they do not interfere with DNA replication.[40]

Targeted Therapy Against the Endothelial Growth Factor Receptor

EGFR is a glycoprotein receptor that belongs to the HER family of receptors.[41] Four membranes of this family have been identified: EGFR, HER-2, HER-3, and HER-4. The main ligand for EGFR and EGF is transforming growth factor beta (TGFβ). Activation of EGFR is complex. Intracellular signaling occurs after receptor activation leads to formation of hetero- and homo-dimers with other members of the EGFR receptor family, including HER-2, HER-3, and HER-4. Subsequent autophosphorylation of the EGFR tyrosine kinase activates downstream signaling. Multiple pathways are involved. Mutation or overexpression of the EGFR can stimulate proliferation, apoptosis, angiogenesis, and metastasis.[41,42] Although both monoclonal antibodies and small molecule TKIs target the same receptor, their mechanisms of action may differ. Antibodies inhibit the EGFR signaling pathways, whereas TKIs work intracellularly. This difference also can lead to different toxicity profiles.

Cetuximab (Erbitux,) is one of two antibodies against EGFR. Once it binds to EGFR, the receptor is internalized and degraded without receptor phosphorylation. This leads to down-regulation of the receptor at the cell surface, inhibits tumor cell proliferation, induces apoptosis, and augments radiosensitivity.[43] HER-1 is overexpressed in 60% to 80% of colorectal cancers. Cetuximab is effective against colorectal cancer, has promising activity in head and neck cancer, and is synergistic with radiation therapy.[44] One of its clinical adverse effects is a characteristic rash that commonly develops over the trunk and face.

Panitumumab (Vectibix), is a fully humanized antibody against EFGR; therefore, it is not neutralized by immune reactions against murine components. It blocks ligand binding and causes receptor internalization, but not degradation.[45]

Gefitinib (Iressa) inhibits the EGFR by blocking the intracellular ATP binding domain and inhibits EGFR tyrosine kinase activity 100% more than other TKIs. Considering the lack of impressive clinical data on this agent, its use is limited to second- and third-line treatment of nonsmall cell lung cancer.[40]

Erlotinib (Tarceva) reversibly inhibits the wild-type EGFR receptor and is approved for metastatic nonsmall cell lung cancer and metastatic pancreatic cancer.

Trastuzumab (Herceptin) affects the HER-2 family of receptors and is indicated for metastatic breast cancer that overexpresses HER-2. It also is given in the adjuvant setting. There is a significant cardiac risk associated with trastuzumab, which is not associated with other targeted agents.

Lapatinib (Tykerb) has dual activity on EGFR and HER-2 receptors, and because it is not cross-resistant with trastuzumab, it is available for use as a second-line agent in the treatment of metastatic HER-2 positive breast carcinoma.

Targeted Therapy Against Vascular Endothelial Growth Factor Receptor

Vascular growth factors stimulate blood vessel formation. VEGF is produced by normal and neoplastic cells and regulates angiogenesis.[46] Angiogenesis is an essential part of tumor growth. Tumors may remain quiescent until proangiogenic factors favor their growth. This usually involves the production of VEGF, platelet-derived growth factors, and basic fibroblast growth factor by the diseased cell. VEGFR has to be overexpressed in tumor cells, and its inhibition is a rational approach to treating malignancy.[47] VEGF, a glycoprotein ligand that belongs to a family of six isoforms, binds transmembrane tyrosine kinase receptors, which activate signal transduction, and increases the permeability of blood vessels. The inhibition of VEGF generally leads to regression of existing tumor blood supply and inhibits the production of new vasculature.

Bevacizumab (Avastin) was the first VEGF inhibitor to be approved by the US Food and Drug Administration (FDA). It is a human monoclonal antibody that binds to and inhibits VEGF, preventing its interaction with receptors (FLT-1 and KDR) that are present on the surface of endothelial cells;[48] this action inhibits cell proliferation. Bevacizumab may also increase access of chemotherapy to cancer cells by decreasing elevated interstitial pressures seen in tumor masses.[49] It binds all VEGF isoforms and causes the regression of tumor vessels and inhibits new vessel formation and apoptosis; as a result, it can lead to destabilization or a response in many solid tumors. Serious toxicities, including gastrointestinal perforation, hemorrhage, and thrombosis, have been reported. Impaired wound healing also has been associated with bevacizumab; therefore, surgery should be 6 to 8 weeks before or after any dose.

Sorafenib (Nexavar), a small molecule VEGF inhibitor, interacts with other receptors, including VEGFR-2 and 3, PDGFR, and c-KIT, and the protein kinase, RAF. Sorafenib also inhibits tumor angiogenesis and has clinical efficacy in renal cell carcinoma.[50]

Targeted Therapy Against the C-KIT Tyrosine Kinase Receptor Pathway

Imatinib (Gleevec) is an oral, small molecule inhibitor of PDGFR and c-KIT. It has a significant role for treating gastrointestinal stromal tumors (GISTs). For tumors that are resistant to imatinib, sunitinib (Sutent) also has potent activity against c-KIT, VEGFR-1 to 3, and PDGFR. Sunitinib also is approved for treating renal cell carcinoma and GISTs.

Colorectal Cancer

Colorectal cancer, the second leading cause of cancer-related mortality in the United States,[51] has a 5-year survival rate for stage 4 disease of less than 5%. This survival has improved with the addition of oxaliplatin and three-drug combination chemotherapy regimens.

Bevacizumab is approved as a first-line agent for stage 4 colorectal cancer. Considering VEGF is expressed in nearly 50% of colorectal cancers,[52] the use of bevacizumab is a rational approach in for treating metastatic colorectal cancer. Bevacizumab results in a higher response rate and increased time to distant progression, and it extends immediate survival more than fluorouracil (5-FU) alone.[53] In a phase 3 trial, 813 chemotherapy-naive patients who had metastatic colorectal cancer received either (1) irinotecan, 5-FU, leucovorin (IFL), plus bevacizumab or (2) IFL plus placebo. Median survival was longer in the first group than the second group (20.3 months versus 15.6 months, respectively), and median progression free survival was also longer (10.6 months versus 6.2 months, respectively). The response rate and duration of response were 44.8% versus 34.8% and 7.1 months versus 10.4 months, respectively.[54] As in other trials with bevacizumab, bleeding, hypertension, and thrombosis occurred at an increased incidence in the bevacizumab arms of this study.

A second agent, cetuximab, is also available for use in the treatment of metastatic colorectal cancer. A study compared irinotecan plus cetuximab versus irinotecan alone, in patients whose disease progressed after irinotecan-based treatment. The combination therapy showed a nearly 23% response rate versus 10.8%, and the time to progression was significantly longer in the combination therapy group, 4.1 versus 1.5 months. There was no statistically significant survival advantage. Toxic effects were more frequent in the combination therapy group.[55] EGFR expression with the tumors did not correlate with clinical response, but at currently, the FDA-approved indication requires that tumors express EGFR.

Breast Cancer

Breast cancer remains the second leading cause of death in women in the United States and the third leading cause of cancer deaths in the United States overall. Twenty percent to 30% of breast cancers over express HER-2, and this correlates with a more aggressive tumor and a poor prognosis.[56]

Trastuzumab initially was approved for metastatic breast carcinoma. The initial study by Cobleigh and colleagues in 1999 showed a 15% response with a 9-month duration of response in heavily pretreated patients.[57] The phase 3 trial that established trastuzumab with chemotherapy for metastatic breast cancer as standard care, randomized 469 patients to receive either chemotherapy (which was paclitaxel or an anthracycline- based regimen) versus chemotherapy plus trastuzumab. Patients treated with trastuzumab had a longer time to progression, higher objective response rate (50% versus 32%), longer duration of response, and longer overall survival (25.1 months versus 20.3 months; $P = .01$).[58]

In 2006, trastuzumab was approved for the adjuvant treatment of HER-2 positive breast cancer.[59] In these trials, patients received doxorubicin and cyclophosphamide followed by paclitaxel after surgical resection, radiation therapy, and endocrine therapy. The patients were randomized to 1 year of trastuzumab versus placebo. The relative risk of recurrence was 52% less in the trastuzumab arm. Trastuzumab also was associated with a 33% increase in overall survival and a 3% to 4% increase in the rate of cardiac dysfunction. There is no consensus regarding the optimal schedule or the duration of therapy with trastuzumab in the adjuvant setting.

Pancreatic Cancer

Pancreatic cancer is the fourth leading cause of death in the United States and claims over 200,000 lives worldwide.[60] Advanced disease has a median survival of 5.7 months, and a 6-month survival rate of 46%.[61,62] Chemotherapy is associated with a 5% response rate. Data suggest that there is a statistically significant decrease in survival in pancreatic cancers that overexpress EGFR.[63] Erlotinib is the only targeted agent that has efficacy against advanced pancreatic cancer. In patients who had advanced or metastatic pancreatic cancer, the median survival rate was 6.4 months with erlotinib plus gemcitabine versus 5.9 months with gemcitabine alone. The 1-year survival rate was significantly better with the erlotinib regimen (23% versus 17%).[64] Despite this statistically significant difference, the clinical significance of a 2-week improvement in median survival with erlotinib is questionable.

Gastrointestinal Stromal Tumors

Ninety percent of GISTs possess an activating mutation of the c-KIT tyrosine kinase. Among the GISTs that harbor no c-KIT mutation, 30% to 50% have a mutation in PDGF that can render the tumor sensitive to imatinib despite a normal c-KIT.[65] One of the initial studies for imatinib with GISTs randomized 147 patients who had documented c-KIT overexpression to either 400 or 600 mg of imatinib daily. Overall, there was a 54% objective response rate and 20% disease stabilization during treatment.[66] Imatinib is also efficacious in the adjuvant setting for GISTs. The clinical trial, ACOSOG-Z 9001, showed that in GISTs measuring more than 3 cm in patients who had an R0/R1 resection, there was a significant improvement in recurrence and survival in the treatment arm.[67] Sunitinib also can be offered when there is disease progression on imatinib.[68]

Hepatocellular Carcinoma

The Study of Heart and Renal Protection (SHARP) trial randomized 602 patients who had advanced (HCC) to sorafenib versus placebo. The sorafenib dose was 400 mg twice daily. Adverse effects included diarrhea and hand–foot syndrome. Sorafenib increased the time to progression from 12.3 weeks to 24 weeks. Overall survival was increased by 3 months, 46 weeks versus 34 weeks.[69]

Cancer Stem Cells: are these Cells the Real Target?

Not all cancer cells within a given tumor have the individual ability to form tumors. In fact, evidence suggests that only a minority of cells within a tumor have the ability to extensively proliferate and develop independent colonies or metastases.[70] These specialized cells are referred to as cancer stem cells. As early as the 1960s, initial experiments with colony forming assays suggested the existence of these cells; however, with limited technologies, it was difficult to establish the cancer stem cell theory over the competing argument that all cells had the same low potential to form colonies. Later, using flow cytometry and specific markers, investigators were able to provide considerable experimental evidence for the existence of cancer stem cells. Specifically, starting with acute myeloid leukemia, investigators showed that, just like normal blood cells, the cells in acute myelogenous leukemia are derived from a small subset of stem cells that give rise to a prominent population of cells with limited clonogenic potential. Similarly, cancer stem cells now have been demonstrated in testicular, brain, colon, and breast cancer.[71]

A growing body of evidence suggests that stem cells are less mitotically active than the nonstem cell population: This in turn suggests that stem cells may be resistant to chemotherapy and radiotherapy.[72,73] Selecting therapies based on their ability to decrease tumor size by means of the elimination of nontumorigenic cancer cells may have led investigators to accept therapies that are not necessarily cytotoxic to stem cells. Treating patients with these therapies might leave residual stem cells and result in local recurrences and distant metastases. Developing cytotoxic therapies that specifically target cancer stem cells may provide a meaningful improvement in cancer treatment. Ideally, these therapies would target tumor stem cells specifically and not normal stem cells from the same tissue. Evidence that this can occur has been demonstrated in leukemia.[74] Now that stem cells can be identified phenotypically for some tumor types, it should be possible to screen for drugs with specific antistem cell toxicity. These novel agents, possibly in addition to standard therapies, may translate response rates into durable remissions.

Table 1
Targeted therapy is valuable for treating many solid tumors[40]

Agent	Mechanism of Action	Cancer
Cetuximab	Epidermal growth factor receptor (EGFR) antibody	Colorectal cancer, squamous cell cancer of the head and neck
Panitumumab	EGFR antibody	Colorectal cancer
Gefitinib	EGFR, tyrosine kinase inhibitor (TKI)	Nonsmall cell lung cancer
Erlotinib	EGFR	Nonsmall cell lung cancer, pancreatic cancer
Trastuzumab	Human epidermal growth factor (HER)-2 antibody	Breast cancer
Lapatinib	HER-2/EGFR, TKI	Breast cancer
Bevacizumab	Vascular endothelial growth factor (VEGF) antibody	Colorectal cancer, nonsmall cell lung cancer, breast cancer, renal cell cancer
Vatalanib	VEGF receptor, platelet-derived growth factor receptor (PDGFR)	Colorectal cancer
Imatinib	C-KIT/PDGFR	Gastrointestinal (GI) stromal tumors
Sunitinib	Multikinase inhibitor	GI stromal tumors
Sorafenib	Multikinase inhibitor	Renal cell, hepatocellular carcinoma, melanoma

SUMMARY

The sequencing of the human genome and the ability to rapidly identify genes and proteins, both normal and mutant, that are involved in tumorigenesis and malignant phenotypes, have changed the ability to understand malignant cells. Understanding these mutations and transformations is allowing physicians to rapidly apply this information to earlier diagnosis, better imaging, and designing targeted agents to alter cells through mechanisms such as growth factor receptor blockade or telomerase inactivation. Current targeted therapies with antibodies and small molecule inhibitors have been effective for metastatic and primary solid tumors, showing increased responses and prolonged survival. These therapies are often well tolerated but have unique toxicity profiles. The cancer surgeon has a pivotal role in the multidisciplinary team to ensure that this evolving knowledge is applied to patients **Table 1.**

REFERENCES

1. McPherson JD, Marra M, Hillier L, et al. A physical map of the human genome. Nature 2001;409(6822):934–41.
2. Venter JC, Adams MD, Myers EW, et al. The sequence of the human genome. Science 2001;291(5507):1304–51.
3. Palacios J, Robles-Frias MJ, Castilla MA, et al. The molecular pathology of hereditary breast cancer. Pathobiology 2008;75(2):85–94.
4. Abdel-Rahman WM, Mecklin JP, Peltomaki P. The genetics of HNPCC: application to diagnosis and screening. Crit Rev Oncol Hematol 2006;58(3):208–20.
5. Galiatsatos P, Foulkes WD. Familial adenomatous polyposis. Am J Gastroenterol 2006;101(2):385–98.

6. Dionigi G, Bianchi V, Rovera F, et al. Medullary thyroid carcinoma: surgical treatment advances. Expert Rev Anticancer Ther 2007;7(6):877–85.

7. Goldenberg DM, Chatal JF, Barbet J, et al. Cancer imaging and therapy with bispecific antibody pretargeting. Update Cancer Ther 2007;2(1):19–31.

8. Olafsen T, Tan GJ, Cheung CW, et al. Characterization of engineered anti-p185HER-2 (scFv-CH3)2 antibody fragments (minibodies) for tumor targeting. Protein Eng Des Sel 2004;17(4):315–23.

9. Sundaresan G, Yazaki PJ, Shively JE, et al. 124I-labeled engineered anti-CEA minibodies and diabodies allow high-contrast, antigen-specific small-animal PET imaging of xenografts in athymic mice. J Nucl Med 2003;44(12):1962–9.

10. Dehdashti F, Picus J, Michalski JM, et al. Positron tomographic assessment of androgen receptors in prostatic carcinoma. Eur J Nucl Med Mol Imaging 2005;32(3):344–50.

11. Peterson LM, Mankoff DA, Lawton T, et al. Quantitative imaging of estrogen receptor expression in breast cancer with PET and 18F-fluoroestradiol. J Nucl Med 2008;49(3):367–74.

12. Virtanen C, Woodgett J. Clinical uses of microarrays in cancer research. Methods Mol Med 2008;141:87–113.

13. Golub TR, Slonim DK, Tamayo P, et al. Molecular classification of cancer: class discovery and class prediction by gene expression monitoring. Science 1999; 286(5439):531–7.

14. Perou CM, Sorlie T, Eisen MB, et al. Molecular portraits of human breast tumours. Nature 2000;406(6797):747–52.

15. Paik S, Shak S, Tang G, et al. A multigene assay to predict recurrence of tamoxifen-treated, node-negative breast cancer. N Engl J Med 2004;351(27):2817–26.

16. Sorlie T, Tibshirani R, Parker J, et al. Repeated observation of breast tumor subtypes in independent gene expression data sets. Proc Natl Acad Sci U S A 2003;100(14):8418–23.

17. Henshall SM, Afar DE, Hiller J, et al. Survival analysis of genome-wide gene expression profiles of prostate cancers identifies new prognostic targets of disease relapse. Cancer Res 2003;63(14):4196–203.

18. Potti A, Mukherjee S, Petersen R, et al. A genomic strategy to refine prognosis in early-stage nonsmall cell lung cancer. N Engl J Med 2006;355(6):570–80.

19. Harris L, Fritsche H, Mennel R, et al. American Society of Clinical Oncology 2007 update of recommendations for the use of tumor markers in breast cancer. J Clin Oncol 2007;25(33):5287–312.

20. zur Hausen H. Viruses in human cancers. Eur J Cancer 1999;35(14):1878–85.

21. Bishop JM. Cellular oncogenes and retroviruses. Annu Rev Biochem 1983;52: 301–54.

22. Alitalo K, Schwab M. Oncogene amplification in tumor cells. Adv Cancer Res 1986;47:235–81.

23. Land H, Parada LF, Weinberg RA. Tumorigenic conversion of primary embryo fibroblasts requires at least two cooperating oncogenes. Nature 1983; 304(5927):596–602.

24. Vogelstein B, Kinzler KW. The multistep nature of cancer. Trends Genet 1993;9(4): 138–41.

25. Harris H. Cell fusion and the analysis of malignancy: the Croonian lecture. Proc Royal Soc London B Biol Sci 1987;179:1.

26. Knudson AG Jr. Mutation and cancer: statistical study of retinoblastoma. Proc Natl Acad Sci U S A 1971;68(4):820–3.

27. Weinberg RA. Cancer: a genetic disorder. In: Mendelsohn J, Howley P, Israel M, et al, editors. The molecular basis of cancer. Phildelphia: Saunders; 2008. p. 3–17.

28. Charames GS, Bapat B. Genomic instability and cancer. Curr Mol Med 2003;3(7): 589–96.
29. D'Andrea A. DNA repair pathways and human cancer. In: Mendelsohn J, Howley P, Israel M, et al, editors. The molecular basis of cancer. Philadelphia: Saunders; 2008. p. 39–57.
30. Cleaver JE. Cancer in xeroderma pigmentosum and related disorders of DNA repair. Nat Rev Cancer 2005;5(7):564–73.
31. Heinen CD, Schmutte C, Fishel R. DNA repair and tumorigenesis: lessons from hereditary cancer syndromes. Cancer Biol Ther 2002;1(5):477–85.
32. Wang W. Emergence of a DNA-damage response network consisting of Fanconi anaemia and BRCA proteins. Nat Rev Genet 2007;8(10):735–48.
33. Cong Y, Shay JW. Actions of human telomerase beyond telomeres. Cell Res 2008;18(7):725–32.
34. De Lange T. Telomere-related genome instability in cancer. Cold Spring Harb Symp Quant Biol 2005;70:197–204.
35. Hahn WC, Meyerson M. Telomerase activation, cellular immortalization and cancer. Ann Med 2001;33(2):123–9.
36. Baylin SB, Herman JG. DNA hypermethylation in tumorigenesis: epigenetics joins genetics. Trends Genet 2000;16(4):168–74.
37. Yang J, Weinberg RA. Epithelial–mesenchymal transition: at the crossroads of development and tumor metastasis. Dev Cell 2008;14(6):818–29.
38. Thiery JP. Epithelial–mesenchymal transitions in tumour progression. Nat Rev Cancer 2002;2(6):442–54.
39. Goh PP, Sze DM, Roufogalis BD. Molecular and cellular regulators of cancer angiogenesis. Curr Cancer Drug Targets 2007;7(8):743–58.
40. Zureikat AH, McKee MD. Targeted therapy for solid tumors: current status. Surg Oncol Clin N Am 2008;17(2):279–301.
41. Grandis JR, Sok JC. Signaling through the epidermal growth factor receptor during the development of malignancy. Pharmacol Ther 2004;102(1):37–46.
42. Baselga J. Why the epidermal growth factor receptor? The rationale for cancer therapy. Oncologist 2002;(7 Suppl 4):2–8.
43. Huang SM, Bock JM, Harari PM. Epidermal growth factor receptor blockade with C225 modulates proliferation, apoptosis, and radiosensitivity in squamous cell carcinomas of the head and neck. Cancer Res 1999;59(8):1935–40.
44. Nait W, Rubin E, Bertino J. Cancer therapeutics. In: Mendelsohn J, Howley P, Israel M, et al, editors. The molecular basis of cancer. Philadelphia: Saunders; 2008. p. 571–82.
45. Yang XD, Jia XC, Corvalan JR, et al. Development of ABX-EGF, a fully human anti-EGF receptor monoclonal antibody, for cancer therapy. Crit Rev Oncol Hematol 2001;38(1):17–23.
46. Folkman J. Angiogenesis. Annu Rev Med 2006;57:1–18.
47. Ferrara N. Vascular endothelial growth factor as a target for anticancer therapy. Oncologist 2004;(9 Suppl 1):2–10.
48. Presta LG, Chen H, O'Connor SJ, et al. Humanization of an antivascular endothelial growth factor monoclonal antibody for the therapy of solid tumors and other disorders. Cancer Res 1997;57(20):4593–9.
49. Willett CG, Boucher Y, di Tomaso E, et al. Direct evidence that the VEGF-specific antibody bevacizumab has antivascular effects in human rectal cancer. Nat Med 2004;10(2):145–7.
50. Wilhelm SM, Carter C, Tang L, et al. BAY 43-9006 exhibits broad spectrum oral antitumor activity and targets the RAF/MEK/ERK pathway and receptor tyrosine

kinases involved in tumor progression and angiogenesis. Cancer Res 2004; 64(19):7099–109.

51. Jemal A, Siegel R, Ward E, et al. Cancer statistics. CA Cancer J Clin 2007;57(1): 43–66.

52. Fernando NH, Hurwitz HI. Targeted therapy of colorectal cancer: clinical experience with bevacizumab. Oncologist 2004;(9 Suppl 1):11–8.

53. Kabbinavar F, Hurwitz HI, Fehrenbacher L, et al. Phase II, randomized trial comparing bevacizumab plus fluorouracil (FU)/leucovorin (LV) with FU/LV alone in patients with metastatic colorectal cancer. J Clin Oncol 2003;21(1):60–5.

54. Hurwitz H, Fehrenbacher L, Novotny W, et al. Bevacizumab plus irinotecan, fluorouracil, and leucovorin for metastatic colorectal cancer. N Engl J Med 2004; 350(23):2335–42.

55. Cunningham D, Humblet Y, Siena S, et al. Cetuximab monotherapy and cetuximab plus irinotecan in irinotecan-refractory metastatic colorectal cancer. N Engl J Med 2004;351(4):337–45.

56. Slamon DJ, Clark GM, Wong SG, et al. Human breast cancer: correlation of relapse and survival with amplification of the HER-2/neu oncogene. Science 1987;235(4785):177–82.

57. Cobleigh MA, Vogel CL, Tripathy D, et al. Multinational study of the efficacy and safety of humanized anti-HER2 monoclonal antibody in women who have HER2-overexpressing metastatic breast cancer that has progressed after chemotherapy for metastatic disease. J Clin Oncol 1999;17(9):2639–48.

58. Slamon DJ, Leyland-Jones B, Shak S, et al. Use of chemotherapy plus a monoclonal antibody against HER2 for metastatic breast cancer that overexpresses HER2. N Engl J Med 2001;344(11):783–92.

59. Romond EH, Perez EA, Bryant J, et al. Trastuzumab plus adjuvant chemotherapy for operable HER2-positive breast cancer. N Engl J Med 2005;353(16):1673–84.

60. Michaud DS. Epidemiology of pancreatic cancer. Minerva Chir 2004;59(2): 99–111.

61. Burris HA III, Moore MJ, Andersen J, et al. Improvements in survival and clinical benefit with gemcitabine as first-line therapy for patients with advanced pancreas cancer: a randomized trial. J Clin Oncol 1997;15(6):2403–13.

62. Diaz-Rubio E. New chemotherapeutic advances in pancreatic, colorectal, and gastric cancers. Oncologist 2004;9(3):282–94.

63. MacKenzie MJ. Molecular therapy in pancreatic adenocarcinoma. Lancet Oncol 2004;5(9):541–9.

64. Moore MJ, Goldstein D, Hamm J, et al. Erlotinib plus gemcitabine compared with gemcitabine alone in patients with advanced pancreatic cancer: a phase III trial of the National Cancer Institute of Canada Clinical Trials Group. J Clin Oncol 2007;25(15):1960–6.

65. Rubin BP, Singer S, Tsao C, et al. KIT activation is a ubiquitous feature of gastrointestinal stromal tumors. Cancer Res 2001;61(22):8118–21.

66. Demetri GD, von Mehren M, Blanke CD, et al. Efficacy and safety of imatinib mesylate in advanced gastrointestinal stromal tumors. N Engl J Med 2002;347(7):472–80.

67. Institute NC. A phase III randomized double-blind study of adjuvant imatinib mesylate (Gleevec; STI571) versus placebo in patients following the resection of primary gastrointestinal stomal tumors (GIST). ACOSOG-Z9001. Available at: http://www.cancer.gov/clinicaltrials/ACOSOG-Z9001.

68. Demetri GD, van Oosterom AT, Garrett CR, et al. Efficacy and safety of sunitinib in patients with advanced gastrointestinal stromal tumour after failure of imatinib: a randomised controlled trial. Lancet 2006;368(9544):1329–38.

69. Llovet J, Ricci S, V M. For the SHARP investigators study group. Sorafenib improves survival in advanced heaptocellular carcinoma (HCC): results of a phase III randomized placebo-controlled trial (SHARP trial). J Clin Oncol 2007;25(Suppl 18S):LBA1.
70. Mimeault M, Hauke R, Mehta PP, et al. Recent advances in cancer stem/progenitor cell research: therapeutic implications for overcoming resistance to the most aggressive cancers. J Cell Mol Med 2007;11(5):981–1011.
71. Buchstaller J, Quintana E, Morrison S. Cancer stem cells. In: Mendelsohn J, Howley P, Israel M, editors. The molecular basis of cancer. Philadelphia: Saunders; 2008. p. 141–54.
72. Bao S, Wu Q, McLendon RE, et al. Glioma stem cells promote radioresistance by preferential activation of the DNA damage response. Nature 2006;444(7120): 756–60.
73. Hermann PC, Huber SL, Herrler T, et al. Distinct populations of cancer stem cells determine tumor growth and metastatic activity in human pancreatic cancer. Cell Stem Cell 2007;1(3):313–23.
74. Yilmaz OH, Valdez R, Theisen BK, et al. Pten dependence distinguishes haematopoietic stem cells from leukaemia-initiating cells. Nature 2006;441(7092): 475–82.

Measuring Outcomes in Oncology Treatment: The Importance of Patient-Centered Outcomes

Aundrea Oliver, MD[a], Caprice C. Greenberg, MD, MPH[a,b,c,*]

KEYWORDS
- Patient-centered outcomes • Patient satisfaction
- Decision regret • Patient preference
- Health-related quality of life • Survey instrument design

The quality of medical care long has been assessed in terms of patient outcomes. Traditional measures such as mortality and morbidity assess the unintended consequences of treatment in a very concrete, measurable way, while survival and recurrence rates similarly depict whether the treatment is achieving its intended goal. Practicing clinicians, however, know that the quality of the care received goes beyond whether the patient lives or dies and whether the cancer recurs or not. Treatment decisions have a very real impact on many aspects of the patient's life beyond those black-and-white outcomes. The problem remains that these concepts can be difficult to define and even more difficult to measure.

In "Crossing the Quality Chasm," the Institute of Medicine defined the six aims of quality healthcare. Care should be safe, effective, patient-centered, timely, efficient, and equitable.[1] This definition clearly illustrates the important role that the patient, including his or her preferences, values, and beliefs, must play in modern health care. The emergence of patient-centered outcomes as a distinct entity further highlights this important paradigm shift. It is no longer adequate to rely on objective data that reflect the providers' point of view. One also must develop concepts and measurement tools that more broadly and reliably capture factors that influence outcome and define

[a] Department of Surgery, Brigham and Women's Hospital, 75 Francis Street, Boston, MA 02115, USA
[b] Center for Surgery and Public Health, Brigham and Women's Hospital, OBC 4-020, 75 Francis Street, Boston, MA 02115, USA
[c] Center for Outcomes and Policy Research, Dana-Farber Cancer Institute, 44 Binney street, SM 271, Boston, MA 02115, USA
* Corresponding author. Division of Breast Surgical Oncology, Brigham and Women's Hospital, 75 Francis Street, Boston, MA 02115.
E-mail address: ccgreenberg@partners.org (C.C. Greenberg).

Surg Clin N Am 89 (2009) 17–25
doi:10.1016/j.suc.2008.09.015
0039-6109/08/$ – see front matter © 2009 Elsevier Inc. All rights reserved.

health from the patient perspective. Patient-centered outcomes research is the study of the relationship of an observational event (outcome) and the treatment provided in the context of the patient.[2]

The paradigm shift is illustrated by the inclusion of patient-centered outcomes in many cooperative group trials.[3] Measures such as quality of life and patient satisfaction are going to play an ever-increasingly prominent role in the assessment of the quality of health care that surgical oncologists provide. Familiarity with patient centered outcomes is imperative. Most surgical oncologists are familiar with the concept of quality of life; however, there are other types of patient-centered outcomes that can be addressed such as patient preference, decision regret, and patient satisfaction. The goal of this article is to provide a broad overview of patient-centered outcomes in oncologic research. It starts with an introduction to these different types of patient-centered outcomes. It then offers an overview of instrument selection and design. Finally, it provides examples of existing approaches to measurement and previously validated instruments for each type of patient-centered outcome.

TYPES OF PATIENT-CENTERED OUTCOMES
Patient Satisfaction

Patient satisfaction is the emotional or cognitive evaluation of a health encounter by a patient as defined by a set of events or experiences. This may be defined by the essential components of the encounter itself (ie, services rendered), or the manner or context in which they are delivered. These definitions highlight the fact that satisfaction is a highly subjective outcome to measure, but important nonetheless. In health care, too often it is forgotten that the patient is a consumer and his or her satisfaction with the health care system and treatment is important in his or her overall experience. Patient satisfaction, therefore, often is used as a tool to assess the quality of care of a health care delivery system, and develop and improve models for patient care. The basic domains assessed in patient satisfaction include: interpersonal aspects, technical quality, accessibility/availability continuity of care delivered, and patient convenience, setting, financial concerns, communication, efficacy, respect, time spent, and concern experienced during the health care encounter.[4,5]

The interpersonal aspects of a health encounter encompass the direct contact between provider and patient. It may include issues of communication, sense of mutual respect, investment of time, or conveyance of personal concern for the patient on the part of the provider. Technical quality primarily refers to the specific proficiency in skill required in a practitioner and intelligence and qualifications of that provider as perceived by the patient. The measures of accessibility and its related endpoints of availability and convenience assess such issues as location (eg, distance traveled for most patients, relationship to public transportation), hours of operation, scheduling (eg, waiting times for an appointment date), accommodations for special needs (eg, teletypewriter [TTY], wheelchair accessible), and in-office waiting time. Continuity includes intraprovider consistency of care and the transfer of information from one provider to another. The setting refers to the physical design of the location of patient care, which can refer to aesthetics and accessibility.

Decision Regret

Regret has been defined as "the negative, cognitively-based emotion that we experience when realizing or imagining that our present situation would have been better had we acted differently."[6] Some scholars further divide regret into dissatisfaction with a decision and its associated outcome on one hand, and disappointment in an outcome caused by a feeling of responsibility for the decision made on the other.[7] The regret is seen as an emotional state of disappointment or sorrow in the former. Self-recrimination, exemplified in the latter, is experienced as the component of regret that describes the degree of responsibility the individual feels for the negative outcome experienced. Decision regret is important in patient-centered outcomes research, in that it can indicate a flaw in information transfer (ie, informed consent and patient education) and treatment decision in the health encounter. Moreover, regret at one point in the treatment encounter can affect future treatment decisions, and the perception of overall quality of life. This construct has been studied extensively in the context of consumer research but has been difficult to capture in health care outcomes, and especially difficult in oncology research in particular. As more medical and surgical treatment options become available and patient-centered healthcare becomes a priority, however, the role of the patient in the treatment decision process increases. This increased patient participation proportionally increases the opportunity for decision regret. In oncologic treatment, very few interventions are curative, and many can have short-term or lifelong morbidity associated with little or no change in overall mortality. One can measure the decision anxiety, degree of responsibility or patient participation, and differences pre- and post outcome in the level of measured regret after an intervention or treatment.[7] Using decision regret measures in conjunction with generic quality-of-life or functional measures may provide a more robust description of the context of decision regret as it relates to outcomes and patient experience.

Patient Preference

Largely discussed in the context of multiple treatment options with equivalent risk–benefit profiles, patient preference is related closely to patient satisfaction and decision regret in outcomes research. It depends upon the assumption of full disclosure of all reasonable treatment options for a given patient in a comprehensible, meaningful way. Only if the patient truly understands his or her treatment options, can she or he form an informed preference for one treatment over other options. Therefore, the measurement of patient preference often is linked tightly to patient education, decision-making analysis including decision regret, and quality-of- life measures. One also can measure patient preference as it pertains to perceived quality of life while undergoing a particular treatment regimen.

Health-Related Quality of Life

Health-related quality of life (HRQOL) describes the experience of different domains of health as modified by both disease and treatment processes.[8] HRQOL is conceptualized as the five different ways in which disease and treatment can impact well-being and quality of life: impairment, functional status, perception of health, social interactions, and duration of life. These constructs are general, abstract concepts that provide a framework for thinking about HRQOL. In order to actually measure HRQOL, more specific, concrete domains of functioning have been defined. These will be discussed under generic measures of HRQOL.

MEASURES

Patient-centered outcomes can be classified into two major categories: generic or disease-specific measures. There are advantages and disadvantages to each type of measure that must be considered. Generic measures are comprehensive and assess the overall impact, independent of specific disease type, treatment, or patient population. Condition-specific measures tend to be more sensitive tools that are designed to capture symptoms that are specific to a given medical condition and the direct effect of a condition on an individual's quality of life. Although it is often ideal to include components of both a generic and disease-specific tool, complexity and cumbersome administration can limit the practicality of this approach. One can modify a generic measure for a specific condition, or add a condition-specific supplement to simplify the tool and expedite administration.

Once one determines the appropriate measurement tool for a particular question, secondary risk adjustment may be required. This includes predisease functional status, baseline functional status at the beginning of treatment, and comorbidities not directly related to the disease in question but which affect overall health and response to treatment. One also may measure disease severity itself for the diagnosis in question. Finally, demographics and psychosocial factors often are included, because they may impact the individual's response to disease or intervention, preference and decision-making, or perception of health.

Generic Versus Condition-Specific Measures

Generic measures are broad measures designed to capture the physical, psychological, and social aspects of health. Their design should allow researchers to assess common denominators that define the effect of treatments on health status and quality of life. Quantity of health refers to the objective measures historically used in outcomes research, which include mortality, morbidity, and survival. The quality of health can be captured by the seven domains of health, which have been defined to measure HRQOL. The seven domains of health are: physical, social, emotional, and cognitive functioning, pain, vitality, and overall well being.[9] These measures are designed to be generic measures of quality of life as it pertains to health; however there are disease-specific questionnaires that may focus on more unique aspects of the domains as they relate to the specific disease process or treatment. As generic measures, however, there are several aspects of each that can be assessed broadly by most measurement tools. Physical functioning primarily refers to physical mobility and independence. Common aspects measured include fitness or physiologic health by clinical or objective measures, basic self-care activities (activities of daily living, ADLs), or more complex self-care activities (instrumental ADLs, IADLs). Social functioning measures often include social role functioning, community involvement, quality of interpersonal relationships, and coping capacity. Emotional functioning describes the range of affective well being, specifically positive and negative emotions and emotional stability. Cognitive functioning measures include memory, reasoning, and orientation to describe range of intellectual ability. Pain often is defined as the degree of debilitating physical discomfort as a sensation, not as a degree of physical functioning. Its measures often capture intensity, frequency, and duration. Vitality simply refers to the patient's general state of well being; however, unlike emotional functioning, it measures sleep quality and quantity, degree of restful sleep, and general energy level. Overall well being is distinct from vitality, social, or emotional functioning, in that it represents the patient's perception of the net balance of all aspects of health-related quality of life. This global measure often refers to the individual's sense of contentment, happiness, or general health status. All of these domains combined generate the overall health-related quality of life. There are several well-validated tools used to assess part or all of these domains in general or in disease-specific terms.

The design of a generic measure of HRQOL requires several specific considerations.[9] First, one must choose which domains of health to measure. This decision will affect the range of measure or the scope and spectrum of performance and change in health status. The measures must have clinical relevance, which provides a context and logic for measurement design and score interpretation. Each domain can be given more or less weight within the overall measurement tool, based on the desired emphasis of the tool. The goal is to design a sensitive (one that is able to capture differences in health status), reliable (one that is consistent and reproducible), and valid (one that measures the constructs it was designed to measure) tool. Finally, practical consideration requires design that allows the investigator to achieve his or her measurement goals while limiting the burden of administration for participants. If the tool is too brief, or administration is too burdensome, it can impact the quality and quantity of information obtained adversely.

Disease-specific measures are designed to focus on the most relevant domains for a particular condition. These measures are either objective (clinical) or subjective (experiential). Unlike generic measures, which look at global changes in health status, disease-specific measures are designed to measure responsiveness or small treatment effects on a particular condition. These tools usually are designed to maximize sensitivity and specificity and focus on signs, symptoms, function, and test results.

Existing Tools Versus Instrument Design

Several generic and condition-specific instruments have been designed and validated previously. It is usually preferable to use a previously validated tool when possible. If such a tool does not exist, it is important to carefully design and validate a new instrument through pilot testing before using it in a large study.

Existing Instruments to Measure Patient-Centered Outcomes

Many of the concepts defined previously naturally interrelate. It is not uncommon for studies that investigate the impact of an intervention on health-related quality of life to also include measures of patient satisfaction, decision regret, and patient preference. A description of the existing approach to measure each patient-centered outcome follows.

Patient satisfaction

The European Organization for Research and Treatment of Cancer (EORTC), an international research organization based in Brussels, Belgium, has served as the epicenter of clinical randomized controlled trials in Europe for over 40 years. The EORTC also has been influential in establishing widely validated quality-of-life measurement tools and tools for patient satisfaction.

The QLQ-INPATSAT32 questionnaire was developed by the EORTC to measure patient satisfaction with inpatient care.[10] This tool was designed to measure the patient satisfaction with the following dimensions of the care experience: provider/support staff technical and interpersonal skills, information availability and provision, information exchange between providers and patient, hospital access, waiting time, general comfort, and satisfaction. This tool was found to have excellent reliability and internal consistency, and was convenient for patients to complete (approximately 15 minutes). Results from the QLQ-PATSAT32 measuring patient satisfaction were compared with the QLQ-C30, a validated quality-of-life tool also developed by the EORTC for patients who have gastric and esophageal cancer. Patient satisfaction and quality of life were found to be independent patient-centered outcomes measuring different components of disease and healthcare. Patients were clearly able to separate their experience of the treatment encounter from their assessment of their quality of life.[11]

Decision regret

Decision regret is rarely the sole outcome measured in oncology. It is often a component of patient satisfaction and decision-making assessments. A simple five-item decision regret scale was developed and has been validated for several treatment modalities including hormone replacement therapy, breast cancer surgery, adjuvant therapy for breast cancer, or treatment for prostate cancer.[7,12] Decision regret was correlated with dissatisfaction with the decision, but it did not measure patient satisfaction with outcome. Waljee and colleagues[13] recently published their study on patient satisfaction and provider trust after breast-conserving therapy. They utilized a shorter six-item patient satisfaction scale, along with the five-item decision regret scale described, a 15-item decisional conflict scale, and an 11-item physician trust scale. As in other studies, the previously mentioned areas were measured in the context of more traditional morbidity measures including postoperative complications, re-excisions, need for completion mastectomy, or poor cosmesis. In this study, dissatisfaction and decision regret correlated strongly with postoperative complications and patient distrust of surgeons. Their study also indicated that decision regret may be linked to preoperative patient education informing patient expectations and investment in the decision-making process. Patients who felt they had shared responsibility in the treatment decision also had outcomes that met with their range of expectations. Davidson and Goldenberg[14] recently published their study investigating decision regret and quality of life in early prostate cancer. Their study also used a combination of quality of life measures, both generic and disease-specific (QLQ-C30, EORTC-PC), the previously described decision regret scale, and a five-item tool to measure the patient's assumed role in decision making. This study revealed that when tested at the time of diagnosis and then again at a significant time after completion of treatment (4 months in this study), decision regret was minimal and did not correlate with adverse outcome. This finding has been consistent with other similar studies in prostate cancer that measured regret up to 2 years after treatment.[15] These studies underline the inter-related nature of patient-centered outcomes and the need for multiple measures to assess for similar but not necessarily associated endpoints.

Patient preference

The premise of patient preference measurement is "the formal measurement of the strength of the preference of patients for a specific treatment or the outcome of such treatment."[16] In order to compare across different disease states, a value or utility usually is attached to each based on its desirability.[9] These utilities function as an adjustment factor for quality of life. In oncology, utilities and probabilities can be combined with length of survival in a single measure of the quantity and quality of life in the respective treatment states. The expected value of each treatment strategy thus is expressed in terms of quality-adjusted life years (QALYs). Such preference weights are important for cost-effectiveness and other decision analyses.

The two most common methods of utility measurement include standard gamble and time trade off.[17-19] The standard gamble method allows the patient to choose between a definite outcome, and a gamble defined as the probability of the best possible outcome (ie, optimal health) versus the probability of the worst possible outcome (ie, death). Time trade off refers to choosing an intervention that may decrease overall life expectancy with a trade off of higher quality of life during that shorter life span. A key component of study design is the identification of the cohort in which preference weighting will be assessed. There is debate about whether it is better to assess preference on a population basis or from patients with firsthand experience with a given condition or treatment.[20,21] These groups are likely to assign different weights to various health states and will impact the study results.

Health-related quality of life

Health-related quality of life is perhaps the most frequently measured patient-centered outcome in clinical oncology. Several generic measures have been developed and validated over time. Commonly used tools include the 36-item Short Form Health Survey (SF-36), Sickness Impact Profile (SIP), and the Nottingham Health Profile (NHP).

The SF-36 is perhaps the best-known method of assessing of HRQOL.[22] It covers the following six domains of health: physical/emotional/social functioning, pain, vitality, and overall well being. There are several different forms related to the SF-36. The SF-36 is so named because it is a shorter version of the longer 149-question Medical Outcomes Study Functioning and Well-Being Profile, the most comprehensive measure of HRQOL. Several shorter versions of the SF-36, most notably the SF-12, have been developed and validated.[23] The SF-36 and related tools were designed for generally healthy populations.

The SIP covers physical, emotional, cognitive, and social functioning, pain, and overall well being.[24] It is a more detailed tool designed to detect subtle changes over time or between groups. The strengths of the SIP are its sensitivity and high reliability; however it is a long and cumbersome tool, which makes it impractical in certain settings.[25] The NHP is a tool that covers the domains of physical, emotional, and social functioning, pain, and vitality.[26] It is intermediate in length compared with the prior two and has been proven to have high reliability and validity in a wide range of health conditions and severity, but lacks some of the sensitivity of the other two measurement tools.

The EORTC QLQ-C30 is perhaps the most common tool used in the oncologic literature to measure health-related quality of life (HRQOL). A recent review article looking at HRQOL, however, found that although the QLQ-C30 predominated as a single validated tool, there were as many studies that used unique unvalidated tools.[27] The EORTC has begun to expand its research to develop more disease-specific tools (eg, QLQ-PAN26 for pancreatic cancer) that can be used as an adjunct to the generic QLQ-C30.[28]

SUMMARY

Patient-centered outcomes research has become an integral part of clinical oncologic research. Since the mid 1980s, there has been a clear paradigm shift toward patient-centered definitions of what constitutes quality healthcare and successful treatment. In surgical oncology, a cure is not always possible. Patient-centered outcomes, however, provide the tools to ensure the highest quality care is provided to prolong life in a meaningful manner as judged by patients.

REFERENCES

1. Institute of Medicine (U.S.), Committee on Quality Of Health Care in America. Crossing the quality chasm: a new health system for the 21st century. Washington: National Academy Press; 2001.
2. Kane RL. Approaching the outcomes question. In: Kane RL, editor. Understanding health care outcomes research. Gaithersburg: Aspen; 1997. p. 3–14.
3. Bottomley A, Aaronson NK, European Organisation for Research and Treatment of Cancer. International perspective on health-related quality-of-life research in

cancer clinical trials: the European Organisation for Research and Treatment of Cancer experience. J Clin Oncol 2007;25(32):5082–6.

4. Maciejewski M, Kawiecki J, Rockwood T. Satisfaction. In: Kane RL, editor. Understanding health care outcomes research. Gaithersburg: Aspen; 1997. p. 67–73.

5. Ware JE, Davies-Avery A, Stewart AL. The measurement and meaning of patient satisfaction. Health Med Care Serv Rev 1978;1:1–15.

6. Zeelenberg M. The use of crying over spilled milk: a note on the rationality and functionality of regret. Philos Psychol 1999;12:325–40.

7. Brehaut JC, O'Connor AM, Wood TJ, et al. Validation of a decision regret scale. Med Decis Making 2003;23(4):281–92.

8. Ware JE. The status of health assessment, 1994. Annu Rev Public Health 1995;16: 327–54.

9. Maciejewski M. Generic measures. In: Kane RL, editor. Understanding health care outcomes research. Gaithersburg: Aspen; 1997. p. 19–48.

10. Brédart A, Coens C, Aaronson N, et al. Determinants of patient satisfaction in oncology settings from European and Asian countries: preliminary results based on the EORTC IN-PATSAT32 questionnaire. Eur J Cancer 2007;43(2):323–30.

11. Avery KN, Metcalfe C, Nicklin J, et al. Satisfaction with care: an independent outcome measure in surgical oncology. Ann Surg Oncol 2006;13(6):817–22.

12. Goel V, Sawka CA, Thiel EC, et al. Randomized trial of a patient decision aid for choice of surgical treatment for breast cancer. Med Decis Making 2001;21(1): 1–6.

13. Waljee JF, Hu ES, Newman LA, et al. Correlates of patient satisfaction and provider trust after breast-conserving surgery. Cancer 2008;112(8):1679–87.

14. Davison BJ, Goldenberg SL. Decisional regret and quality of life after participating in medical decision making for early stage prostate cancer. BJU Int 2003; 91(1):14–7.

15. Potosky AL, Legler J, Albertsen PC, et al. Health outcomes after prostatectomy or radiotherapy for prostate cancer: results from the prostate cancer outcomes study. J Natl Cancer Inst 2000;92:1582–92.

16. Stiggelbout AM, de Haes JC. Patient preference for cancer therapy: an overview of measurement approaches. J Clin Oncol 2001;19(1):220–30.

17. Froberg DG, Kane RL. Methodology for measuring health states–II: scaling methods. J Clin Epidemiol 1989;42(5):459–71.

18. Johnson EJ, Steffel M, Goldstein DG. Making better decisions: from measuring to constructing preferences. Health Psychol 2005;24(Suppl 4):S17–22.

19. Young JM, Solomon MJ, Harrison JD, et al. Measuring patient preference and surgeon choice. Surgery 2008;143(5):582–8.

20. Froberg DG, Kane RL. Methodology for measuring health states—III: population and context effects. J Clin Epidemiol 1989;42(6):585–92.

21. Frost MH, Bonomi AE, Ferrans CE, et al. Patient, clinician, and population perspectives on determining the clinical significance of quality-of-life scores. Mayo Clin Proc 2002;77:488–94.

22. Ware JE, Sherbourne CD. The MOS 36-item short-form health survey (SF-36). I. Conceptual framework and item selection. Med Care 1992;30(6):473–83.

23. Ware JE, Kosiknski M, Keller SD. A 12-item short form health survey: construction of scales and preliminary tests of reliability and validity. Med Care 1996;34(3): 220–3.

24. Bergner M, Bobbit RA, Carter WB, et al. The sickness impact profile: development and final revision of a heath status measure. Med Care 1981;8:787–805.

25. Bergner M. Development, testing, and use of the sickness impact profile. In: Walker SR, Rosser RM, editors. Quality-of-life assessment: key issues in the 1990s. Boston: Kluwer Publishing; 1993. p. 95–109.

26. Hunt SM, McKenna SP, McEwan JA. A quantitative approach to perceived health status: a validation study. J Epidemiol Community Health 1980;34:281–5.

27. Goodwin PJ, Black JT, Bordeleau LJ, et al. Health-related quality-of-life measurement in randomized clinical trials in breast cancer—taking stock. J Natl Cancer Inst 2003;95(4):263–81.

28. de Haes J, Curran D, Young T, et al. Quality-of-life evaluation in oncological clinical trials—the EORTC model. The EORTC Quality of Life Study Group. Eur J Cancer 2000;36(7):821–5.

Surgical Palliation: Getting Back to Our Roots

Alan A. Thomay, MD[a], David P. Jaques, MD[b], Thomas J. Miner, MD[c],*

KEYWORDS

- Surgical palliation • Palliative triangle
- Advanced malignancy • Quality of life

To cure sometimes, to relieve often, to comfort always
    Folk saying dating back to the fifteenth century, inscribed on the statue of
Dr. Edward Livingston Trudeau at Saranac Lake, New York[1]

Those who carefully study history become acutely aware of the cyclical nature of human understanding and behavior. As a species, we reveal the same strengths and weaknesses time and time again, repeat the same triumphs, and make the same mistakes over and over. In medicine, the discipline of palliation, which has its origins in the beginning of medical care, represents another example of history repeating itself. Early on, the focus of care in medicine was solely on alleviating pain and suffering because "cures" were not readily available. With the remarkable scientific and industrial advances of the twentieth century, modern physicians began to believe that achieving a cure was the only acceptable form of medical therapy. The health care profession as a whole began to acknowledge new cures, all the while eschewing patient comfort. As more and more physicians become reacquainted with the fact that death is a natural part of life,[2] this practice will no longer be acceptable.

Surgeons have been at the forefront of the movement toward palliative care for decades, as palliative procedures in the past have centered on three areas that often present as surgical emergencies: obstruction, bleeding, and perforation. Attention has been focused more recently on alleviating the more chronic complaints of individual patients, such as pain, nausea, vomiting, inability to eat, anemia, and jaundice. Palliative operations (representing 12.5% of all surgical procedures performed in

[a] Department of Surgery, The Alpert Medical School of Brown University, Rhode Island Hospital, 593 Eddy Street–APC 4, Providence, RI 02903, USA
[b] Department of Surgery, Washington University School of Medicine, Barnes-Jewish Hospital, 1 Barnes-Jewish Hospital Plaza, St. Louis, MO 63110, USA
[c] Surgical Oncology, Department of Surgery, The Alpert Medical School of Brown University, Rhode Island Hospital, 593 Eddy Street–APC 4, Providence, RI 02903, USA
* Corresponding author.
E-mail address: tminer@usasurg.org (T.J. Miner).

Surg Clin N Am 89 (2009) 27–41
doi:10.1016/j.suc.2008.10.005
surgical.theclinics.com
0039-6109/08/$ – see front matter © 2009 Elsevier Inc. All rights reserved.

one series)[3] are commonly performed to alleviate symptoms when cure is not possible. It is considered inappropriate to select a palliative procedure based on a desire for longer survival.[4,5] Thus, surgical palliation can be defined as the application of procedures with the primary intention of improving the quality of life or relieving symptoms caused by an incurable disease. The intent behind the procedure is what makes palliative surgery a discipline and transforms a palliative operation into a tool to accomplish a goal.

An examination of the history of surgical palliation can help us chart the future of the field. The term *palliative care* was coined in 1973 by the Canadian surgeon Balfour Mount, often recognized as the father of palliative care in North America, as a way to avoid using the more familiar term *hospice*, which had a negative connotation to many of his patients and colleagues.[6] Many current operations and operations used until recently to achieve a surgical "cure" can trace their roots back to procedures designed to alleviate symptomatic and often painful diseases. The most famous example is the William S. Halsted radical mastectomy, which was first used in 1882 to manage pain emanating from locally advanced and ulcerating breast cancers, but was found to be effective in sometimes curing cancer. The radical mastectomy quickly became the gold standard for the treatment of breast cancer and remained so until the mid 1970s.[7] Similarly, coronary artery bypass grafting was first advocated for the symptomatic relief of angina pectoris, but then was found to have survival benefits, and now is a common procedure both for relieving symptoms and extending survival.[6]

Despite medicine's established role in palliation, many physicians are ill-prepared to administer palliative care. Surgical training in palliation is cursory and the quantity and quality of peer-reviewed[8] and surgical textbook[5] literature is generally lacking. When considering the appropriate and effective use of palliative procedures, a surgeon is often confronted with a full range of multidisciplinary treatment options and technical considerations that could potentially relieve some of the symptoms caused by an advanced malignancy. In the palliative phase of care, one must not allow attempts to improve overall survival outweigh efforts aimed at minimizing morbidity and relieving symptoms. While no surgeon wishes to crush a patient's and family's hope for cure, the surgeon also has a responsibility to present realistic goals and expectations so a terminal patient may die with dignity and without undue suffering and pain. This position represents a shift in the classic treatment paradigm and gets back to the roots of medicine, where quality of life often was much more important than quantity. It forces surgeons to constantly reevaluate and rebalance the difficult medical and ethical question of cancer cure versus patient care.

This article provides an overview of the surgical approach to patients who may benefit from palliative care. While the article's details lend themselves to the treatment of complications secondary to advanced malignancies, the data herein can also be extrapolated to other chronic, terminal diseases. Guidelines for patient selection are discussed, using currently available outcomes data as a platform for the critical decision-making process. Suggestions for a multidisciplinary team approach are offered, using the palliative triangle as the ideal model of communication and cooperation. Finally, methods for measuring success are detailed, along with proposals for how to better equip the surgeons of tomorrow with the knowledge and experience needed to tackle these difficult and intimate problems.

WHAT IS KNOWN

Past attempts at describing palliation unfortunately have been based upon anecdotal experiences and individual expectations. Advances in surgical palliative care will depend upon accurate analyses of outcomes data and quality-of-life assessments. To facilitate a dialog with an individual patient, surgeons must be armed with current, reliable, reproducible, and global data from which they can base their individual treatment decisions. However, few verifiable, high-powered, prospective trials are currently available to provide the necessary information. A recent review of the surgical literature on palliative procedures found that most studies were retrospective and focused primarily on procedure risks rather than potential benefits. In those studies available, validated methods for quality-of-life and pain assessment were used only sporadically.[8]

What is well known, however, is that physicians traditionally have been poor at communicating to patients about end-of-life issues and medical care. Indeed, many terminally ill patients spend their final days in fear that they will lose control of their lives and suffer prolonged, painful, and impersonal deaths. At most institutions, surgeons are renowned for rarely discussing "code status" and end-of-life issues with patients or family before even the most complex of operations. This issue garnered mainstream recognition in 1995 with the publication of the results from the Study to Understand Prognoses and Preferences for Outcomes and Risks of Treatments (SUPPORT) trial.[9] Phase I of this study observed that 50% of physicians did not respect or know their patients preferences for end-of-life care and 40% of patients had severe and potentially treatable pain for the several days before their deaths. The interventional arm (phase II), designed to advocate for the individual patient, failed to improve care or patient outcomes. The SUPPORT trial made it painfully obvious that further investigation into the modern health care system was needed to provide better end-of-life care.

Recent data from the surgical literature are now providing some of the critical data required to make difficult clinical decisions regarding surgical palliation. A prospective analysis of 1022 palliative procedures from the Memorial-Sloan Kettering Cancer Center (MSKCC)[10] demonstrated initial symptom resolution in 80% of patients, although further interventions were required for new (25%) or recurrent (25%) symptoms. The procedures were either operative (70%) or endoscopically (30%) based, and were performed electively in 82%, urgently in 16%, and emergently in 2%. **Table 1** summarizes by organ system the most common palliative operations performed. Symptomatic improvement was noted within 30 days in those patients who experienced progress in their clinical condition. Palliative procedures were associated with significant morbidity (40%) and mortality (10%) and with limited anticipated survival (approximately 6 months). Furthermore, poor palliative outcomes were associated with patients who had poor performance status, poor nutrition, weight loss, and no previous cancer therapy. Although predictable symptom relief following palliative procedures can be expected in carefully selected patients, recurrence or the development of additional symptoms limits the durability of the intervention.

Because of the morbidity and mortality associated with palliative operations in terminally ill patients, it has been suggested that anticipatory surgery should be performed for impending problems when patients are more fit for operation. Such preemptive palliation contradicts the surgical aphorism that "it is impossible to palliate the asymptomatic patient," and suggests that improved clinical outcomes can be expected from procedures performed for anticipated symptoms.[11] This question was examined with data from the MSKCC palliative database as described in **Fig. 1**. Preemptive palliative procedures were performed in 107 (13%) of the 823 patients undergoing a palliative procedure, with prevention of the anticipated symptom noted in 84% of those patients. Rates of operative morbidity (29%), mortality (11%), and treatment for debilitating additional symptoms (24%) were similar to those seen in patients having palliative procedures for active symptoms. **Figs. 2** and **3** demonstrate that

Table 1
Symptom resolution for the most common palliative operations by organ system

Organ System	Number of Procedures (%)	Symptom	Most Common Operative Procedure	Number of Patients	Number of Symptoms Resolved (%)
Gastrointestinal	516 (50)	Upper obstruction	Gastrojejunostomy	28	21 (75)
		Mid/lower obstruction	Small bowel resection/bypass	33	30 (91)
		Jaundice	Billiary bypass	30	27 (90)
Neurologic	218 (21)	Neurologic	Resection of brain metastases	125	97 (78)
Cardiorespiratory	108 (11)	Dyspnea	Pleurodesis	32	27 (84)
Skin/musculoskeletal	101 (10)	Bone pain/instability	Repair pathologic fracture	53	46 (87)
		Wound/tumor hygiene	Excision of tumor for local control	18	15 (83)
Genitourinary	79 (8)	Obstruction	Ureteral stents	41	31 (76)

The most common presenting symptoms for each of five organ systems are listed, along with the most common palliative procedure performed for each. Effective symptom resolution was achieved in greater than 75% of all symptomatic patients.

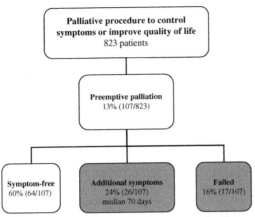

Fig. 1. Outcomes of preemptive palliative procedures. Preemptive palliative procedures were performed on 107 patients in anticipation of specific symptom development (eg, pain, obstruction). Following a preemptive palliative procedure, 84% of patients never developed the anticipated symptom complex. Although 60% of patients remained symptom-free for the remainder of their lives, 24% encountered additional debilitating symptoms that required a subsequent palliative procedure.

although greater overall survival was associated with preemptive palliation (309 days versus 181 days, $P = .002$), there was no significant difference in symptom-free survival between the groups (200 days versus 155 days, $P = .2$). These findings suggest that the good intentions of preemptive palliation may be rewarded by the prevention of anticipated symptoms and are associated with longer overall survival. Morbidity and treatment for additional symptoms diminish potential benefits and offer a cautionary note regarding careful patient selection when considering palliation of the asymptomatic patient.[12]

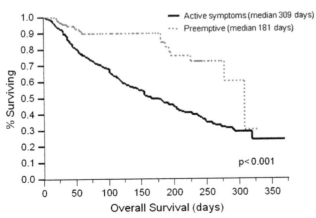

Fig. 2. Overall survival in patients undergoing preemptive palliative procedures. Kaplan-Meier curve demonstrating that palliative procedures performed preemptively were associated with improved overall survival. Performance status, nutritional status, and preemptive palliation were independently associated with longer median survival on multivariate analysis ($P < .001$, Kaplan-Meier estimation).

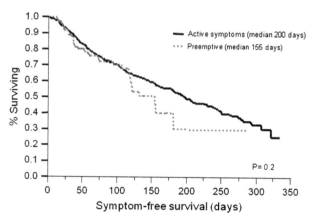

Fig. 3. Symptom-free survival in patients undergoing preemptive palliative procedures. Kaplan-Meier curve demonstrating that preemptive palliative procedures were not associated with a significant improvement in symptom-free survival. Although anticipated symptoms were frequently prevented, symptoms associated with treatment-related complications or the development of new complaints were commonly encountered as a patient's diseases progressed ($P = .2$, Kaplan-Meier estimation).

Symptomatic improvement also is frequently associated with palliative operations for locally recurrent rectal cancer. In an earlier study, bleeding (40%) and obstruction (70%) often improved after surgery, but effective pain control (20%) was difficult to achieve.[13] The durability of symptom relief was limited, as many patients had recurrence of their initial symptoms or developed additional symptoms, making a completely symptom-free clinical course uncommon. In patients who presented with an asymptomatic recurrence, less than half remained symptom-free at death or the completion of follow-up. This study also demonstrated that symptom relief in patients with locally recurrent rectal cancer is associated with resection of all gross local disease. When resection of local disease is not possible, symptom relief, although not as durable, can be achieved with the careful application of additional palliative procedures on an as-needed basis.

Another study analyzed noncurative gastrectomies with a partitioned survival analysis to compare the impact of potential benefits associated with palliative surgery.[14] This technique analyzes treatments by defining relevant clinical health states and comparing their duration with regard to treatment, toxicity, and relapse. Although regularly used to evaluate chemotherapy trials, it is also well suited to evaluate surgical palliation in which treatment-related toxicity plays such an important role in clinical decision making. Duration in the TWiST (time without symptoms or toxicity) state decreased in patients who experienced a major postoperative complication (8.5 months versus 2.1 months, $P = .04$). Because palliative gastrectomies are associated with significant perioperative morbidity and mortality, palliative resections should be performed only in carefully selected patients with severe symptoms.

The absence of a firm, evidence-based foundation for clinical practice often results in variations in care for the patient with advanced cancer, as recommendations can vary amongst providers, specialties, and geographic regions. The therapeutic window for palliative intervention is small. If that brief period is allowed to pass without an intervention, potential beneficial treatment opportunities can easily be lost, possibly leading to the use of other therapies that may be more harmful to the patient's dignity, comfort, and quality of life. Future outcomes research on palliative procedures will, it is hoped, determine the optimal time for intervention for a wide array of clinical scenarios. Surgeons must be committed to treatment based on scientific evidence, rather than individual habits or preferences, even if the evidence seems to suggest overtreatment or undertreatment.

THE SURGEON'S ROLE IN PALLIATION
The Palliative Triangle

Decisions regarding the use of surgical procedures for the palliation of symptoms caused by advanced malignancies require the highest level of surgical judgment. Regardless of the anatomic site leading to the need for palliative intervention, decisions over surgical palliation must consider the medical prognosis of the cancer, the availability and success of nonsurgical treatments, and the individual patient's quality and expectancy of life. Therapy for symptoms must remain flexible and individualized because the disease, as it progresses, will make a continuous impact on the specific needs of the patient. Optimal palliative decision making is facilitated through effective interactions among the patient, family members, and the surgeon through a dynamic relationship described by the term *palliative triangle* (**Fig. 4**).

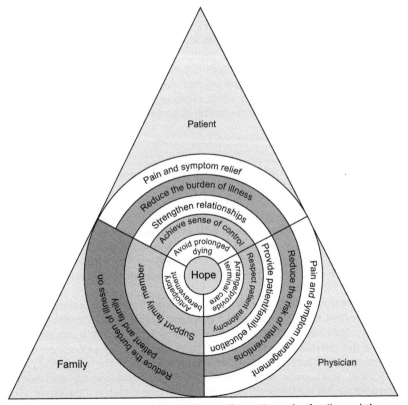

Fig. 4. The palliative triangle. Interactions among the patient, the family, and the surgeon guide individual decisions regarding palliative care. Hope for achievable goals is advanced as each participant of the palliative triangle fulfills specific obligations.

Through the dynamics of the triangle, the patient's complaints, values, and emotional support are considered against known medical and surgical alternatives. Outcomes data obtained through reports on surgical palliation as presented in this article can be especially useful for surgeons seeking to dispense accurate information regarding chance of success, procedure-related durability, the possibility for complications, and anticipated survival. Patients, family members, and surgeons may at times have unrealistic individual expectations. The dynamics of the palliative triangle help to moderate such beliefs and guide the decision-making process toward the best possible choice for the patient. This strong relationship also may explain the observation that patients tend to be highly satisfied with surgeons following palliative operations. That includes patients experiencing no demonstrable benefit from surgery and those experiencing serious complications. These patients were satisfied because the surgeon was there for them at this difficult time of great need; discussed the risks, benefits, and alternatives of all of their choices; and remained engaged with them throughout the remainder of their lives.[15]

Even though the thoughtfulness, judgment, and time required to make such complicated palliative decisions are appreciated by patients and families, some physicians and surgeons shy away from this process with the explanation that they do not want to take away "hope" from those battling cancer. Clearly, it is inappropriate to suggest that an operation with palliative intent will prolong survival. Rather than focus on what cannot be provided (cure), emphasis must be placd on those things that can be realistically delivered. It is reasonable for the patient with advanced cancer to hope for good quality of life, symptom resolution, technically superior palliative operations, dignity, and compassion. As the palliative triangle suggests, the successful surgeon places this definition of hope at the center of a patient's overall care. Through continued personal interactions, each participant in the palliative triangle contributes to making a unique decision, recognizing that varying procedures will have different goals for every individual. Although identical procedures can be performed for similar clinical problems, whether it is right or wrong depends on the unique circumstances of each patient.

Getting to "No"

The last 2 decades have seen medical practice move away from the classical paternalistic pattern toward one of patient autonomy. The discipline has evolved to recognize that surgical treatment options are not right for every patient, and care must be individualized in the multidisciplinary manner that is most appropriate for a specific patient. Thus, rather counterintuitively, there will be times when the most appropriate decision a surgeon can make in the treatment of a terminal patient is *not* to perform an operation. This means saying "no" to a significant number of patients for whom the risks of surgery too much outweigh reasonable expectations of benefits.

A thorough search of the available literature reveals that patient selection is the single most important factor in successful palliation, owing to the significant morbidity and mortality from palliative procedures. The goal is to identify those patients who will achieve the greatest benefit from any given therapy. Considerations relating to the medical condition and performance status of the patient, the extent and prognosis of the cancer, knowledge of the natural history of the primary and secondary symptoms, potential durability of the procedures, and quality-of-life expectations of the individual patient will aid this determination. This is where surgical judgment is imperative, because these problems cannot be thought of in terms of right or wrong. With so little research into this field, global answers that fit a predetermined algorithm are presently nonexistent. However, evidence from the largest prospective trial to date shows patients with poor performance status, poor nutrition, and no experience with previous cancer therapy will respond poorly to palliative procedures.[10]

The palliative surgeon must also anticipate, understand, and address a patient's and family's expectations about the proposed procedure. In going forward, surgeons must be very cautious never to promise an outcome that cannot realistically be delivered. When recognizing those patients who are at risk for procedure-related complications or death, or for whom a particular procedure is unlikely to provide an idealized benefit, surgeons should understand that saying "no" is appropriate. If communicated effectively, the patient will ultimately understand that this does not represent abandonment or failure on the part of the surgeon, but rather a team approach to minimizing symptoms without sacrificing quality of life.

A Multidisciplinary Approach to an Individualized Decision

In the era of informed consent, terminally ill patients can easily find themselves overwhelmed by the endless number of decisions they are required to make to be responsible for and guide their own care. They are presented with numerous treatment options, lists of potential complications, and estimates on prognosis, and it is expected that they come to a logical conclusion without the benefit of a doctor's understanding of the disease process. While preserving patient autonomy is exceedingly important to the modern medical practice, if not done correctly, the patient can be left feeling alone and abandoned. In stark contrast, palliative care emphasizes solidarity and community among the patient, the patient's family, and the entire medical team. By confronting the issues head-on as part of a team, the terminally ill patient can expect to hear the following: "You have lived well. The entire medical team wants to help you die well, and on your terms."

Proper surgical palliation aims to incorporate the principles of hospice care into the acute setting and, therefore, requires a multidisciplinary approach. Individual surgeons, as they continue to maintain a leadership role in the care of patients, have a multitude of resources from which they can draw. Surgeons can receive guidance from their surgical mentors, as well as from the American College of Surgeons,[16] which created the Surgical Palliative Care Task Force in 1998 to facilitate the introduction of precepts and techniques of palliative care. In addition, surgeons can look to their internal medicine colleagues for help in tackling difficult ethical issues and symptom complexes. Hospice and palliative medicine was officially recognized as a specialty by the American Board of Medical Specialties in September 2006. Today, more than 1300 hospitals nationwide provide palliative care programs[17] and 65 hospital-based palliative care fellowship programs now operate in the United States.[18]

Modern surgeons cannot stop there. Through their leadership, surgeons must use the expertise of anyone and everyone who can help each patient reach the decision best suited for him or her. The nursing and patient care staffs are vital parts of the team, as they have the most direct contact with the patient and can observe for new symptoms as well as monitor and treat pain. Chaplains can help ensure that a course of treatment is in line with the patient's spiritual beliefs. Pharmacists and nutritionists can help to overcome the complex medication interactions and side effects so common in the elderly and terminally ill. Massage, physical, and occupational therapists may all provide physical comfort and temporary rehabilitation. Finally, hospital and insurance administrators can aid in navigating the health care system, so that patients and families can be free to spend meaningful days together without worrying over the cost of care at the end of life.[19,20]

ACCURATELY MEASURING SUCCESS

One of the reasons progress in surgical palliation has been slower than expected is that measuring the success of any given therapy has traditionally been quite difficult. Outcome measurements in cancer research focus mainly on the gold standards of 30-day mortality and overall 5-year survival. These statistics become irrelevant to terminally ill patients, whose primary concerns are to live as well as possible in the time they have remaining. In a review of the surgical literature on palliation, Miner and colleagues[8] noted that only 17% of all papers dealing with palliative procedures addressed patient quality of life, and only 40% of those used a validated, previously published research tool. The remainder discussed palliation only in anecdotal and subjective experience-related terms. In this subset of patients, the importance of quality-of-life assessments cannot be overstated, and is often underappreciated by the treating physician.[21–23] These data demonstrate what many already knew: Changing the physician mindset from quantity to quality of life represents the biggest barrier to successful, mainstream palliative care.

Validated and reproducible study instruments are readily available in the literature for use in investigations into palliative procedures. These surveys have all been rigidly designed, stringently tested, and shown to be easy to administer, brief, reliable, valid, and responsive to changes in a patient's clinical condition. The Functional Assessment of Cancer Therapy is a 33-item general cancer quality-of-life measure for evaluating patients receiving cancer treatment.[24] The Functional Living Index for Cancer is a 10-minute questionnaire that uses 22 questions detailing physical well-being and ability, emotional state, sociability, family situation, and nausea.[25] The Edmonton Symptom Assessment System specifically targets symptoms common in cancer patients, including pain, tiredness, nausea, depression, anxiety, drowsiness, appetite, well-being, and shortness of breath.[26] Finally, the Memorial Symptom Assessment Scale inquires about 24 common symptoms and asks patients to determine how often they experience the symptom, along with the severity and the amount of distress it caused them.[27] Each of these study tools can provide reliable and translatable data for future trials of palliative procedures.

The treatment of pain in terminally ill patients can be difficult, as these patients tend to have an increased pain severity along with varying levels of tolerance to narcotics. However, the successful treatment of a patient's pain begins with adequate and accurate recognition of pain location, duration, and intensity. Several simple, yet certifiable and reliable, pain scales are available and can be readily used in clinical practice. Numeric and verbal rating scales ask the patient to identify how much pain they are having by choosing a number from 0 (no pain) to 10 (the worst pain imaginable). The visual analog scale is a straight line with the left end of the line representing no pain and the right end of the line representing the worst pain; patients are asked to mark on the line where they think their pain is.[28] The Faces Pain Scale uses six faces with different expressions on each face and the patient is asked to choose the face that best describes how he or she is feeling.[29] An added benefit of this rating scale is that it can be used by people as young as 3 years.

For investigative purposes, several more detailed survey pain-assessment scales are available. The McGill Pain Questionnaire was developed in 1975 as a way to evaluate a patient experiencing significant pain, as well as to monitor the pain over time and determine the effectiveness of any intervention.[30] The survey asks patients to describe what their pain feels like, how strong it is, and how it changes over time. The Memorial Pain Assessment Card, a condensed survey of pain symptoms, can be completed by experienced patients in under 20 seconds.[31] The card can distinguish pain intensity from pain relief and from general psychologic distress, and was shown to be practically equivalent to a full battery of detailed surveys.

Yet, the absence of an established evidence base in many areas of palliative care is due, at least in part, to major challenges investigators face in designing palliative care trials. Palliative care research faces both ethical and methodological challenges that extend far beyond those of standard research trials.[32,33] Unique ethical issues include the vulnerability of the terminally ill population, high rates of mental incapacity and emotional distress, which create challenges to informed consent, conflict of interest within the dual roles of the clinician-researcher, and difficulty in properly assessing risks and benefits of a particular procedure.[32–36] Research challenges include barriers to collaborative research across specialties; difficulties with recruitment, attrition and compliance;[37] and unclear standards for the types of "best care" practices that should be used. Such problems threaten the credibility of palliative medicine as it struggles to maintain an evidence base on par with those of other specialties. As Casarett[38] best explains:

As long as the randomized controlled trial is the standard by which effectiveness is judged, the field whose interventions have not been proven by this test is at risk of being relegated to second-class status in the medical hierarchy.

Although it is possible to construct an excellent randomized prospective trial to study palliative care, as demonstrated by the International Conference on Malignant Bowel Obstruction,[33] the usefulness of such trials in the palliative care field cannot match those in trials related to other clinical problems. In palliative medicine, the value of a procedure is defined by the individual needs of specific patients, not the overall superiority of a specifically prescribed treatment regimen given to carefully defined patient groups. Because of the appropriate and required emphasis on individualized and patient-specific decision making in palliative medicine, it must be recognized that the role and requirement for the randomized prospective clinical trial is problematic.[39,40] Such trials would provide valuable information important to patient counseling and decision making, but not information useful to constructing generalized algorithms or treatment plans. This emphasis on care tailored for each individual—a central component of palliative medicine—will continue to challenge researchers and practitioners who strive to provide well-constructed and thoughtful studies. In suggesting improvements to palliative care research, many have said the use of multidisciplinary teams of researchers is essential and have called for mixed methods of research. The use of both deductive and inductive methods of inquiry and measurement will result in a much more robust understanding of the topic.[41]

CONTINUING THE TREND

Continuing along the path toward excellent palliative care requires diligent attention to the education of future surgeons in palliative decision-making and communication skills. This then begs the following question: How do you teach residents and medical students to make these difficult, personal, and individualized decisions? With the restrictions to residency training secondary to managed-care and work-hour regulations, surgical training programs have become algorithm based. While this likely works with the old surgical adage of "see one, do one, teach one," all too often residents looking for guidance in the proper conversations of palliative care never get the opportunity to "see one." Robert Milch summed up this idea best in his talk on palliative care in surgical resident education at the American College of Surgeons Clinical Congress in 2003:[42]

If you think about it, demonstration of competency in communication skills is much like performing an operation. We would never think of sending an untutored, unmentored, unsupervised house officer into an operating room to do a procedure never seen, modeled, or performed before, and about which he had only read in a book. Yet this sort of demand for communication skills is one on which we place our house officers all the time, and they have not been taught good communication skills. And very often they have not seen it modeled or mentored.

The vast majority of surgical training programs have no set curriculum for teaching palliative care. However, in one study, 47 general surgery residents from Brown University were surveyed and all felt that managing end-of-life issues are valuable skills for a surgeon and would be a useful and important part of their training.[43] The study was based upon a pilot curriculum in palliative surgical care designed specifically for residents. Presented over three 1-hour sessions, the curriculum included didactic sessions, group discussion, and role-playing scenarios and residents were asked to complete pretest, posttest, and 3-month follow-up surveys. At pretest, only 9% of residents believed they had previously received adequate training in palliation during their residency and only 57% stated they felt comfortable speaking to a patient about end-of-life issues. At posttest and 3-month follow-up, however, these goals were met for 85% of residents. While not designed for mastery of this complex topic, this study demonstrated that surgeons can be introduced effectively to palliative care early in their careers with only a brief time commitment. When used correctly, lessons such as these in conversation and advanced decision making can provide a building block to successful palliation spanning an entire career.[44–46]

WHERE TO GO FROM HERE

The surgical aspects of palliation are complex and require knowledge of complicated disease processes, a wide array of palliative treatment options, potential therapeutic pitfalls, and, most importantly, the individual patient's preferences. Surgeons must become well schooled in the risk assessment of patients before initiating multidisciplinary strategies supported by evidence in the literature. Such factors as symptom severity, the degree of symptom resolution, the timing and choice of procedure, the durability of the intervention, associated complications, and patient preferences all play major roles in determining the overall benefit of the palliative operation. When a cure is not possible, surgeons must get away from focusing on treating the disease and remember to care for the individual patient.

Incorporating palliation into a surgical practice takes time, effort, experience, understanding, and compassion. Surgeons must take the time to evaluate each symptom and therapeutic procedure individually and avoid the trap of making palliation algorithm-based. Obtaining experience requires only time and a desire to improve care. While surgical palliative literature is scarce, the surgeon should make the best use of what's available for data to underpin treatment decisions. Surgeons would benefit by residency curricula that give more emphasis to palliative care so that surgeons learned these lessons early in their professional development.

The root of palliative care lies in the compassion a physician has for his or her terminally ill patient and sensitivity the physician has for the patient's physical, emotional, and spiritual turmoil. The surgeon's responsibility is to lead a team of health care professionals in providing adequate pain and symptom relief, with realistic expectations of benefit, without crushing a patient's hope for reasonably good quality of life in his or her remaining days. The appropriate application of palliative procedures in well-selected patients can provide some of the most useful and effective forms of symptom relief available. In those who are not suitable for operative intervention, a surgeon can remain at the bedside and make it known that *cure* and *care* are not mutually exclusive surgical concepts. Indeed, as inscribed on the statue of Trudeau, it should be remembered that the best care a physician can provide is "to comfort always."

REFERENCES

1. Russell IJ. Consoler toujours—to comfort always. J Musculoskel Pain 2000;8(3): 1–5.
2. McCue JD. The naturalness of dying. JAMA 1995;273(13):1039–43.
3. Krouse RS, Nelson RA, Farell BR, et al. Surgical palliation at a cancer center: incidence and outcomes. Arch Surg 2001;136:773–8.
4. McCahill LE, Krouse RS, Chu DZ, et al. Decision making in palliative surgery. J Am Coll Surg 2002;195:411–22.
5. Easson AM, Crosby JA, Librach SL. Discussion of death and dying in surgical textbooks. Am J Surg 2001;182:34–9.
6. McCahill LE, Dunn GP, Mosenthal AC, et al. Palliation as a core surgical principle: part 1. J Am Coll Surg 2004;199(1):149–60.
7. Halstead WJ. The results of radical operations for the cure of cancer of the breast. Ann Surg 1907;46:1–27.
8. Miner TJ, Jaques DP, Tavaf-Motamen H, et al. Decision making on surgical palliation based on patient outcome data. Am J Surg 1999;177(2):150–4.
9. The SUPPORT Principal Investigators. A controlled trial to improve care for seriously ill hospitalized patients. The Study to Understand Prognoses and Preferences for Outcomes and Risks of Treatments (SUPPORT). JAMA 1995;274(20): 1591–8.
10. Miner TJ, Brennan MF, Jaques DP. A prospective, symptom related, outcomes analysis of 1022 palliative procedures for advanced cancer. Ann Surg 2004; 240(4):719–26.
11. Cady B. Basic principles in surgical oncology. Arch Surg 1997;132(4):338–46.
12. Miner TJ, Jaques PP. The role of pre-emptive palliation in advanced cancer. Ann Surg Oncol 2006;5:173s.
13. Miner TJ, Jaques DP, Paty PB, et al. Symptom control in patients with locally recurrent rectal cancer. 2003;10(1):72–79.
14. Miner TJ, Karpeh MS. Gastrectomy for gastric cancer: defining critical elements of patient selection and outcome assessment. Surg Oncol Clin N Am 2004;13(3): 455–66.
15. Miner TJ, Jaques DP, Shriver CD. A prospective evaluation of patients undergoing surgery for the palliation of an advanced malignancy. Ann Surg Oncol 2002; 9(7):696–703.
16. American College of Surgeons. The Surgical Palliative Care Task Force of the Division of Education page. Available at: http://www.facs.org/palliativecare/main.html. Accessed August 1, 2008.
17. Center to Advance Palliative Care (CAPC) page. Available at: http://www.capc.org/. Accessed August 1, 2008.
18. American Academy of Hospital and Palliative Medicine (AAHPM). Fellowship program directory page. Available at: http://www.aahpm.org/index.html. Accessed August 1, 2008.
19. Singer PA, Lowy FH. Rationing, patient preferences, and cost of care at the end of life. Arch Intern Med 1992;152:478–80.
20. Silberman G. Cancer palliation: economic and societal implications. Cancer Treat Rev 1993;19(Suppl A):97–102.

21. Osoba D. Lessons learned from measuring health-related quality of life in oncology. J Clin Oncol 1994;12:608–16.
22. Fayers PM, Jones DR. Measuring and analyzing the quality of life in cancer clinical trials: a review. Stat Med 1983;2:429–46.
23. Strain JJ. The evolution of quality of life evaluations in cancer therapy. Oncology 1990;4:22–6.
24. Cella DF, Tursky DS, Gray G, et al. The functional assessment of cancer therapy scale: development and validation of the general measure. J Clin Oncol 1993; 11:570–9.
25. Schipper H, Clinch J, McMurray A, et al. Measuring the quality of life of cancer patients: the functional living index—cancer: development and validation. J Clin Oncol 1984;2:472–83.
26. Bruera E, Kuehn N, Miller MJ, et al. The Edmonton Symptom Assessment System (ESAS): a simple method for the assessment of palliative care patients. J Palliat Care 1991;7:6–9.
27. Portenoy RK, Thaler HT, Kornblith AB, et al. The Memorial Symptom Assessment Scale: an instrument for the evaluation of symptom prevalence, characteristics and distress. Eur J Cancer 1994;30A(9):1326–36.
28. Collins SL, Moore RA, McQuay HJ. The visual analogue pain intensity scale: What is moderate pain in millimetres? Pain 1997;72(1–2):95–7.
29. Bieri D, Reeve RA, Champion GD, et al. The Faces pain scale for the self-assessment of the severity of pain experienced by children: development, initial validation, and preliminary investigation for ratio scale properties. Pain 1990;41(2):139–50.
30. Holroyd KA, Holm JE, Keefe F, et al. A multicenter evaluation of the McGill pain questionnaire: results from more than 1700 chronic pain patients. Pain 1992;48: 301–11.
31. Fishman B, Pasternak S, Wallenstein SL, et al. The Memorial Pain Assessment Card: a valid instrument for the evaluation of cancer pain. Cancer 1987;60: 1151–8.
32. Krouse RS, Easson AM, Angelos P. Ethical considerations and barriers to research in surgical palliative care. J Am Coll Surg 2003;196:469–74.
33. Krouse RS. The International Conference on Malignant Bowel Obstruction: a meeting of the minds to advance palliative care research. J Pain Symptom Manage 2007;34(1S):S1–6.
34. Mount B, Cohen R, MacDonald N, et al. Ethical issues in palliative care research revisited. Panminerva Med 1995;9:165–70.
35. Casarett DJ, Knebel A, Helmers K. Ethical challenges of palliative care research. J Pain Symptom Manage 2003;25:S3–5.
36. Easson AM, Lee KF, Brasel K, et al. Clinical research for surgeons in palliative care: challenges and opportunities. J Am Coll Surg 2003;196(1):141–51.
37. Jordhoy MS, Kaasa S, Fayers P, et al. Challenges in palliative care research; recruitment, attrition and compliance: experience from a randomized controlled trial. Panminerva Med 1999;13:299–310.
38. Casarett D. 'Randomize the first patient:' old advice for a new field. AAHPM Bulletin 2002;2:4–5.
39. Storey CP. Randomized trials in palliative care: trying trials. J Palliat Med 2004;7: 393–4.
40. Penrod JD, Morrison RS. Randomized trials in palliative care: challenges for palliative care research. J Palliat Med 2004;7:398–402.
41. Fineberg IC, Grant M, Aziz NM, et al. Prospective integration of cultural consideration in biomedical research for patients with advanced cancer: recommendations

from an international conference on malignant bowel obstruction in palliative care. J Pain Symptom Manage 2007;34(1S):S28–39.

42. McCahill LE, Dunn GP, Mosenthal AC, et al. Palliation as a core surgical principle: part 2. J Am Coll Surg 2004;199(2):321–34.

43. Klaristenfeld DD, Harrington DT, Miner TJ. Teaching palliative care and end-of-life issues: a core curriculum for surgical residents. Ann Surg Oncol 2007;14(6): 1801–6.

44. Huffman JL. Educating surgeons for the new golden hours: honing the skills of palliative care. Surg Clin North Am 2005;85(2):383–91.

45. Bradley CT, Brasel KJ. Core competencies in palliative care for surgeons: interpersonal and communication skills. Am J Hosp Palliat Care 2007–2008;24(6): 499–507.

46. Buckman R. Communication skills in palliative care: a practical guide. Neurol Clin 2001;19:989–1004.

Multimodal Treatment for Head and Neck Cancer

Miriam N. Lango, MD

KEYWORDS

- Head and neck squamous carcinoma • Multimodal treatment
- Organ preservation • Radiation

Head and neck cancer is a relatively uncommon malignancy, comprising 2% to 3% of all cancers diagnosed in the United States. In 2008, an estimated 47,560 patients were diagnosed with head and neck cancer, and an estimated 11,260 died of the disease. Fortunately, the incidence of smoking-related cancers appears to be declining in North America and Western Europe, possibly related to a decrease in smoking in these areas.

EPIDEMIOLOGY

Smoking increases the risk of head and neck squamous cell carcinoma tenfold, in a dose-dependent fashion. The association with smoking is strongest for laryngeal cancer, whereas the synergism between smoking and ethanol abuse is strongly linked to the development of hypopharyngeal cancer. Historically, smoking has been associated in the development of 80% to 90% of head and neck squamous cell carcinomas. The age-adjusted incidence of head and neck cancer has declined since the mid-1980s. Reductions in incidence are not uniform across all tumor sites however. In contrast to the decline in age-adjusted incidences of oral cavity, laryngeal, and hypopharyngeal cancers, a 2% increased incidence of base of tongue cancer and a 4% increase in tonsil cancer has been found.[1] In addition, these cancers now are diagnosed more often in patients younger than 45 and in patients without the usual risk factors. Although the cause is unknown, there is mounting evidence that the human papilloma virus (HPV) is the etiologic agent responsible. The incidence of HPV-related oropharyngeal cancer has increased dramatically over the last 30. The observed improvement in clinical outcome for patients with oropharyngeal cancer over this period has been attributed to favorable tumor biology of HPV-related oropharyngeal malignancy[1,2]

TUMOR SITES

Head and neck cancers arise in the oral cavity (tongue and floor of mouth), oropharynx (base of tongue and tonsil), larynx (supraglottic and glottic larynx), and hypopharynx

Department of Surgical Oncology, Fox Chase Cancer Center, 333 Cottman Avenue, Philadelphia, PA 19011, USA
E-mail address: miriam.lango@fccc.edu

Surg Clin N Am 89 (2009) 43–52
doi:10.1016/j.suc.2008.09.018
0039-6109/08/$ – see front matter © 2009 Elsevier Inc. All rights reserved.

surgical.theclinics.com

(pyriform sinuses and postcricoid region). Cancers of the larynx, hypopharynx, and floor of mouth are most strongly linked with a history of smoking (with or without alcohol abuse), while oral cavity and oropharyngeal cancers in patients without such risk factors are not uncommon.

MANAGEMENT OF HEAD AND NECK CANCER

In general, early stage disease may be managed with single modality treatment, while advanced stage disease is managed with multimodality treatment. Unfortunately, with the exception of glottic larynx and oral tongue cancers, most head and neck cancers remain asymptomatic until late in the disease course. As a result, most patients present with advanced-stage disease, with locally advanced disease or regional spread of cancer.

The management of head and neck cancer has changed over the last 20 to 30 years. Historically, most advanced-stage head and neck cancers were treated with surgery followed by radiation. Traditional surgical techniques, however, rarely resulted in functional organ preservation. Surgery for laryngeal and hypopharyngeal cancers most commonly involved total laryngectomy or laryngopharyngectomy with loss of natural speech, while oropharyngeal tumor extirpation frequently involved mandibulectomy or mandibulotomy approaches, and pharyngeal resections were associated with significant cosmetic and functional deficits. Until recently, cancer control using primary radiation was believed to be inferior to that of surgery, and radiation was itself associated with significant side effects. Nevertheless, incremental improvements in the nonsurgical management of laryngeal and hypopharyngeal cancer have led to primary radiation-based approaches being the preferred treatment for advanced-stage laryngeal, hypopharyngeal, and oropharyngeal cancers. In contrast, many significant morbidity associated with primary radiation to the oral cavity has led surgery to be the primary treatment modality for oral cavity carcinomas at most institutions.

ORAL CAVITY CANCER

Early cancers of the oral cavity (stages 1 and 2) may be treated with primary surgery or radiation with equivalent effectiveness, although primary surgery is favored at most institutions, and allows for a graded therapeutic approach permitting the use of adjuvant treatment in patients who have adverse pathologic features. For stage 1 and 2 oral tongue cancers less than 2 mm thick, partial glossectomy will be curative most of the time. The risk of occult regional spread of cancer increases when the primary cancer has a thickness greater than 2 mm, and observation of the neck in such patients, has been associated with treatment failure in almost 50% of patients,[3] suggesting elective neck dissection is warranted. Patients who have adverse pathologic features on pathologic review of the surgical specimen require additional treatment.[4]

Advanced stage oral cavity squamous carcinomas require multimodal treatment. At most institutions, radiation or chemoradiation therapy follows surgical ablation. Tumor extirpation most often is performed directly through the mouth. Mandibular resection may be required if cancer is fixed to the mandible or if bony erosion is identified. Following surgical ablation, various reconstructive options are available. For large resections, microvascular free-tissue transfer effectively restores soft tissue loss, and generates good cosmetic and functional results. Oral cavity resections may result in variable alterations in speech, but swallowing usually is well preserved, even when large resections are performed.

Most patients who have advanced staged oral cavity cancers will require adjuvant treatment. Pathologic findings following surgical resection determine the need for and intensity of adjuvant treatment. In the presence of multiple positive nodes, perineural invasion, or angiolymphatic invasion, adjuvant radiation is recommended. In the presence of positive surgical margins or extracapsular spread in metastatic lymph nodes, more aggressive management may be recommended. Adjuvant concurrent chemoradiation has been found to diminish locoregional recurrence and improve survival relative to radiation alone in such high-risk patients.[5-7]

OROPHARYNGEAL CANCER

Oropharyngeal cancer treatment may involve primary surgical or radiotherapeutic approaches. For locally advanced disease (T3-4) or metastatic disease (N2-3), combined modality treatment generally is needed. No randomized studies for oropharyngeal cancer comparing primary surgery versus radiation have been done. Traditionally, these tumors were removed through the mouth if such an approach yielded sufficient exposure, but more often, external approaches were required. Mandibulotomy (splitting of the jaw) provided excellent exposure, but was associated with significant morbidity. Lateral pharyngotomy and transhyoid approaches were possible in select cases but resulted in dysphagia and the need for a temporary tracheotomy. To obtain adequate surgical margins, relatively large resections of apparently normal muscle and soft tissue were required. Functional outcomes were especially poor with total glossectomy, which frequently necessitated total laryngectomy to prevent life-threatening aspiration. In the absence of significantly improved local control with surgery, it became increasingly difficult to justify the perceived functional and cosmetic alterations following traditional radical surgery. As a result, nonsurgical approaches, perceived as being less morbid, have been increasingly employed for the management of oropharyngeal cancer.

Primary Radiotherapeutic Approaches for Oropharyngeal Cancer

To enhance locoregional control with radiation for locally advanced head and neck cancer, treatment intensification was pursued vigorously and tested in clinical trials over the last 30 years. Studies of accelerated and hyperfractionated radiotherapy demonstrated an improvement in locoregional control and survival.[8-10] Locoregional control was improved further by the addition of chemotherapy.[11] In 1987, the Radiation Therapy Oncology Group, and the Eastern Cooperative Oncology group in 1992 reported favorable results from combining standard radiation with concurrent high-dose cisplatin (100 mg/m^2) given every 3 weeks during radiation for unresectable head and neck cancers. The use of high-dose concurrent cisplatin with radiotherapy was associated with an improvement in locoregional control and survival in patients with unresectable cancers. This approach subsequently was tested in resectable cancers, where it improved locoregional control but not survival.[12,13] Other chemoradiation schemes also have shown promise. Local control in patients who have locally advanced disease remains suboptimal, however. In one study of oropharyngeal cancer treated with induction chemotherapy with carboplatin and paclitaxel followed by concurrent chemoradiation with paclitaxel, although an overall 3-year locoregional control rate of 82% was reported, greater than half of patients classified as T4 relapsed locally. In general, local recurrence remains a common site of failure. It is unclear that the aggressive use of multiagent systemic therapy, prior to or during radiation, will have an effect on this endpoint.[15]

Surgery After Radiotherapy

After the completion of radiation, a determination of the response to radiation both at the primary site and neck is necessary, but hampered by treatment-related changes. Imaging of the neck using a CT scan 4 weeks after the completion of radiation has been found helpful in identifying patients with residual cancer in the neck who would benefit from neck dissection.[16] Findings on imaging studies of the primary site have been less reliable. Early operative restaging of the primary site performed 4 to 8 weeks after radiation has been associated with improved outcomes for patients requiring surgical salvage.[17] Although the morbidity of surgery after failure of radiation is considerable and oncologic outcomes variable,[9,18,19] effective salvage with acceptable operative complications has been reported.[17,20,21]

Treatment-Related Toxicity

The intensification of nonoperative management has been associated with a dramatic increase in acute treatment-related toxicity and mortality.[22] Gastrostomy tube placement is needed in most patients undergoing intensive treatment with chemoradiation as a result of inadequate oral intake caused by severe (grades 3 and 4) mucositis. Many centers advocate prophylactic feeding tube placement in head and neck cancer patients to prevent the rapid weight loss associated with aggressive treatment with chemoradiation. Reported treatment-related mortality rates of 2% to 5% are not uncommon.[5,14,23] Such reports are all the more striking, because subjects in clinical trials tend to be relatively young and healthy. Trotti and colleagues[22] identified systematic under-reporting of acute and late adverse events in head and neck cancer clinical trials, favoring high intensification treatment schemes. Aggressive chemoradiation regimens may not be tolerated well by average head and neck cancer patients, who as a group are not as motivated as those enrolling in clinical trials. Results of clinical trial results thus may not be generalizable, and clinical judgment is required when treating individual patients with head and neck cancer.

Novel strategies to ameliorate some of the chronic effects of radiation such as xerostomia and chronic dysphagia have been explored. Persistent xerostomia, virtually universal in patients treated with radiation, is ameliorated by using intensity-modulated radiotherapy (IMRT) to spare salivary glands from radiation toxicity, with patients reporting improvement in quality of life.[24] The need to spare the contralateral parotid gland in patients requiring bilateral neck radiation is now an accepted indication for IMRT. Chronic dysphagia is common in oropharyngeal cancer patients treated with chemoradiation, with most patients being unable to resume unmodified regular diets.[14] Silent aspiration is highly prevalent in this patient population.[25] The use of chemoradiation also has been associated with an increased incidence of prolonged feeding tube dependence, with 5% to 25% of patients requiring nutritional support long after the completion of radiation. Using IMRT to spare specific structures important for swallowing function such as the pharyngeal constrictors or esophagus appears promising and is an active area of investigation.[26]

The toxicity profiles of biologic agents make them attractive alternatives to traditional chemotherapeutic agents. Of the large number of agents currently under investigation, the epidermal growth factor receptor antagonist cetuximab has been studied most. A recent clinical trial of radiation therapy for advanced-stage head and neck cancer revealed improved survival in the group treated with concurrent cetuximab. Interestingly, the survival benefit was confined to patients receiving altered radiation fractionation. In the absence of a standard chemoradiation arm, results of this study are difficult to interpret. Nevertheless, the use of biologic agents in combination with or as substitute for traditional chemotherapy with radiation is likely to continue to increase.

Oropharyngeal Cancer and Human Papilloma Virus

The relative incidence of oropharyngeal cancer has increased, particularly in subjects less than 45 years old.[27] This increase in incidence has been accompanied by a decline in mortality and an increased prevalence of HPV in oropharyngeal tumor specimens.[28] Although mortality from oropharyngeal cancer has declined, mortality rates for patients with oral cavity and laryngeal cancers have remained stagnant or increased.[29] There is mounting evidence that HPV may be causally related to these observations. Patients who have HPV-related oropharyngeal cancers are believed to have an improved prognosis. In a prospective trial of 96 oropharyngeal cancer patients treated with chemoradiation, the overall 2-year survival was 95% for patients who had HPV- positive tumors, compared with 62% for patients who had HPV-negative tumors ($P = .005$).[30] Risk stratification by HPV status likely will serve as the basis for treatment modification in future clinical trials for patients who have oropharyngeal cancer.

LARYNGEAL AND HYPOPHARYNGEAL CANCER

The indications for total laryngectomy have decreased over the last 20 years, as larynx preserving therapies have become standard of care. Laryngeal-preserving surgeries including open partial laryngectomy, and transoral approaches have yielded excellent control of disease in patients who have localized disease (T1-2N0). At this time, most patients with locally advanced disease or bulky nodal disease are treated with concurrent chemoradiation. The use of larynx-preserving surgery for advanced disease is currently an active area of investigation.[31]

Primary Radiation for Laryngeal Cancer

In the United States, most patients who have advanced-stage laryngeal or hypopharyngeal cancer are treated with chemoradiation. Until the early 1990s, the standard treatment for locally advanced (T3-4) laryngeal cancer and hypopharyngeal cancer was total laryngectomy and laryngopharyngectomy, respectively. A landmark study conducted by the Department of Veterans Affairs Laryngeal Cancer Study Group[32] demonstrated the feasibility of a chemoradiation approach for laryngeal preservation. In this study, patients with stage 3 and 4 laryngeal cancers were randomized to induction chemotherapy using cisplatin and 5-fluorouracil followed by radiation for responders or an immediate laryngectomy. Using such an approach, the larynx was preserved in 64% of those treated with induction chemotherapy, without a difference in survival between groups. The European Organization for Research and Treatment (EORTC) conducted a phase 3 trial for hypopharyngeal carcinoma with a similar design.[33] Induction chemotherapy selected a subset of patients who had advanced-stage pyriform sinus cancer for organ preservation without any apparent decrease in survival. A subsequent trial, the Radiation Therapy Oncology Group (RTOG) 91-11 trial,[13] randomized patients who had laryngeal cancer to one of three groups: induction chemotherapy followed by radiation, concurrent chemoradiation using cisplatin, or radiation alone. In this study, concurrent chemoradiation improved locoregional control and larynx preservation compared with the other two arms. The morbidity of nonsurgical treatments of laryngeal cancer however was significant in this trial, and associated with a 3% risk of treatment-related death. The addition of chemotherapy to radiation was associated with a greater than threefold increase in acute toxicity burden without an improvement in survival.[22] Thus, organ preservation comes at a cost.

Indications for Total Laryngectomy

Primary laryngectomy remains the best treatment option for some patients who have advanced laryngeal cancer. Patients who have laryngeal cancer must be capable of compliance and have an adequate performance status to undergo chemoradiation. Patients who have locally advanced larynx cancer, with cartilaginous destruction and organ dysfunction are also poor candidates for chemoradiation. Anatomic organ preservation in a patient who will remain tracheotomy tube- and gastrostomy tube-dependent is senseless. Care of the laryngectomy stoma is simpler, associated with less pain, and has little or no aspiration or problems with foul tracheal secretions.

Total laryngectomy also is indicated as salvage after failure of nonsurgical treatments. At this time, failure of previous therapy may be the most common indication for total laryngectomy. Salvage laryngectomy has been associated with an increased risk of wound complications, relative to those performed before radiation. Major wound complications have been reported in 27% of patients, with a range between 5% and 48% in a recent review of the literature.[21] Similarly, pharyngocutaneous fistulas have been reported in 15% to 80% of patients undergoing salvage laryngectomy, although the wound complication rates, fistula rates, and oncologic outcomes appear to be influenced by surgeon and hospital experience. Fistula may result in rupture of the carotid artery, a catastrophic and usually fatal complication of surgery in this setting, rarely seen in the absence of antecedent radiation. Referral of such complex patients to high-volume centers is recommended.

LARYNGEAL PRESERVATION SURGERY AND MINIMALLY INVASIVE SURGERY FOR HEAD AND NECK CANCER

Surgical extirpation may be accomplished with laryngeal preservation for many patients who have laryngeal cancer. For T1-2 and select T3 and T4 laryngeal cancers, avoidance of a permanent tracheal stoma is possible using laryngeal conservation surgery, which includes several procedures, including supraglottic partial laryngectomy, supracricoid partial laryngectomy, and others. In a supracricoid partial laryngectomy with cricohyoidepiglottopexy or cricohyoidopexy as described by Laccourreye,[34,35] resection of the endolarynx is followed by impaction of the cricoid cartilage and hyoid bone. Acutely, the surgery is associated with swallowing impairment and aspiration. As a result, a temporary tracheotomy is required. Because the entire endolarynx is resected, wide surgical resection margins frequently are obtained, achieving high local control rates. Dufour reported laryngeal preservation rates of 90% and local control rates of 91% for 118 T3N0-3 laryngeal cancers.[36] In general, larynx-preserving surgery is not offered to patients who are anticipated to require adjuvant radiation for tumor control, since radiation exacerbates airway edema and swallowing dysfunction, and increases the risk of chondronecrosis. Open partial laryngectomy, including supracricoid partial laryngectomy, are successfully used in the salvage setting with acceptable oncologic and functional outcomes in properly selected patients.[37,38]

In contrast to laryngeal preservation surgery, performed through incisions in the neck, minimally invasive surgical approaches involve tumor ablation performed through the mouth. Typically, transoral approaches are associated with restricted surgical exposure. By means of technologic advances, many of these limitations have been overcome. The evolution of minimally invasive surgery for tumors of the upper aerodigestive tract began with the development of the CO_2 laser coupled to an operative microscope initially described by Strong and Jako in 1972.[39] The subsequent development of bivalved laryngoscopes and specialized endoscopic instrumentation enabled larger tumors from various aerodigestive tract sites to be removed transorally. Steiner and colleagues[40–42] reported effective local control following endoscopic CO_2 laser resection for laryngeal, base of tongue, and hypopharyngeal cancers. Surgical resections were customized for the extent of the primary tumor. Transoral laser surgery was compared with Mohs micrographic surgery for cutaneous malignancies, in which tumor transection, followed by narrow margin extirpation with preservation of noninvolved tissue, was associated with high rates of local tumor control. Tracheotomies and feeding tubes rarely were required. Transoral robotic surgery using the daVinci Surgical System has been adapted for use in the head and neck, for extirpation of various upper aerodigestive tract cancers.[43–45] The angled telescopes and wristed instruments used with robotic surgery significantly improve exposure and access. The use of the photonic gap band fiber, a flexible carbon dioxide laser fiber, has the potential to further enhance tumor extirpation. The CO_2 laser cuts through tissues with little bleeding or charring, and transmission through a flexible fiber enables laser delivery to previously inaccessible sites.[46] Recovery from minimally invasive surgery is generally rapid. Bleeding in the postoperative period is while infrequent may be severe.

Functional outcomes following minimally invasive surgery are better than those following open approaches. For patients treated with minimally invasive surgery who do not require adjuvant treatment with radiation, rehabilitation from surgery is generally prompt and functional outcomes are expected to be excellent. The long-term functional outcomes of patients who require radiation and chemotherapy due to the presence of adverse pathologic features, or advanced stage disease, are not likely to be as favorable. Many patients requiring additional therapy could have been treated with primary radiation, albeit to a higher radiation dose. Does surgery contribute to local control? How much of a decrease in the intensity of adjuvant treatment yields a clinically significant difference in quality of life? Rigorous assessments of therapeutic trials incorporating surgery are lacking. Long-standing barriers to randomized clinical trials involving surgery, including patient preferences and institutional biases, will continue to pose challenges. A multicenter database registry with a well-defined cohort and standardized clinical protocol as described by Higgins and colleagues[47] creating a well-defined study population would be a good start. In the absence of data, the role of minimally invasive surgery for advanced-stage head and neck cancer remains ill-defined.

SUMMARY

The multimodal treatment of head and neck cancer has been associated with improvements in locoregional control and organ preservation, but at the cost of significant acute and chronic toxicity. Various strategies to describe and quantify outcomes in a meaningful way, devise methods to diminish acute and late effects, and enhance quality of life are under investigation. Risk stratification may allow treatment modification based on tumor biology. The ultimate goal includes improved survival with preservation of function and quality of life.

REFERENCES

1. Sturgis EM, Cinciripini PM. Trends in head and neck cancer incidence in relation to smoking prevalence: an emerging epidemic of human papillomavirus-associated cancers? Cancer 2007;110(7):1429–35.

2. Ernster JA, Sciotto CG, O'Brien MM, et al. Rising incidence of oropharyngeal cancer and the role of oncogenic human papilloma virus. Laryngoscope 2007; 117(12):2115–28.

3. Spiro RH, Huvos AG, Wong GY, et al. Predictive value of tumor thickness in squamous carcinoma confined to the tongue and floor of the mouth. Am J Surg 1986; 152(4):345–50.

4. Sparano A, Weinstein G, Chalian A, et al. Multivariate predictors of occult neck metastasis in early oral tongue cancer. Otolaryngol Head Neck Surg 2004; 131(4):472–6.

5. Cooper JS, Pajak TF, Forastiere AA, et al. Postoperative concurrent radiotherapy and chemotherapy for high-risk squamous cell carcinoma of the head and neck. N Engl J Med 2004;350(19):1937–44.

6. Bernier J, Domenge C, Ozsahin M, et al. Postoperative irradiation with or without concomitant chemotherapy for locally advanced head and neck cancer. N Engl J Med 2004;350(19):1945–52.

7. Bernier J, Cooper JS, Pajak TF, et al. Defining risk levels in locally advanced head and neck cancers: a comparative analysis of concurrent postoperative radiation plus chemotherapy trials of the EORTC (#22931) and RTOG (# 9501). Head Neck 2005;27(10):843–50.

8. Horiot JC, Le Fur R, N'Guyen T, et al. Hyperfractionation versus conventional fractionation in oropharyngeal carcinoma: final analysis of a randomized trial of the EORTC cooperative group of radiotherapy. Radiother Oncol 1992;25(4):231–41.

9. Bourhis J, Overgaard J, Audry H, et al. Hyperfractionated or accelerated radiotherapy in head and neck cancer: a meta-analysis. Lancet 2006;368(9538):843–54.

10. Parsons JT, Mendenhall WM, Cassisi NJ, et al. Hyperfractionation for head and neck cancer. Int J Radiat Oncol Biol Phys 1988;14(4):649–58.

11. Brizel DM, Albers ME, Fisher SR, et al. Hyperfractionated irradiation with or without concurrent chemotherapy for locally advanced head and neck cancer. N Engl J Med 1998;338(25):1798–804.

12. Adelstein DJ, Lavertu P, Saxton JP, et al. Mature results of a phase III randomized trial comparing concurrent chemoradiotherapy with radiation therapy alone in patients with stage III and IV squamous cell carcinoma of the head and neck. Cancer 2000;88(4):876–83.

13. Forastiere AA, Goepfert H, Maor M, et al. Concurrent chemotherapy and radiotherapy for organ preservation in advanced laryngeal cancer. N Engl J Med 2003;349(22):2091–8.

14. Machtay M, Rosenthal DI, Hershock D, et al. Organ preservation therapy using induction plus concurrent chemoradiation for advanced resectable oropharyngeal carcinoma: a University of Pennsylvania phase II trial. J Clin Oncol 2002; 20(19):3964–71.

15. Vokes EE, Stenson K, Rosen FR, et al. Weekly carboplatin and paclitaxel followed by concomitant paclitaxel, fluorouracil, and hydroxyurea chemoradiotherapy: curative and organ-preserving therapy for advanced head and neck cancer. J Clin Oncol 2003;21(2):320–6.

16. Liauw SL, Mancuso AA, Amdur RJ, et al. Postradiotherapy neck dissection for lymph node-positive head and neck cancer: the use of computed tomography to manage the neck. J Clin Oncol 2006;24(9):1421–7.

17. Yom SS, Machtay M, Biel MA, et al. Survival impact of planned restaging and early surgical salvage following definitive chemoradiation for locally advanced squamous cell carcinomas of the oropharynx and hypopharynx. Am J Clin Oncol 2005;28(4):385–92.

18. Temam S, Pape E, Janot F, et al. Salvage surgery after failure of very accelerated radiotherapy in advanced head-and-neck squamous cell carcinoma. Int J Radiat Oncol Biol Phys 2005;62(4):1078–83.
19. Bourhis J, Lapeyre M, Tortochaux J, et al. Phase III randomized trial of very accelerated radiation therapy compared with conventional radiation therapy in squamous cell head and neck cancer: a GORTEC trial. J Clin Oncol 2006; 24(18):2873–8.
20. Weber RS, Berkey BA, Forastiere A, et al. Outcome of salvage total laryngectomy following organ preservation therapy: the radiation therapy oncology group trial 91–11. Arch Otolaryngol Head Neck Surg 2003;129(1):44–9.
21. Goodwin WJ Jr. Salvage surgery for patients with recurrent squamous cell carcinoma of the upper aerodigestive tract: when do the ends justify the means? Laryngoscope 2000;110(3 Pt 2 Suppl 93):1–18.
22. Trotti A, Pajak TF, Gwede CK, et al. TAME: development of a new method for summarising adverse events of cancer treatment by the Radiation Therapy Oncology Group. Lancet Oncol 2007;8(7):613–24.
23. de Castro G Jr, Snitcovsky IM, Gebrim EM, et al. High-dose cisplatin concurrent to conventionally delivered radiotherapy is associated with unacceptable toxicity in unresectable, nonmetastatic stage IV head and neck squamous cell carcinoma. Eur Arch Otorhinolaryngol 2007;264(12):1475–82.
24. Pacholke HD, Amdur RJ, Morris CG, et al. Late xerostomia after intensity-modulated radiation therapy versus conventional radiotherapy. Am J Clin Oncol 2005;28(4):351–8.
25. Langerman A, Maccracken E, Kasza K, et al. Aspiration in chemoradiated patients with head and neck cancer. Arch Otolaryngol Head Neck Surg 2007; 133(12):1289–95.
26. Feng FY, Kim HM, Lyden TH, et al. Intensity-modulated radiotherapy of head and neck cancer aiming to reduce dysphagia: early dose–effect relationships for the swallowing structures. Int J Radiat Oncol Biol Phys 2007;68(5):1289–98.
27. Shiboski CH, Schmidt BL, Jordan RC. Tongue and tonsil carcinoma: increasing trends in the U.S. population ages 20–44 years. Cancer 2005;103(9):1843–9.
28. Dahlstrand H, Lindquist W, Ye T, et al. Human papillomavirus (HPV) as a risk factor for the increase in incidence of tonsillar cancer and its expression of E6 and E7. Presented at: ASCO Annual Meeting Proceedings. Chicago, May 30–June 3 2008, 2008.
29. Carvalho AL, Nishimoto IN, Califano JA, et al. Trends in incidence and prognosis for head and neck cancer in the United States: a site-specific analysis of the SEER database. Int J Cancer 2005;114(5):806–16.
30. Fakhry C, Westra WH, Li S, et al. Improved survival of patients with human papillomavirus-positive head and neck squamous cell carcinoma in a prospective clinical trial. J Natl Cancer Inst 2008;100(4):261–9.
31. Agrawal A, Moon J, Davis RK, et al. Transoral carbon dioxide laser supraglottic laryngectomy and irradiation in stage I, II, and III squamous cell carcinoma of the supraglottic larynx: report of Southwest Oncology Group phase 2 trial S9709. Arch Otolaryngol Head Neck Surg 2007;133(10):1044–50.
32. Induction chemotherapy plus radiation compared with surgery plus radiation in patients with advanced laryngeal cancer. The Department of Veterans Affairs Laryngeal Cancer Study Group. N Engl J Med 1991;324(24):1685–90.
33. Lefebvre JL, Chevalier D, Luboinski B, et al. Larynx preservation in pyriform sinus cancer: preliminary results of a European Organization for Research and Treatment of Cancer phase III trial. EORTC Head and Neck Cancer Cooperative Group. J Natl Cancer Inst 1996;88(13):890–9.

34. Laccourreye H, Laccourreye O, Weinstein G, et al. Supracricoid laryngectomy with cricohyoidopexy: a partial laryngeal procedure for selected supraglottic and transglottic carcinomas. Laryngoscope 1990;100(7):735–41.

35. Laccourreye H, Laccourreye O, Weinstein G, et al. Supracricoid laryngectomy with cricohyoidoepiglottopexy: a partial laryngeal procedure for glottic carcinoma. Ann Otol Rhinol Laryngol 1990;99(6 Pt 1):421–6.

36. Dufour X, Hans S, De Mones E, et al. Local control after supracricoid partial laryngectomy for advanced endolaryngeal squamous cell carcinoma classified as T3. Arch Otolaryngol Head Neck Surg 2004;130(9):1092–9.

37. Deganello A, Gallo O, De Cesare JM, et al. Supracricoid partial laryngectomy as salvage surgery for radiation therapy failure. Head Neck 2008;30(8):1064–71.

38. Marioni G, Marchese-Ragona R, Lucioni M, et al. Organ-preservation surgery following failed radiotherapy for laryngeal cancer. Evaluation, patient selection, functional outcome, and survival. Curr Opin Otolaryngol Head Neck Surg 2008; 16(2):141–6.

39. Strong MS, Jako GJ. Laser surgery in the larynx. Early clinical experience with continuous CO 2 laser. Ann Otol Rhinol Laryngol 1972;81(6):791–8.

40. Steiner W, Ambrosch P, Hess CF, et al. Organ preservation by transoral laser microsurgery in piriform sinus carcinoma. Otolaryngol Head Neck Surg 2001; 124(1):58–67.

41. Steiner W, Fierek O, Ambrosch P, et al. Transoral laser microsurgery for squamous cell carcinoma of the base of the tongue. Arch Otolaryngol Head Neck Surg 2003;129(1):36–43.

42. Ambrosch P, Kron M, Steiner W. Carbon dioxide laser microsurgery for early supraglottic carcinoma. Ann Otol Rhinol Laryngol 1998;107(8):680–8.

43. Weinstein GS, O'Malley BW Jr, Snyder W, et al. Transoral robotic surgery: supraglottic partial laryngectomy. Ann Otol Rhinol Laryngol 2007;116(1):19–23.

44. Weinstein GS, O'Malley BW Jr, Snyder W, et al. Transoral robotic surgery: radical tonsillectomy. Arch Otolaryngol Head Neck Surg 2007;133(12):1220–6.

45. O'Malley BW Jr, Weinstein GS, Snyder W, et al. Transoral robotic surgery (TORS) for base of tongue neoplasms. Laryngoscope 2006;116(8):1465–72.

46. Holsinger FC, Prichard CN, Shapira G, et al. Use of the photonic band gap fiber assembly CO2 laser system in head and neck surgical oncology. Laryngoscope 2006;116(7):1288–90.

47. Higgins KM, Wang JR. State of head and neck surgical oncology research— a review and critical appraisal of landmark studies. Head Neck 2008;30:1636–42.

The Role of Minimally Invasive Treatments in Surgical Oncology

Mark S. Choh, MD[a,b], James A. Madura II, MD[c,d],*

KEYWORDS
- Laparoscopy • Endoscopy • Cancer
- Minimally invasive surgery

Surgical extirpation of malignancy remains the only hope for cure and the best means of palliation for many forms of cancer. The evolutions of anesthesia, blood product transfusion, and reconstructive techniques enable the modern surgeon to resect nearly anything. But at what cost and what benefit? How many times has a perfectly executed surgical procedure been rebuked by unfavorable tumor biology in the form of early and extensive recurrence? The true revolution of minimally invasive intervention for cancer will occur as the genetic and cellular mechanisms of malignancy are revealed, allowing directed therapy at this level. In the mean time, minimally invasive is synonymous with laparo-endoscopic surgical techniques. These techniques have altered the way surgery is performed for both benign and malignant diseases radically.

Since the introduction of fiber-optic endoscopy in the 1960s and the widespread introduction of laparoscopic cholecystectomy in the 1980s, there has been a huge increase in the use of minimally invasive surgical modalities in clinical practice. The incorporation of these techniques into routine practice has led to the innovation and development of surgical endoscopic techniques in other fields, such as thoracoscopy and transanal endoscopic microsurgery (TEM), and more recent developments, such as robotic surgery and natural orifice transluminal endoscopic surgery (NOTES).

The implementation of these techniques for oncologic indications in surgical practice has progressed at a much slower pace, however. In general, the surgical community has been hesitant to use minimally invasive techniques as part of cancer

---

[a] Department of General Surgery, Rush University Medical Center, 1725 West Harrison Avenue, Chicago, IL 60612, USA
[b] Department of Minimally Invasive and Robotic Surgery, University of Illinois-Chicago, 840 S. Wood Street, Suite 435E, Chicago, IL 60612 USA
[c] Department of Surgery, John H. Stroger Hospital of Cook County, 1901 West Harrison Avenue, Chicago, IL 60612, USA
[d] Department of General Surgery, Rush University Medical Center, 1725 West Harrison Avenue, Suite 818, Chicago, IL 60612, USA
* Corresponding author. Department of General Surgery, Rush University Medical Center, 1725 West Harrison Avenue, Suite 818, Chicago, IL 60612.
E-mail address: james_madura@rush.edu (J.A. Madura).

Surg Clin N Am 89 (2009) 53–77
doi:10.1016/j.suc.2008.09.017
0039-6109/08/$ – see front matter © 2009 Published by Elsevier Inc.

surgical.theclinics.com

treatments, because of concerns that a minimally invasive surgical approach will compromise the oncologic principles of the treatment. For most of the malignancies addressed, these issues deal with the adequacy of resection of the primary tumor, along with the ability to perform a similar extent of lymphadenectomy to an open case. Although many laparoscopic or thoracoscopic operations for benign disease have shown a clinical benefit in terms of improved cosmesis, less postoperative pain, shorter return of bowel function, shorter length of hospitalization, and quicker return to normal activity, those benefits are minimized if it means a lesser cancer operation is performed or if tumor dissemination occurs as a result of pneumoperitoneum.

Although it is established that diagnostic laparoscopy is beneficial in improving diagnosis and patient outcomes in certain malignancies, there are only a handful of examples where the minimally invasive surgical treatment of cancer has been accepted widely. Colon cancer is the most notable, with several large, prospective, multicenter randomized control trials demonstrating similar oncologic outcomes with its corresponding open surgical treatment. No other malignancy has had trials of the magnitude of the Clinical Outcomes of Surgical Therapy (COST) and Conventional versus Laparoscopic-Assisted Surgery in patients with Colon Cancer (CLASICC) trials to demonstrate the efficacy of minimally invasive techniques to treat cancer. The oncologic outcomes with video-assisted thoracic surgery (VATS) lobectomy for early stage lung cancer have been similar to those with open thoracotomy with reduction in pain and debility; however, thoracic surgeons have been slow to adopt VATS lobectomy into their practice.

For many malignancies, however, there is a paucity of literature examining minimally invasive treatments. For some, such as adrenal cortical carcinomas, the rarity of the disease itself prevents the development of a large enough study to adequately compare the two treatments. For others, such as pancreatic cancer, the technical difficulty of the laparoscopic treatment would preclude most surgeons from incorporating the operation into practice. And just as with any disease process and subsequent treatment, there exist regional differences on a local, national, and international level that make it difficult to generalize data. As technology continues to expand with new techniques and applications, one must measure these interventions against the results of standard therapy. Can new technology achieve the same, or better results and what is the real benefit and cost to patients and the system?

COLON CANCER

Colorectal cancer is the third most commonly diagnosed cancer and the second leading cause of cancer-related death for both men and women in the United States. Most patients diagnosed with colorectal cancer undergo surgical resection as the primary modality of treatment. In 1991, Jacobs and colleagues[1] reported the first laparoscopic resection of a sigmoid colon cancer. From then on, experience with laparoscopic techniques for colon resection increased rapidly.

Reports of port site recurrences, including one series that reported port site metastases in 3 of 14 patients, led to hesitancy on the part of surgeons to use laparoscopy for oncologic resections, however.[2,3] This led to several randomized controlled trials comparing the oncologic outcomes of the use of laparoscopic-assisted and open resections for colon cancer. The results of these trials have quelled initial fears of using laparoscopy for colon cancer, and provide some of the strongest evidence for the use of minimally invasive techniques for oncologic indications.

Studies examining short-term outcomes of laparoscopic colectomy for cancer have been consistent, demonstrating longer operative times, but less blood loss, less postoperative pain and use of narcotic analgesia, quicker return of bowel function, and shorter length of hospitalization.[4–7] These studies also have shown equivalent perioperative morbidity and mortality rates[5–7] and in some cases, improved results, especially with higher-volume centers.[4,8] Studies assessing the adequacy of oncologic resection, such as lymph node harvest, margins, and length of vascular pedicle also showed no significant difference between open and laparoscopic resections.[4–9]

Lacy and colleagues[4] first published the results of a single-institution randomized controlled trial of 219 patients undergoing laparoscopic-assisted and open colon resections in 2002. This trial from Barcelona actually demonstrated a significant improvement in cancer-related survival (91% versus 79%, $P = .03$) and a trend toward improvement in overall survival (82% versus 74%, $P = .14$) at 5 years. This difference in survival was explained by an improvement in survival among resections in patients who had stage 3 tumors.

The Barcelona trial led the way to three larger multicenter randomized controlled trials comparing laparoscopic and open resections for colon cancer. The most recognized is the COST trial,[5] which enrolled and randomized 872 patients to undergo resection by 66 surgeons from 48 institutions in North America. The initial report of outcomes of the COST trial revealed no difference in 3-year overall survival (86% in laparoscopic group versus 85% in open group, $P = .51$) and recurrence rates (16% versus 18%, $P = .32$). A more recent report of 5-year outcomes revealed similar outcomes for disease-free 5-year survival (69.2% versus 68.4%, $P = .94$), overall 5-year survival (76.4% versus 74.6%, $P = .93$), and recurrence rates (19.4% versus 21.8%, $P = .25$).[10]

Two other large, multi-institution, randomized controlled trials from Europe have helped support the short- and long-term results of the COST trial. The 3-year outcomes of the COLOR trial,[6] a multicenter randomized controlled trial from Europe, have yet to be published. The CLASICC trial[7,11] included 794 patients from 27 United Kingdom centers and was unique in that it included patients with both colon and rectal cancer. In addition, it randomized patients at a ratio of 2:1 laparoscopic to open. When examining the 413 patients in the colon cancer group only, there was no difference at 3 years in local recurrence (8.6% in laparoscopic group versus 7.9% in open group, $P = .76$), distant recurrence (15.2% versus 14.3%, $P = .74$), overall survival, or disease-free survival. The data in the rectal cancer group will be discussed in a separate section.

Although early reports noted port site recurrences as high as 4%,[12] port site and wound recurrences reported in the large randomized studies were low (0.9% to 1.9%) and comparable to historical rates of abdominal wall recurrences in open resections.[4,5,11,13] Various methods have been used to prevent wound implants during specimen retrieval, such as wound protection, gasless laparoscopy, wound excision, peritoneal irrigation; none have been studied extensively in human trials.

Available data support the use of laparoscopic resections for colon cancer. That being said, surgeons must approach each patient on a case-by-case basis. Indications for resection must remain the same as with open surgery, and accurate preoperative localization by means of barium enema, CT colonography, or endoscopic tattooing is imperative, because palpation of the tumor is not as reliable with laparoscopy. Adherence to oncologic principles of proximal ligation of the primary arterial supply, adequate margins, and a lymphadenectomy of at least 12 lymph nodes[14,15] are mandatory. Failure to achieve these oncologic principles during laparoscopic resection mandates conversion to an open resection.

In addition, laparoscopic colon resection must be performed by surgeons comfortable with laparoscopy if the results from these clinical trials are to be expected. The surgeons in both the COST and COLOR trials had performed at least 20 colon resections. The number of cases required to become competent depends on the individual surgeon and his or her prior laparoscopic experience.

RECTAL CANCER

Although proximal tumors of the intraperitoneal rectum can be approached similarly to a distal colon cancer, most rectal cancers are a separate entity, with different preoperative staging and operative and treatment strategies. Therefore, the applicability of minimally invasive techniques to rectal cancer also must be examined separately. Advances in the treatment of rectal cancers such as the standardization of total mesorectal excision (TME), the introduction of TEM, and the use of neoadjuvant chemoradiation therapy have improved outcomes;[16] however, surgical resection remains the mainstay of curative treatment for rectal cancer. Similar to colon cancer, there is a growing body of literature supporting the use of laparoscopy and TEM as acceptable and possibly preferred methods of surgical resection for rectal cancers.

Laparoscopic Resection of Rectal Cancer

In 2004, Leung and colleagues[17] published results of a randomized trial comparing 403 laparoscopic and open resections of sigmoid and proximal rectal cancers, excluding tumors less than 5 cm from the dentate line. Findings with short-term outcomes were similar to those in the colon cancer literature with significantly longer operating room times (189.9 versus 144.2 minutes, $P<.001$), but less blood loss (169 versus 238 mL, $P = .06$), postoperative narcotic use, and shorter time to first flatus, bowel movement, and oral intake (all $P<.001$) noted in the laparoscopic group. Hospital stay and time to resumption of normal activity were also significantly shorter. Conversion occurred in 23.2% of patients, with immediate conversion in the 34 cases where local invasion was noted. There was no significant difference in the rates of postoperative mortality or complications. Of note, direct costs were higher in the laparoscopic group ($9297 versus $7194, $P<.001$). Short-term outcomes data from the CLASICC study mentioned previously[7] support these results.

Short-term measures of the adequacy of oncologic resection in these studies raise some concerns. Although distal margins in the Leung trial[16] were similar between the laparoscopic and open groups, there was a trend toward a lower lymph node yield in the laparoscopic group (11.1 versus 12.1, $P = .18$). Similar results were found in a more recent prospective, nonrandomized analysis by Strohlein and colleagues;[18] the lymph node harvest in the laparoscopic group was significantly less than in the open group (13.5 versus 16.9, $P = .001$), although this may be explained partially by a slightly higher rate of the use of neoadjuvant therapy in the laparoscopic group (20.2% versus 14.2%). In addition, a higher, although statistically nonsignificant rate of positive circumferential margins was found in the CLASSIC trial[7] among patients undergoing anterior resection (12% versus 6%, $P = .19$).

These short-term markers of resection adequacy, however, have not resulted in differences in long-term oncologic outcomes. In the Leung study,[17] there were no differences in 5-year overall survival (76.1% in laparoscopic group versus 72.9% in open group, $P = .61$), disease free survival (75.3% versus 78.3%, $P = .45$), or local recurrence (6.6% versus 4.1%, $P = .37$). Similarly, the higher rates of positive radial margins with the laparoscopic anterior resection group in the CLASICC study[18,19] did not result in a higher rate of local recurrence as initially hypothesized (7.8% versus 7.0%, $P = .70$). In addition, 3-year overall survival and disease-free survival rates were similar in the laparoscopic and open groups.

In the Strohlein study,[18] similar results were noted; however, a significant improvement in 5-year survival was noted in patients undergoing laparoscopic deep anterior resection ($P = .035$). Some authors have postulated that the improved magnification of the endoscopic camera allows for a more precise dissection of the mesorectum with better preservation of the autonomic nerve plexus and other structures.[7,11] This is supported by the higher proportion of complete TME resections in the CLASICC study (77% versus 66%).[7] A recent Cochrane systematic review of the literature comparing laparoscopic versus open TME resections[20] found similar long-term outcomes in the two groups.

Most of literature does not include patients who underwent neoadjuvant radiation as part of their treatment, and the presence of postradiation changes may make a laparoscopic dissection more difficult. More recent literature supports similar short-term outcomes with laparoscopic TME after neoadjuvant therapy;[19,21] however, long-term oncologic outcomes for patients in this group are still pending.

Literature currently supports the use of laparoscopy for the resection of rectal cancer. Surgical principles that apply to open resections must still be followed, however; these include removal of the blood and lymphatics up to the origin of the superior rectal artery or inferior mesenteric artery, a distal margin of 1 to 2 cm, and total mesorectal excision. As with colon cancer, surgeon experience must be adequate to tackle laparoscopic resection of rectal tumors. In addition, unique patient factors such as pelvic anatomy, obesity, and the possibility of a bulky uterus may prohibit laparoscopic intervention from a technical standpoint.

Transanal Endoscopic Microsurgery

TEM, a technique used as an extension of local transanal excision, was developed by Karl Buess in the mid-1980s.[22] The system consists of a 40 mm diameter proctoscope, an optical stereoscope, and an insufflation mechanism to create a pneumorectum working space, along with four working ports for instrument access (**Fig. 1**). This results in superior visualization and maneuverability that allows surgeons to access lesions in the rectum that previously were inaccessible with conventional transanal excision techniques.

TEM initially was used for the excision of benign polyps that were unresectable by means of colonoscopy; since then, numerous series have examined the use of TEM

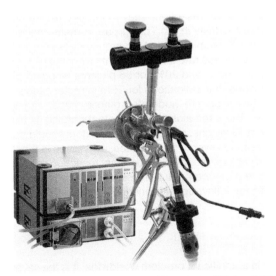

Fig. 1. Transanal endoscopic microsurgery setup. (*Courtesy of* Richard Wolf Medical Instruments Corporation, Vernon Hills, IL; with permission.)

for rectal cancer as an alternative to a major abdominal operation, particularly in T1 tumors. The rationale behind local excision of these tumors is that they have an extremely low risk of nodal involvement. A review by Hermanek and colleagues[23] of 1588 rectal tumors revealed that well differentiated to moderately differentiated pT1 tumors had a 3% risk of positive lymph nodes; therefore, a major resection involving lymphadenectomy is unlikely to provide additional benefit. Endorectal ultrasound or MRI using endorectal coils, however, can identify suspicious lymph nodes preoperatively, with 60% to 92% accuracy, and these should be used as part of a routine preoperative work-up.[24,25]

It is clear that in experienced hands, TEM can be performed safely with low morbidity rates. In comparing TEM with traditional anterior resection, Winde and colleagues[26] found significantly less blood loss, lower operative times, use of analgesia, and shorter length of hospitalization in the TEM group. Most complications are minor and include self-limiting bleeding, tenesmus, fecal soilage, and urinary retention. In a review of 334 patients undergoing TEM, Mentges and colleagues[27] reported a 0.3% mortality rate and a 5.5% rate of major complications such as hemorrhage requiring intervention, entry into the peritoneum causing sepsis, and rectovaginal fistula. Studies examining functional results after TEM have shown short-term dysfunction when measured by either manometry or surveys, but improvement in these symptoms over the long term.[28,29]

With respect to oncologic outcomes, most authors report good-to-excellent results, with low recurrence rates, and long-term survival numbers similar to those of open resection. Duhan-Floyd and Saclarides[30] reported a series of 53 patients undergoing TEM for pT1 rectal cancers, with a 7.5% recurrence rate. All patients underwent open resection of their recurrences, and no disease-related deaths were noted. Winde and colleagues[26] conducted a small prospective, randomized controlled trial of 52 patients with uT1N0 rectal cancer who were randomized to undergo either TEM-assisted resection or open anterior resection. Although local recurrence rates were higher in the TEM group (4.2% versus 0%), there was no difference in 5-year survival. With respect to more advanced tumors, Lezoche and colleagues[31] randomized 40 patients with T2N0 rectal carcinomas who underwent neoadjuvant chemoradiation therapy to either TEM or laparoscopic anterior resection. They found two recurrences in each group, with no cancer-related mortality in the TEM group. A meta-analysis of 22 studies by Suppiah and colleagues[32] examining local recurrence rates after TEM for rectal cancer reported a 6% local recurrence rate for 552 patients who had pT1 cancer, 14% for 174 patients who had pT2 cancer, and 20% for 56 patients who had pT3 lesions.

Most authors conclude that indications for TEM in rectal cancer include uT1N0 lesions that are well differentiated to moderately differentiated, with no evidence of lymphovascular invasion. There remains some debate regarding its use in higher-risk T1 and well differentiated T2 lesions. More advanced tumors should not be resected with TEM for curative intent; however, it can be a feasible option in these patients if significant comorbidities precluding a major abdominal resection are present. Salvage resection of local recurrences can result in excellent long-term disease-free survival rates; therefore diligent follow-up of patients undergoing resection by means of TEM is mandatory.

ESOPHAGUS

Esophageal cancer is a significant problem worldwide; it is the seventh most common cause of cancer death, and 13,900 new cases are diagnosed in the United States each year.[33] Surgical resection is the only hope for cure; however, a large proportion of patients is unresectable at the time of presentation. Even with resection, prognosis is poor, with 40% of patients dying in the first year after surgery and 5-year disease-free survival rates of 27%.[34,35]

It can be difficult to assess the potential benefits and outcomes of minimally invasive approaches to esophageal resection, since there is no consensus on the optimal open approach to esophageal resection. Some larger studies have shown an improvement in perioperative morbidity with the transhiatal approach to esophagectomy,[36,37] and other studies have shown no significant difference.[38] Data from other centers suggest that the transthoracic approach results in a more complete lymphadenectomy.[34] In addition, studies have shown that outcomes may be related more to hospital and surgeon volume than the surgical approach.[39] Because no agreed-upon standard of resection has been determined for the traditional open approach to esophagectomy, it is difficult to evaluate outcomes after minimally invasive approaches to esophageal resection.

A myriad of minimally invasive techniques for esophagectomy have been described. An initial report by McAnema and colleagues[40] in 1994 described the thoracoscopic-assisted mobilization of the esophagus combined with an open abdominal approach. Following this, DePaula and colleagues[41] in 1995 demonstrated the feasibility of laparoscopic transhiatal esophagectomy. Since then, numerous approaches to minimally invasive esophagectomy have been described, including thoracoscopic-assisted esophageal resection, laparoscopic transhiatal resection, hand-assisted laparoscopic transhiatal resection, and three-field, combined thoracoscopic/laparoscopic resection.[42–47]

Examination of short-term outcomes after minimally invasive esophagectomy (MIE) has demonstrated different approaches to be safe and feasible with outcomes equivalent to traditional open approaches. In a series of 46 patients undergoing MIE, mostly by means of a three-field technique, Nguyen and colleagues[44] demonstrated a mortality (4.3%), major complication (17.4%), and anastomotic leak (8.7%) rates that were similar to those of historical controls.[48] In a retrospective review comparing 332 MIE cases (309 thoracoscopic-assisted with open laparotomy, 23 total MIE) with 114 open cases, Smithers and colleagues[49] demonstrated less blood loss, less time in the thorax, and a shorter length of stay with the minimally invasive approaches, with no increase in lymph node harvest, complication rates, or mortality.

Luketich and colleagues[45] have reported the largest series of total MIE to date. Using a combined thoracoscopic/laparoscopic/cervical three-field technique, he reported short- and long-term outcomes on 222 patients undergoing MIE. Short-term outcomes were also similar to historical series, with a 30-day mortality rate of 1.4% and an anastomotic leak rate of 11.7%. Mean hospital stay was 7 days, however, much less than in open series.[48]

As with any oncologic indication for minimally invasive surgery (MIS), concerns about adequacy of oncologic resection with MIE exist. There are no randomized trials comparing open and minimally invasive approaches for esophageal cancer; however, reported case series have promising results that suggest that oncologic outcomes after MIE may be similar to those of open series. Braghetto and colleagues[39,50] reported a consecutive series of 166 patients undergoing esophagectomy for cancer. Three-year survival rates were 93.8% for stage 1 disease and 54% for stage 2a disease among patients undergoing MIE, and there was no significant difference when compared with patients in the open group. Similarly, in the Smithers group,[49] there was no significant difference in survival when the open, thoracoscopic-assisted, and total MIE groups were compared stage for stage for 3-year survival. The Luketich series[45] included 185 patients undergoing MIE for cancer, and 3-year survival rates for stage 1, 2a, 2b, and 3 patients were

65%, 41%, 45%, and 17%. The small numbers in all these series make it difficult to make any definitive conclusions; however, the data suggest that survival outcomes with MIE may be similar to those after traditional approaches to resection.

With experience and improved technology, the hope is that minimally invasive approaches may improve short-term outcomes by eliminating the need for either a thoracotomy requiring lung collapse and rib spreading, or a major laparotomy, while providing at least equivalent, if not improved survival outcomes over traditional open approaches. Although further work must be done to determine the optimal approach to esophageal resection, it is clear that minimally invasive approaches to esophageal resection will play a major role in the treatment of esophageal cancer for years to come.

STOMACH

Gastric cancer is the second leading cause of cancer-related deaths worldwide; however, it only ranks 13th on the list in the United States.[51] Although it is decreasing in incidence, it continues to be one of the deadliest gastrointestinal malignancies, with over 30% of patients presenting with stage 4 disease, overall 5- year survival less than 40%, and the ability to perform a curative resection in as few as 20% of patients in Western series.[52] Despite the grim prognosis, surgical intervention must be aggressive and attentive to oncologic principles, because an R0 resection is the most important prognostic factor for resectable gastric cancer.[53–55]

MIS applied to gastric cancer has the potential to improve patient quality of life over traditional open surgery. There is no doubt that upper abdominal surgeries reap great benefit from MIS as documented in cholecystectomy, antireflux and diaphragmatic surgery, splenectomy, and bariatric surgery. Patients experience less pain after MIS compared with open surgeries in the upper abdomen because of the absence of upper abdominal incisions and aggressive, prolonged retraction needed for traditional surgical exposures. This translates to less pulmonary embarrassment and faster recovery, which has been documented after laparoscopic gastrectomy for benign and malignant disease.[56,57] Endoscopic and laparoscopic resections of benign and low malignant potential lesions (such as gastrointestinal stromal tumors, GIST) have been received with little controversy and are considered preferred approaches in centers where the expertise is available. The same concerns that prefaced the wide acceptance of laparoscopic colon surgery for malignancy have slowed the adoption of MIS approaches to gastric cancer, however; These include: adequate surgical margin, lymph node harvest, effect on pattern of recurrence, and long-term survival data. Facility with advanced endoscopic and laparoscopic techniques and desire of traditional surgical oncologists to adopt new technology likely have roles in the limited widespread application also.

Currently, a range of MIS options for gastric adenocarcinoma are being performed around the world, including endoscopic mucosal resection (EMR), intragastric mucosal resection, laparoscopic wedge resection, and partial and total laparoscopic or laparoscopic-assisted gastric resections. Choice of approach should have the patient's best chance for curative resection in mind.

Endoscopic Mucosal Resection for Gastric Cancer

In Asia, where there is a high prevalence of gastric cancer, aggressive screening practices have led to more frequent identification of early gastric cancer (EGC). The gold standard for the treatment of early gastric cancer remains gastrectomy with lymph node dissection, with 5-year survival rates in the 96% to 99% range.[58–60] Outcomes after endoscopic resection of early gastric cancers are similar to those after operative treatment in these, mainly Japanese series. One must keep in mind that gastric cancer in North America is thought to be a different entity, often found at a more advanced stage with less favorable histology. Therefore, endoscopic therapy for gastric cancer has not found widespread use in Western centers.

EGC is defined by the Japanese classification system as cancer that does not invade beyond the submucosa (T1) regardless of lymph node involvement.[61] The ideal candidates for EMR within this group are those patients whose risk of lymph node involvement is minimal. Although there have been no prospective randomized trials comparing operative and endoscopic resections for early gastric techniques, large retrospective series have identified commonly accepted indications for EMR: well differentiated, intestinal type carcinoma that is limited to the mucosa. Tumors must have no evidence of ulceration and be 20 mm or less in elevated types and 10 mm or less in depressed or flat types.[62] When these criteria are met, and no lymphovascular invasion is seen on final pathologic examination, incidence of lymph node involvement is less than 0.4%.[63]

More recently, expanded criteria have been proposed, based on large retrospective series examining characteristics of EGC and risk of lymph node metastases.[64,65] These indications include nonulcerated, well differentiated mucosal tumors of any size and ulcerated mucosal tumors of up to 30 mm. In addition, they include nonulcerated lesions with microscopic (less than or equal to 500 μm) invasion into the submucosa. Survival rates after EMR using the expanded criteria have been excellent; in a series of 714 patients undergoing EMR, 146 (20%) diagnosed using the extended indications, 3-year overall and disease-specific survival rates were 99.2% and 93.7%, respectively.[66]

Numerous methods have been used for EMR of EGC, from fulguration to wide excision using a submucosal technique. The benefit of EMR over fulguration is that it provides a complete pathologic specimen for accurate depth staging and does not exclude the possibility of further surgical therapy should the need for it arise. Endoscopic resection techniques include strip biopsy, double snare polypectomy, and cap-fitted endoscopic resection. More recently, the use of endoscopic submucosal dissection (ESD) techniques has given endoscopists the ability to resect larger cancers as a single specimen, resulting in a higher rate of curative resection in some series.[66] In addition, intragastric mucosal resection techniques using the transgastric deployment of laparoscopic instruments have been described.[67]

Laparoscopic Resection for Gastric Cancer

Laparoscopic surgery for gastric cancer is the logical extension of nearly 20 years of laparoscopic surgery on the stomach for benign diseases such as peptic ulcer disease, gastroesophageal reflux, and bariatric procedures.[68,69] Regardless of one's commitment to lesser or more radical surgical intervention for gastric cancer, all of the proposed operations done in conventional open surgery can be, and have been, performed laparoscopically. The first laparoscopically assisted Billroth I gastrectomy for EGC was performed in 1991 as reported by Katano and colleagues[70] in 1994. The preliminary results of 10 patients undergoing laparoscopically assisted total gastrectomy were reported in 1995 to be equivalent to open surgery with the benefits of less pain and faster recovery.[71] Laparoscopic extended lymphadenectomy and pancreaticosplenectomy subsequently have been published.[72,73] Data are maturing that confirm the initial impression of equivalent oncologic results and the benefits of the MIS approach. Five-year results of a randomized prospective trial comparing 59 patients subjected to open or laparoscopic subtotal gastrectomy showed no statistical difference in number of lymph nodes resected, mortality, morbidity, or overall and disease-free survival with the benefits of reduced blood loss, shorter time to resumption of oral intake, and earlier discharge from hospital attributed to the laparoscopic approach.[74] The authors' own data confirm the ability to achieve adequate lymph node retrieval and margins even in advanced gastric cancers.[75] MIS techniques now are being applied in palliative resections also. To the authors' knowledge, none of the early concerns for port site recurrence, dissemination of tumor, or inadequate tumor clearance have materialized.

The technical aspects of MIS gastrectomy involve stapling, multifield procedures, multiple anastomoses, and dealing with unexpected anatomy and challenges. The learning curve is quite shallow (meaning it takes a large number of cases to become proficient). It is therefore likely that the widespread application of MIS to gastric cancer will be slow to occur.

PANCREAS

Of all the operations in general surgery, resections of the pancreas are among the most complex, requiring an extensive dissection of a retroperitoneal organ with an intimate relationship with numerous major vascular structures and often a complex reconstruction involving the alimentary and biliary tracts. Performing pancreatic resections, whether at the head or tail, therefore, remains among the most technically challenging operations that can be performed in a minimally invasive fashion. In addition, fewer than 20% of adenocarcinomas of the pancreas are considered resectable for cure,[76,77] and the poor prognosis of this disease makes it difficult to assess the clinical benefits of laparoscopy in pancreatic cancer. Although there is generalized support for using diagnostic laparoscopy and laparoscopic ultrasound as a means to assess resectability of pancreatic tumors,[78,79] most of the literature involving resections of the pancreas for oncologic indications remains anecdotal.

Both laparoscopic distal pancreatectomy and laparoscopic pancreaticoduodenectomy (LPD) first were reported in 1994.[80,81] An early report by Gagner, who performed the first laparoscopic Whipple procedure, questioned the clinical benefit of laparoscopic pancreatic resection, reporting long operative times and high complication rates, with minimal benefit in short-term outcomes, such as hospital stay.[82] More recent reports, however, have confirmed the feasibility of laparoscopic pancreatic resections and supported some benefits in short-term postoperative outcomes. Conversion rates for laparoscopic resection have been between 0% and 20%.[83–85] Edwin and colleagues[83] reported on 32 patients who underwent either enucleation or distal pancreatectomy, with or without splenectomy, with a short median hospital stay (5.5 days) and postoperative need for opioid analgesia (2 days). Complications were reported at 38%; however, most of the complications reported were minor. Mabrut and colleagues[84] reported the results of a multicenter, retrospective review of 127 patients undergoing laparoscopic pancreas resections; most (79%) undergoing distal pancreatectomy. Mean operating times were reasonable at 190 minutes, and median postoperative hospital stay was 7 days, which was significantly less when compared with the group undergoing open resection after conversion. Pancreas-related complication rates were 31%, comparable to published results on open resections.[86]

Similarly, the feasibility of LPD is being supported by recent literature. Various techniques and approaches have been reported, including hand-assisted and robot-assisted techniques, as well as using a minilaparotomy for the reconstructive portion of the operation.[82,87–91] Indications and short-term outcomes of currently published case series are listed in **Table 1**. Although operative times are quite lengthy, there does seem to be a trend toward shorter times with more experience. Hospital stay is difficult to

Table 1
Short-term outcomes of laparoscopic pancreaticoduodenectomy

Author	Number of Patients	Operative Details	Conversion	Diagnosis	Operative Time (Min)	Length of Stay (Days)	Complication Rate
Gagner et al, 1997	10	Laparoscopic pylorus-preserving PD	40%	Pancreatic adenocarcinoma–4 Ampullary cancer–3 Chronic pancreatitis–2 Cholangiocarcinoma–1	510	22.3	50%
Giulianotti et al, 2003	8	Robot-assisted PD	12.5%	Pancreatic adenocarcinoma–3 Mucinous cystadenoma–2 Cholangiocarcinoma–2 Ampullary carcinoma–1	490	NR	37%
Dulucq et al, 2006	22	13 total laparoscopic 9 laparoscopic-assisted	13.6%	Pancreatic adenocarcinoma–11 Ampullary cancer–3 Chronic pancreatitis–2 Duodenal adenocarcinoma–2 Other–4	287	16.2	32%
Palanivelu et al, 2007	42	Laparoscopic pylorus-preserving PD	0%	Ampullary Ca–24 Pancreatic adenocarcinoma–9 Pancreatic cystadenoma–4 Cholangiocarcinoma–3 Chronic pancreatitis–2	370	10.2	31%
Pugliese et al, 2008	19	6 total laparoscopic 7 laparoscopic assisted	31%	Pancreatic adenocarcinoma–11 Ampullary carcinoma–4 Cholangiocarcinoma–3 Mesenchymal tumor–1	461	18	37%

Abbreviations: Ca, cancer; PD, pancreaticoduodenectomy.

analyze because of the wide variation in the approach to postoperative management. That being said, complication rates in the later series seem to be similar to those published in larger studies of the standard open pancreaticoduodenectomy.[92]

There have been no studies, however, that specifically have examined long-term oncologic outcomes after laparoscopic pancreatic resections. Palanivelu and colleagues[89] reported the largest series, 42 patients, to date. Of these, 40 were performed for malignant indications with close follow-up. Median survival for the total group was 49 months, and 5-year survival was 30.7% for ampullary carcinoma and 19.1% for pancreatic adenocarcinoma.

It is clear that performing laparoscopic pancreatic resections requires a significant amount of experience and technical expertise. If performed by skilled and practiced surgeons with proper indications, it is definitely feasible; however, the true clinical benefit remains to be seen. As technological advances in endoscopy, robotics, and surgical instrumentation improve, the use of laparoscopy in pancreatic surgery will continue to grow.

LIVER

Like the pancreas, liver resection, whether performed open or laparoscopically, remains one of the more complex operations performed in surgery. Because of significant risks of bleeding, difficulty in obtaining hemostasis, and risk of major morbidity because of bile leakage, incomplete resection, and air embolism, many surgeons have shied away from implementing minimally invasive techniques for resecting hepatic malignancies. Since the first report of a laparoscopic partial hepatectomy by Gagner and colleagues in 1992,[93] however, there has been a steady increase in international experience with wedge resection, minor anatomic resections, and even major hepatic resections for both benign and malignant disease. Technological innovations in intraoperative ultrasound, ultrasonic dissection techniques, and endoscopic linear staplers have made laparoscopic liver resections not only feasible, but also beneficial to patients when performed by surgeons with appropriate expertise and experience.

A recent meta-analysis by Simillis and colleagues[94] examined short-term outcomes of studies comparing laparoscopic hepatic resections (LHR) and open hepatic resections (OHR) for benign and malignant neoplasms. An examination of eight studies comprising 409 hepatic resections (165 [40.3%] laparoscopic, 244 [59.7%] open) found significant decreases with LHR in operative blood loss (-123 mL, 95% CI, -179 to -67 mL, $P<.001$), duration of hospital stay (-2.6 days, 95% CI, -3.8 to -1.4 days, $P<.001$), and period to first oral intake (-0.5 days, 95% CI, -1.0 to 0.0 days, $P = .05$). In addition, there were no significant differences in postoperative mortality or complications. These differences were all similar when studies matched for the presence of malignancy were analyzed.

Most commonly, liver resections for malignancy involve resection of either hepatocellular carcinoma (HCC) or metastases from colorectal cancer (CRM). Although there are only a handful of studies examining the oncologic outcomes of LHR for malignancy, early data suggest comparable survival rates to open resections.

Although controversial, orthotopic liver transplantation may offer the highest recurrence-free survival rates in patients who have HCC.[95] Limited organ availability and strict indications for transplantation, however, limit its availability as a treatment option. Newer techniques such as transarterial chemoembolization (TACE), ethanol injection, and radiofrequency ablation frequently are used in select cases of HCC. Surgical resection, however, remains the primary modality of treatment for many patients. Kaneko and colleagues[96] examined 30 cases of LHR for HCC, all of whom underwent either left lateral segmentectomy or partial hepatectomy. When compared with 28 control cases based on similar preoperative criteria, there was no difference in 5-year overall survival (61% versus 62%, not significant [NS]) or disease-free survival (31% versus 29%, NS). Vibert and colleagues[97] reported data on 113 laparoscopic liver resections (including major hepatectomies), 65 of them for malignant disease (16 for HCC, 41 for CRM, and 8 for other metastatic disease). With respect to HCC, overall survival and disease-free survival at 3 years were 66% and 68%, respectively, numbers that compare with open results. More recently, Chen and colleagues[98] reported a series of 116 patients undergoing LHR for HCC, including 19 patients undergoing major resection of more than two segments. Five-year overall survival rates were similar in the minor (two or less segments) and major (three or more segments) resection groups (59.4% and 61.7%).

Resection of isolated CRM after resection of the primary tumor has been shown to improve survival rates when appropriate timing and patient selection are employed.[99] In the study by Vibert and colleagues,[97] follow-up data were available in 30 patients who underwent LHR for CRM; all patients underwent adjuvant systemic chemotherapy. Although 14 recurrences were noted, overall survival was excellent, at 87% at 3 years, with a disease-free survival rate of 51% at 3 years.

These data suggest that the use of LHR for malignant neoplasms improves short-term outcomes with similar long-term oncologic results. Because of the increased risk of major bleeding complications and the inability to gain rapid hemostasis with the laparoscopic approach, it is imperative that a surgeon is familiar with the various laparoscopic instruments and techniques that are required for a safe laparoscopic liver resection. In addition, patient-related factors such as cirrhosis, ascites, adhesions, anatomic anomalies, and tumor-related factors such as size, location, and relationship to major vascular structures must be taken into account when selecting candidates for LHR.

ADRENALECTOMY

Although there has not been a large, prospective, randomized controlled trial comparing laparoscopic versus open adrenalectomy, there have been numerous well-designed retrospective and prospective nonrandomized studies demonstrating a dramatic benefit in clinical outcomes such as postoperative pain, cosmesis, return of bowel function, and length of hospitalization, along with no significant increase, and in some cases, a decrease in complication rates.[100–102] Since the introduction of laparoscopic adrenalectomy (LA) in 1992,[103] data have led to LA becoming the gold standard for resecting benign adrenal lesions and incidentalomas, based on a 2002 consensus statement published by the National Institutes of Health (NIH).[104] The approach to malignant lesions of the adrenal gland is not as straightforward, however.

The indications for adrenalectomy have not changed with the recent popularization of laparoscopic adrenalectomy. Functioning tumors, lesions with an increased risk of malignancy, and in some cases, solitary metastatic lesions to the adrenal gland are indications for resection of the adrenal gland. Lesions greater than 6 cm should be considered for resection, and lesions of intermediate size (4 to 6 cm) should be evaluated on an individual basis based on patient's age and comorbidities, as well as suspicious features on imaging (irregular borders, heterogenous lesions with calcification or necrosis, and invasion of surrounding structures).

Adrenal Cortical Carcinoma

Primary adrenal cortical carcinoma (ACC) is an extremely rare and aggressive tumor. These tumors account for approximately 0.1% of all adrenal lesions and 4% of surgically resected specimens,[105] and they have dismal prognosis. Reported 5-year survival rates are between 22% and 26%,[106,107] and locoregional recurrence rates are 30% after traditional open resection.[108] Because of the rarity of this tumor, there are only a handful of case series that discuss the role of laparoscopy in resecting primary ACC. An early report by Suzuki and colleagues[109] discussed a case of peritoneal dissemination and mortality of a patient who underwent laparoscopic adrenalectomy for ACC. Since then, series examining patients with ACC have reported locoregional recurrence rates ranging from 0% to 100%; however, a combined examination of these reports resulted in rates of 26% for local recurrences and 32% for peritoneal recurrences (**Table 2**), rates that approximate those from larger open studies. Reported survival rates are also similar; Porpiglia and colleagues[110] reported a series of 13 patients undergoing resection for malignancy, seven with ACC. At a mean follow-up of 30 months, there was only one death; five patients had no evidence of recurrent disease. Nocca and colleagues[111] compared nine patients undergoing resection for ACC. Four patients undergoing laparoscopic resection with a mean tumor size of 85 mm had a mean survival of 42.3 months compared with five patients undergoing open resection with a mean tumor size of 122 mm with a mean survival of 29.7 months.

Isolated Adrenal Metastasis

The adrenal glands are a common site of metastasis for several malignancies, including melanoma, colon, renal, and lung cancers. Numerous reports have demonstrated improved survival after resection of solitary adrenal metastases.[112,113] As surgeons became more comfortable using laparoscopy for resection of benign adrenal lesions, experience began to grow with laparoscopic resections for metastatic disease.

An early report by Heniford and colleagues[114] reported ten patients undergoing laparoscopic adrenalectomy for malignancy, nine with metastatic lesions, with no locoregional recurrences at a mean follow-up of 8.3 months. In a series of 31 patients, Moinzadeh and Gill[115] reported 26 with adrenal metastasis; 53% of patients were alive at a median follow-up of 42 months. Five-year estimated Kaplan-Meier survival was 40%. More recently, Strong and colleagues[116] from Memorial Sloan Kettering reported their experience with the resection of 94 patients who had isolated adrenal metastases. Laparoscopic resection was used for 31 patients, and there was no difference in local recurrence, margin status, disease-free survival, or overall survival between the open and laparoscopic groups, although the mean size of the laparoscopic tumors was smaller in the open group.

These data suggest that oncologic outcomes after laparoscopic adrenalectomy for primary ACC or metastatic adrenal lesions may be acceptable given appropriate preoperative indications for laparoscopic resection. There does not seem to be a size limitation on laparoscopic resection, as long as adequate local resection and negative margins can be achieved.

MINIMALLY INVASIVE THYROID SURGERY FOR THYROID CANCER

Papillary and follicular carcinomas of the thyroid both have extremely favorable prognosis, with a high definitive cure rate and low mortality.[117,118] Surgical resection remains the mainstay of treatment, although there is some controversy on the optimal extent of thyroid resection, and the role of central neck dissection without a preoperative suspicion of lymph node metastases. The use of endoscopic techniques in the neck may seem unconventional; however, surgeons are using minimally invasive techniques to perform thyroid resections, for benign and malignant conditions.

Table 2
Reported recurrence after laparoscopic adrenalectomy for adrenal cortical carcinoma

| First Author | Institution/Location | Year | Total with Adrenal Cortical Carcinoma | Number of Patients | | | Follow-Up (Months) |
				Local Recurrence	Peritoneal Recurrence	Distant Recurrence	
Ushiyama	Hamamatsu/Japan	1997	1	1	0	0	19
Hamoir	Liege/Belgium	1998	1	0	1	0	6
Foxius	Louvain/Belgium	1999	1	0	1	0	6
Valeri	Firenze/Italy	2002	1	1	NR	NR	8
Porpiglia	Orbassano/Italy	2002	4	0	0	NR	19*
MacGillivray	Maine Medical Center/United States	2002	1	0	0	1	42
Henry	Marseilles/France	2002	6	0	0	1	28*
Kebebew	University of California San Francisco/United States	2002	6†	2	NR	1	40‡
Zeh	Johns Hopkins/United States	2003	4	1	NR	1	24*
Prager	University of Vienna/Austria	2004	2	0	0	0	60, 27
Moinzadeh	Cleveland Clinic/United States	2005	6	2	NR	NR	21
Gonzalez	MDACC	2005	6	3	5	4	15*
Total	—	—	39	10/39 (26%)	7/22 (32%)	8/28 (29%)	—

Abbreviations: NR, not reported; MDACC, M.D. Anderson Cancer Center.
* Median
† One case converted to open after diagnostic laparoscopy
‡ Mean
Adapted from Gonzalez RJ, Shapiro S, Sarlis N, et al. Laparoscopic resection of adrenal cortical carcinoma: a cautionary note. Surgery 2005;138:1083; with permission.

One of the difficulties in assessing oncologic outcomes with minimally invasive thyroid surgery is the wide variation in techniques used. Techniques described include minimizing incision length to 2.5 to 3.5 cm, video-assisted techniques using a small 1.0 to 1.5 cm central or lateral neck incision, and completely endoscopic techniques by means of the chest, breast, or axilla (on one or both sides). All of these techniques have been examined with or without the use of CO_2 insufflation and skin-lifting techniques.[119–124] Benefits of these approaches are mainly cosmetic, with reduced incisions that in some cases are moved to more inconspicuous areas. Studies have shown reduced postoperative pain and reductions in postoperative hospital stay[123,125] when compared with traditional open surgery.

Most surgeons' indications for endoscopic thyroid surgery are quite strict: thyroid nodules of 3.0 to 3.5 cm or less, no previous neck radiation or operation, and no evidence of thyroiditis. The size or volume of the thyroid appears to be the biggest limiting factor for minimally invasive thyroid surgery.[123] With these indications, however, complication rates have been comparable, with permanent recurrent laryngeal nerve injury rates between 0 and 2.8%[119,121–123,125] and permanent hypocalcemia between 0% and 1.0%,[119,120,122,125] rates that are similar to conventional thyroid surgery.[126]

There have been no reports of long-term oncologic outcome after video-assisted thyroid resections for malignancy. Reports using secondary short-term measures of the oncologic adequacy of resection have shown promising results. Chung and colleagues[125] analyzed 103 patients undergoing endoscopic surgery by means of a bilateral breast and axillary approach and found no difference between 3-month serum thyroglobulin levels when compared with 198 patients undergoing open thyroidectomy. In a small, prospective study of patients undergoing resection for papillary carcinoma, Miccoli and colleagues[127] randomized 33 patients to open or video-assisted thyroid resection and found no postoperative difference in radioactive iodine uptake or mean thyroglobulin level at follow-up.

In addition, smaller case series have demonstrated the feasibility of adding central lymph node dissection in conjunction with video-assisted thyroid surgery for patients who have papillary thyroid carcinoma or positive RET oncogene mutations undergoing prophylactic thyroidectomy,[128–130] and even a lateral lymph node dissection.[131] The lack of long-term analyses of survival and recurrence rates, however, should lead to hesitancy with labeling these techniques as a definitive oncologic operation. The excellent prognosis and long-term survival for most thyroid cancer patients likely will be unaffected by the application of MIS.

VIDEO-ASSISTED THORACIC SURGERY FOR LUNG CANCER

Like many advanced minimally invasive surgical techniques, the use of VATS for lung cancer has been slow to replace open procedures. First described in the early 1990s,[132,133] it is estimated that only 5% of the 40,000 lobectomies performed each year in the United States are being done using thoracoscopic techniques.[134] The literature has shown, however, that the use of VATS has significant advantages with respect to short-term outcomes, and recent results show the longer-term oncologic outcomes after VATS lobectomy for early nonsmall cell lung cancer (NSCLC) are similar to those after traditional open resection.

Numerous reports have demonstrated that VATS lobectomy is safe and feasible. Perioperative mortality rates are low, between 0.5% and 2.7%, with low conversion rates in the largest series.[135–137] Complication rates vary based on authors' experience and definition of complications; however, in the largest published series of 1100 patients undergoing VATS lobectomy, McKenna and colleagues[134] reported a 15.3% complication rate. The most common complications reported in larger series are similar to those reported in the open literature and include atrial arrhythmias, pneumonia, persistent air leak, and myocardial infarction. Reports of short-term outcomes after VATS lobectomy demonstrate the thoracoscopic approach has resulted in low operative blood loss with no significant change in operative time,[138] less postoperative pain, and earlier return to baseline function[139,140] In a small retrospective cohort study examining longer-term quality-of-life measures, Suguira and colleagues[138] noted that after at an average of 12 months after surgery, none of the patients undergoing VATS lobectomy complained of post-thoracotomy pain, while 26.7% of those undergoing traditional thoracotomy still were taking narcotics for chest wall pain.

More importantly, long-term oncologic data after VATS lobectomy for lung cancer demonstrate excellent outcomes. The cohort of 500 patients reported by Onaitis and colleagues[135] included 416 patients who had NSCLC, and 2-year survival rates for stage 1 and stage 2 disease were 85% and 77%. Kaplan-Meier survival curves for 976 patients who had NSCLC in the series by McKenna and colleagues[134] are shown in **Fig. 2**. Although there have been no large multicenter randomized trials comparing VATS lobectomy with open resection, a small, prospective trial by Sugi and colleagues[141] randomized 100 patients who had clinical stage 1a lung cancer to either VATS lobectomy or traditional resection. Two patients in the VATS group were converted to thoracotomy, resulting in 52 patients in the open group and 48 patients in the VATS group. There was no significant difference in 3- and 5-year overall survival rates between the two groups (93% and 85% in the open group, 90% and 90% in the VATS group).

Current data support the use of thoracoscopic techniques for resection of early stage lung cancer. Improved short-term outcomes related to decreased postoperative pain, less blood loss, and a shorter length of hospital stay and return to preoperative function likely are related to the avoidance of a rib-spreading thoracotomy. In addition, studies have shown an immunologic benefit with VATS, resulting in decreased

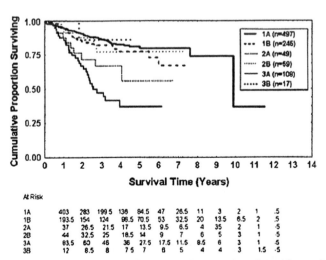

Fig. 2. Overall survival by disease stage for 976 patients undergoing video-assisted thoracic surgery lobectomy for nonsmall cell lung cancer. (*From* McKenna RJ, Houck W, Fuller CB. Video-assisted thoracic surgery lobectomy: experience with 1100 cases. Ann Thorac Surg 2006;81:423; with permission.)

cytokine release and improved lymphocyte function,[142,143] although the clinical benefit of these findings has yet to be examined thoroughly. The routine use of VATS should be limited to single lobe resections in patients who have either clinical stage 1 or 2 lung cancer, and appropriate work-up for the presence of locally invasive or metastatic disease is mandatory. More involved resections, such as sleeve lobectomies and pneumonectomies have been reported, but data are sparse, and these operations should only be performed in high-volume, experienced centers with careful monitoring and reporting of outcomes.

SUMMARY

Laparoscopic and minimally invasive techniques will continue to penetrate and transform all areas of surgery, including oncology. Long-term data will likely prove that minimally invasive techniques are equivalent in oncologic outcomes without deleterious effects. Physicians must continue to insist that these operations are performed for the same indications and accomplish the same surgical goals as traditional operations while providing significant benefit to patients to justify the inevitable increase in expense. New skill sets and technology demand attention to training and credentialing to assure safe patient outcomes.

REFERENCES

1. Jacobs M, Verdeja JC, Goldstein HS. Minimally invasive colon resection (laparoscopic colectomy). Surg Laparosc Endosc 1991;1:144–50.
2. Berends FJ, Kazemier G, Bonjer HJ, et al. Subcutaneous metastases after laparoscopic colectomy. Lancet 1994;344:58.
3. Vukasin P, Ortega AE, Greene FL, et al. Wound recurrence following laparoscopic colon cancer resection: results of the American society of colon and rectal surgeons laparoscopic registry. Dis Colon Rectum 1996;39:S20–3.
4. Lacy AM, Garcia-Valdecasa JC, Delgado S, et al. Laparoscopy-assisted colectomy vs. open coloectomy for the treatment of nonmetastatic colon cancer: a randomized trial. Lancet 2002;359:2224–9.
5. The COST Study Group. A comparison of laparoscopically assisted and open colectomy for colon cancer. N Engl J Med 2004;350:2050–9.
6. Veldkamp R, Kuhry E, Hop Wc, et al. Colon Cancer Laparoscopic or Open Resection Study Group. Laparoscopic surgery versus open surgery for colon cancer: short-term outcomes of a randomized trial. Lancet Oncol 2005;6:477–84.
7. Guillou PJ, Quirke P, Thorpe H, et al. Short-term endpoints of conventional versus laparoscopic-assisted surgery in patients with colorectal cancer (MRC CLASICC trial): multicentre, randomized controlled trial. Lancet 2005;365:1718–26.
8. Kuhry E, Bonjer HJ, Haglind E, et al. COLOR Study Group. Impact of hospital case volume on short-term outcome after laparoscopic operation for colonic cancer. Surg Endosc 2005;19:687–92.
9. Liang JT, Huang KC, Lai HS, et al. Oncologic results of laparoscopic versus conventional open surgery for stage II or III left-sided colon cancers: a randomized controlled trial. Ann Surg Oncol 2007;14:109–17.
10. Fleshman J, Sargent DJ, Green E, et al. Laparoscopic colectomy for cancer is not inferior to open surgery based on 5-year data from the COST Study Group trial. Ann Surg 2007;246:655–64.
11. Jayne DG, Guillou PJ, Thorpe H, et al. Randomized trial of laparoscopic-assisted resection of colorectal carcinoma: 3-year results of the UK MRC CLASICC Trial Group. J Clin Oncol 2007;25:3061–8.

12. Wexner SD, Cohen SM. Port metastases after laparoscopic colorectal surgery for cure of malignancy. Br J Surg 1995;82:295–8.
13. Reilly WT, Nelson H, Schroeder G, et al. Wound recurrence following conventional treatment of colorectal cancer: a rare but perhaps underestimated problem. Dis Colon Rectum 1996;39:200–7.
14. National quality forum endorsed commission on cancer measures for quality of cancer care for breast and colorectal cancers. Available at: http://www.facs.org/cancer/qualitymeasures.html. Accessed August 1, 2008.
15. NCCN Clinical Practice Guidelines in Oncology: colon cancer (2008). Available at: http://www.nccn.org/professionals/physician_gls/PDF/colon.pdf. Accessed January 21, 2008.
16. Tijandra JJ, Kilkenny JW, Buie WD, et al. The Standards Practice Task Force, The American Society of Colon and Rectal Surgeons. Practice parameters for the management of rectal cancer. Dis Colon Rectum 2005;48:411–23.
17. Leung KL, Kwok SPY, Lam SCW, et al. Laparoscopic resection of rectosigmoid carcinoma: prospective randomized trial. Lancet 2004;363:1187–92.
18. Strohlein MA, Grutzner KU, Jauch KW, et al. Comparison of laparoscopic vs. open access surgery in patients with rectal cancer: a prospective analysis. Dis Colon Rectum 2008;51:385–91.
19. Rosati R, Bona S, Romario UF, et al. Laparoscopic total mesorectal excision after neoadjuvant chemoradiotherapy. Surg Oncol 2007;16(Suppl 1):583–9.
20. Breukink S, Pierie J, Wiggers T. Laparoscopic versus open total mesorectal excision for rectal cancer. Cochrane Database Syst Rev 2006;CD005200.
21. Breukink S, Pierie JP, Grond AJ, et al. Laparoscopic vs. open total mesorectal excision: a case–control study. J Colorect Dis 2005;20:428–33.
22. Buess G, Kipfmuller K, Hack D, et al. Technique of transanal endoscopic microsurgery. Surg Endosc 1988;2:71–5.
23. Hermanek P, Gall FP. Early (microinvasive) colorectal carcinoma: pathology, diagnosis, surgical treatment. Int J Colorectal Dis 1986;1:79–84.
24. Knaebel HP, Koch M, Feise T, et al. Diagnostics of rectal cancer: endorectal ultrasound. Recent Results Cancer Res 2005;165:46–57.
25. Schaffzin DM, Wong WD. Endorectal ultrasound in the preoperative evaluation of rectal cancer. Clin Colorectal Ca 2004;42:124–32.
26. Winde G, Nottberg H, Keller R, et al. Surgical cure for early rectal carcinoma (T1). Transanal endoscopic microsurgery vs. anterior resection. Dis Colon Rectum 1998;41:526–7.
27. Mentges B, Buess G, Schaefer D, et al. Local therapy of rectal tumors. Dis Colon Rectum 1996;39:886–92.
28. Kreis ME, Jehle EC, Haug V, et al. Functional results after transanal endoscopic microsurgery. Dis Colon Rectum 1996;39:1116–21.
29. Cataldo PA, O'Brien S, Olsen T. Transanal endoscopic microsurgery: a prospective evaluation of functional results. Dis Colon Rectum 2005;48:1366–71.
30. Floyd ND, Saclarides TJ. Transanal endoscopic microsurgical resection of pT1 rectal tumors. Dis Colon Rectum 2005;49:164–8.
31. Lezoche E, Guerrieri M, Paganini AM, et al. Transanal endoscopic versus total mesorectal laparoscopic resections of T2-N0 low rectal cancers after neoadjuvant treatment: a prospective randomized trial with a 3-years minimum follow-up period. Surg Endosc 2005;19:751–6.
32. Suppiah A, Maslekar S, Alabi A, et al. Tranasanal endoscopic microsurgery in early rectal cancer: time for a trial? Colorectal Disease 2008;10:314–29.

33. Jemal A, Murray T, Samuels A, et al. Cancer statistics, 2003. CA Cancer J Clin 2003;53:5–26.
34. Hulscher JB, van Sandick JW, de Boer AG, et al. Extended transthoracic compared with limited transhiatal resection for adenocarcinoma of the esophagus. N Engl J Med 2002;21:1662–9.
35. Muller JM, Erasm H, Stelzner M, et al. Surgical therapy of oesophageal cancer. Br J Surg 1990;77:845–57.
36. Hulscher JBF, van Sandick JW, de Boer AGEM, et al. Extended transthoracic resection compared with limited resection for adenocarcinoma of the esophagus. N Engl J Med 2002;347:1662–9.
37. Orringer MB, Marshall B, Iannettoni MD. Transhiatal esophagectomy for treatment of benign and malignant esophageal disease. World J Surg 2001;25:196–203.
38. Rentz J, Bull D, Harpole D, et al. Transthoracic versus transhiatal esophagectomy: a prospective study of 945 patients. J Thorac Cardiovasc Surg 2003; 125:1114–20.
39. Birkmeyer JD, Siewers AE, Finlayson EVA, et al. Hospital volume and surgical mortality in the United States. N Engl J Med 2002;346:1128–37.
40. McAnema OJ, Rogers J, Williams NS. Right thoracoscopically assisted oesophagectomy for cancer. Br J Surg 1994;81:236–8.
41. DePaula AL, Hashiba K, Ferriera ET, et al. Laparoscopic transhiatal esophagectomy with esophagogastroplasty. Surg Laparosc Endosc 1995;5:1–5.
42. Smithers BM, Gotley DC, McEwan D, et al. Thoracoscopic mobilization of the esophagus. A 6- year experience. Surg Endosc 2001;15:176–82.
43. Bonavina L, Bona D, Binyom PR, et al. A laparoscopy-assisted surgical approach to esophageal carcinoma. J Surg Res 2004;117:52–7.
44. Nguyen NT, Roberts P, Follette DM, et al. Thoracoscopic and laparoscopic esophagectomy for benign and malignant disease: lessons learned from 46 consecutive procedures. J Am Coll Surg 2003;197:902–13.
45. Luketich JD, Alvelo-Rivera M, Buenaventura PO, et al. Minimally invasive esophagectomy: outcomes in 222 patients. Ann Surg 2003;238:486–94.
46. Bizekis C, Kent MS, Luketich JD, et al. Initial experience with minimally invasive Ivor–Lewis esophagectomy. Ann Thorac Surg 2006;82:402–6.
47. Suzuki Y, Urashima M, Ishibashi Y, et al. Hand-assisted laparoscopic and thoracoscopic surgery (HALTS) in radical esophagectomy with three-field lymphadenectomy for thoracic esophageal cancer. Eur J Surg Oncol 2005;31:1166–74.
48. Orringer MB, Marshall B, Iannettoni MD. Transhiatal esophagectomy: clinical experience and refinements. Ann Surg 1999;230:392–400.
49. Smithers BM, Gotley DC, Martin I, et al. Comparison of the outcomes between open and minimally invasive esophagectomy. Ann Surg 2007;245:232–40.
50. Braghetto I, Csendes A, Cardemil G, et al. Open transthoracic or transhiatal esophagectomy versus minimally invasive esophagectomy in terms of morbidity, mortality and survival. Surg Endosc 2006;20:1681–6.
51. Ries LAG, Melbert D, Krapcho M, et al. SEER Cancer Statistics Review, 1975–2005, based on November 2007 SEER data submission, posted to the SEER web site, 2008. Bethesda: National Cancer Institute; 2008. Available at: http://seer.cancer.gov/csr/1975_2005/. Accessed July 7, 2008.
52. Sugarbaker PH, Yu W, Yonemura Y. Gastrectomy, peritonectomy, and perioperative intraperitoneal chemotherapy: the evolution of treatment strategies for advanced gastric cancer. Semin Surg Oncol 2003;21:233–48.
53. Allum WH, Powell DJ, McKonkey CC, et al. Gastric cancer: a 25 year review. Br J Surg 1989;76:535–40.

54. Maruyama K, Okabayashi K, Kinoshita Y. Progress in gastric cancer surgery in Japan and its limits of radicality. World J Surg 1987;11:418–25.

55. Persiani R, D'Ugo D, Rausei S, et al. Prognostic indicators in locally advanced gastric cancer (LAGC) treated with preoperative chemotherapy and D2 gastrectomy. J Surg Oncol 2005;89:227–36.

56. Shimizu S, Uchiyama A, Mizumoto K, et al. Lparoscopically assisted distal gastrectomy for early gastric cancer: is it superior to open surgery? Surg Endosc 2000;14:27–31.

57. Adachi Y, Suematsu T, Shiraishi N, et al. Quality of life after laparoscopy-assisted billroth I gastrectomy. Ann Surg 1999;229:49–54.

58. Sano T, Sasako M, Kinoshita T, et al. Recurrence of early gastric cancer: follow-up of 1475 patients and review of Japanese literature. Cancer 1993;72:3174–8.

59. Sasako M, Kinoshita T, Maruyama K, et al. Prognosis of early gastric cancer. Stom Int 1993;28:139–46.

60. Itoh H, Oohata Y, Nakamura K, et al. Complete 10-year postgastrectomy follow-up of early gastric cancer. Am J Surg 1989;158:14–6.

61. Association JGC. Japanese classification of gastric carcinoma. Kyoto (Japan); 1998. p. 10–24.

62. Tada M, Tanaka Y, Matsuo N, et al. Mucosectomy for gastric cancer. Current status in Japan. J Gastroenterol Hepatol 2000;15:D98–102.

63. Yamao T, Shirao K, Ono H, et al. Risk factors for lymph node metastases from intramucosal gastric carcinoma. Cancer 1996;77:602–6.

64. Gotoda T, Yanagisawa A, Sasako M, et al. Incidence of lymph node metastasis from early gastric cancer: estimation with a large number of cases at two large centers. Gastric Cancer 2000;3:219–25.

65. Soetikno R, Kaltenbach T, Yeh R, et al. Endoscopic mucosal resection for early cancers of the upper gastrointestinal tract. J Clin Oncol 2005;23:4490–8.

66. Oda I, Saito D, Tada M, et al. A multicenter retrospective study of endoscopic resection for early gastric cancer. Gastric Cancer 2006;9:262–70.

67. Ohashi S, Yoden Y, Kanno H. Laparoscopic intragastric surgery with interventional endoscopy: a new concept in lap surgery. Surg Endosc 1994;8:497.

68. Mouret P, Froncois Y, Vignal J, et al. Laparoscopic treatment of perforated peptic ulcer. Am J Surg 1990;77:1006.

69. Trus TL, Hunter JG. Minimally invasive surgery of the esophagus and stomach. 1997;173:242–55.

70. Kitano S, Iso Y, Moriyama M, et al. Laparoscopy-assisted billroth I gastrectomy. Surg Laparosc Endosc 1994;4:146–8.

71. Huscher CG, Napolitano C, Chiodini S, et al. Laparoscopy-assisted gastrectomy for cancer: initial experience. Bologna, Italy: Monduzzi Editore; 1995. p. 1215–9.

72. Azagra JS, Goergen M, De Simone P, et al. Minimally invasive surgery for gastric cancer. Surg Endosc 1999;13:351–7.

73. Uyama I, Sugioka A, Fujita J, et al. Laparoscopic total gastrectomy with distal pancreatosplenectomy and D2 lymphadenectomy for advanced gastric cancer. Gastric Cancer 1999;2:230–4.

74. Huscher C, Mingoli A, Sgarzini G, et al. Laparoscopic versus open subtotal gastrectomy for distal gastric cancer: five-year results of a randomized prospective trial. Ann Surg 2005;241:232–7.

75. Lin S, Madura J, Velasco J. Laparoscopic surgery for advanced gastric adenocarcinoma.

76. Ettinghausen SE, Schwartzentruber DJ, Sindelar WF. Evolving strategies for the treatment of adenocarcinoma of the pancreas: a review. J Clin Gastroenterol 1995;21:48–60.
77. Sener SF, Fremgen A, Menck HR, et al. Pancreatic cancer: a report of treatment and survival trends for 100,313 patients diagnosed from 1985–1995 using the National Cancer Database. J Am Coll Surg 1999;189:1–7.
78. Tilleman EHBM, Busch ORC, Bemelman WA, et al. Diagnostic laparoscopy in staging pancreatic carcinoma: developments during the past decade. J Hepatobiliary Pancreat Surg 2004;11:11–6.
79. Stefanidis D, Grove KD, Schwesinger WH, et al. The current role of staging laparoscopy for adenocarcinoma of the pancreas: a review. Ann Oncol 2006;17: 189–99.
80. Cuschieri A. Laparoscopic surgery of the pancreas. J R Coll Surg Edinb 1994; 53:764–7.
81. Gagner M, Pomp A. Laparoscopic pylorus-preserving pancreaticoduodenectomy. Surg Endosc 1994;8:408–10.
82. Gagner M, Pomp A. Laparoscopic pancreatic resection: is it worthwhile? J Gastrointest Surg 1997;1:20–6.
83. Edwin B, Mala T, Mathisen O, et al. Laparoscopic resection of the pancreas: a feasibility study of the short-term outcome. Surg Endosc 2004;18:407–11.
84. Mabrut JY, Fernandez-Cruz L, Azagra JS, et al. Laparoscopic pancreatic resection: results of a multicenter European study of 127 patients. Surgery 2005;137:597–605.
85. Melotti G, Butturini G, Piccoli M, et al. Laparoscopic distal pancreatectomy: results on a consecutive series of 58 patients. Ann Surg 2007;246:77–82.
86. Lillemoe KD, Kaushal S, Cameron JL, et al. Distal pancreatectomy: indications and outcomes in 235 patients. Ann Surg 1999;229:693–700.
87. Kimura Y, Hirata K, Mukaiya M, et al. Hand-assisted laparoscopic pylorus-preserving pancreaticoduodenectomy for pancreatic head disease. Am J Surg 2005;189:734–7.
88. Dulucq JL, Wintringer P, Mahajna A. Laparoscopic pancreaticoduodenectomy for benign and malignant diseases. Surg Endosc 2006;20:1045–50.
89. Palanivelu C, Jani K, Senthilnathan P, et al. Laparoscopic pancreaticoduodenectomy: technique and outcomes. J Am Coll Surg 2007;205:222–30.
90. Pugliese R, Scandroglio I, Sansonna F, et al. Laparoscopic pancreaticoduodenectomy: a retrospective review of 19 cases. Surg Laparosc Endosc Percutan Tech 2008;18:13–8.
91. Giulianotti PC, Coratti A, Angelini M, et al. Robotics in general surgery: personal experience in a large community hospital. Arch Surg 2003;138:777–84.
92. Yeo CJ, Cameron JL, Sohn TA, et al. Pancreaticoduodenectomy with or without extended retroperitoneal lymphadenectomy for periampullary adenocarcinoma: comparison of morbidity and mortality and short-term outcome. Ann Surg 1999; 229:613–22.
93. Gagner M, Rheault M, Ducu J. Laparoscopic partial hepatectomy for liver tumor. Surg Endosc 1992;6:97–8.
94. Simillis C, Constantinides VA, Tekkis PP, et al. Laparoscopic versus open hepatic resections for benign and malignant neoplasms—a meta-analysis. Surgery 2007;141:203–11.
95. Llovet JM, Burroughs A, Bruix J. Hepatocellular carcinoma. Lancet 2003;362: 1907–17.
96. Kaneko H, Takagi S, Otsuka Y, et al. Laparoscopic liver resection of hepatocellular carcinoma. Am J Surg 2005;189:190–4.

97. Vibert E, Perniceni T, Levard H, et al. Laparoscopic liver resection. Br J Surg 2005;93:67–72.
98. Chen HY, Juan CC, Ker CG. Laparoscopic liver surgery for patients with hepatocellular carcinoma. Ann Surg Oncol 2008;15:800–6.
99. Fong Y, Fortner J, Sun RL, et al. Clinical score for predicting recurrence after hepatic resection for metastatic colorectal cancer: analysis of 1001 consecutive cases. Ann Surg 1999;230:309–18.
100. Prinz RA. A Comparison of laparoscopic and open adrenalectomies. Arch Surg 1995;130:489–92.
101. Brunt LM, Doherty GM, Norton JA, et al. Laparoscopic adrenalectomy compared to open adrenalectomy for benign adrenal neoplasms. J Am Coll Surg 1996;183:1–10.
102. Schell SR, Talamini MA, Udelsman R. Laparoscopic adrenalectomy for nonmalignant disease: improved safety, morbidity, and cost-effectiveness. Surg Endosc 1999;13:30–4.
103. Gagner M, Lacroix A, Bolte E. Laparoscopic adrenalectomy in Cushing's syndrome and pheochromocytoma. N Engl J Med 1992;327:1033.
104. National Institutes of Health. Management of the clinically inapparent adrenal mass (incidentaloma). 2002. State-of-the-science conference statement. Available at: http://consensus.nih.gov/2002/2002AdrenalIncidentalomasos021html.htm. Accessed February 4–6, 2002.
105. Young WF Jr. Management approaches to adrenal incidentalomas. A view from Rochester, Minnesota. Endocrinol Metab Clin North Am 2000;29:159–85.
106. Luton JP, Cerdas S, Billaud L, et al. Clinical features of adrenocortical carcinoma, prognostic factors, and the effect of mitotane therapy. N Engl J Med 1990;322:1195–201.
107. Tritos NA, Cushing GW, Heatley G, et al. Clinical features and prognostic factors associated with adrenocortical carcinoma: Lahey Clinic Medical Center experience. Am Surg 2000;66:73–9.
108. Gonzalez RJ, Shapiro S, Sarlis N, et al. Laparoscopic resection of adrenal cortical carcinoma: a cautionary note. Surgery 2005;138:1078–86.
109. Suzuki K, Ushiyama T, Mugiya S, et al. Hazards of laparoscopic adrenalectomy in patients with adrenal malignancy. J Urol 1997;158:2227.
110. Porpiglia F, Fiori C, Tarabuzzi R. Is laparoscopic adrenalectomy feasible for adrenocortical carcinoma or metastasis? BJU Int 2004;94:1026–9.
111. Nocca D, Aggarwal R, Mathieu A, et al. Laparoscopic surgery and corticoadrenalomas. Surg Endosc 2007;21:1373–6.
112. Kim SH, Brennan MF, Russo P, et al. The role of surgery in the treatment of clinically isolated adrenal metastasis. Cancer 1998;82:389–94.
113. Lo CY, van Heerden JA, Soreide JA, et al. Adrenalectomy for metastatic disease to the adrenal glands. Br J Surg 1996;83:528–31.
114. Heniford BT, Arca MJ, Walsh RM, et al. Laparoscopic adrenalectomy for cancer. Semin Surg Oncol 1999;16:293–306.
115. Moinzadeh A, Gill IS. Laparoscopic radical adrenalectomy for malignancy in 31 patients. J Urol 2005;173:519–25.
116. Strong VE, D'Angelica MA, Tang L, et al. Laparoscopic adrenalectomy for isolated adrenal metastasis. Ann Surg Oncol 2007;14:3392–400.
117. Schlumberger MJ. Papillary and follicular thyroid carcinoma. N Engl J Med 1998;338:298–306.
118. De Groot LJ, Kaplan EL, McCormick M, et al. Natural history, treatment, and course of papillary thyroid carcinoma. J Clin Endocrinol Metab 1990;71:414–24.

119. Timon C, Miller IS. Minimally invasive video-assisted thyroidectomy: indications and technique. Laryngoscope 2006;116:1046–9.
120. Shimizu K. Minimally invasive thyroid surgery. Clin Endocrinol Metab 2001;15: 123–37.
121. Inabnet WB, Jacob BP, Gagner M. Minimally invasive endoscopic thyroidectomy by a cervical approach. Surg Endosc 2003;17:1808–11.
122. Miccoli P, Berti P, Materazzi G, et al. Minimally invasive video-assisted thyroidectomy: five years of experience. J Am Coll Surg 2004;199:243–8.
123. Perigli G, Cortesini C, Qirici E, et al. Clinical benefits of minimally invasive techniques in thyroid surgery. World J Surg 2008;32:45–50.
124. Kitigawa W, Shimizu K, Akasu H, et al. Endoscopic neck surgery with lymph node dissection for papillary carcinoma of the thyroid using a totally gasless anterior neck skin lifting method. J Am Coll Surg 2003;196:990–4.
125. Chung YS, Choe JH, Kang KH, et al. Endoscopic thyroidectomy for thyroid malignancies: comparison with conventional open thyroidectomy. World J Surg 2007;31:2302–6.
126. Randolph GW. Surgery of the thyroid and parathyroid glands. Philadelphia: Saunders; 2003. p. 434–9.
127. Miccoli P, Elisei R, Materazzi G, et al. Minimally invasive video-assisted thyroidectomy for papillary carcinoma: a prospective study of its completeness. Surgery 2002;132:1070–4.
128. Miccoli P, Elisei R, Berti P, et al. Video-assisted prophylactic thyroidectomy and central compartment nodes clearance in two RET gene mutation adult carriers. J Endocrinol Invest 2004;27:557–61.
129. Bellantone R, Lombardi CP, Raffaelli M, et al. Central neck lymph node removal during minimally invasive video-assisted thyroidectomy for thyroid carcinoma: a feasible and safe procedure. J Laparoendosc Adv Surg Tech 2004;12:181–5.
130. Miccoli P, Elisei R, Donatini G, et al. Video-assisted central compartment lymphadenectomy in a a patient with a positive RET oncogene: initial experience. Surg Endosc 2007;21:120–3.
131. Miccoli P, Materazzi G, Berti P. Minimally invasive video-assisted lateral lymphadenectomy: a proposal. Surg Endosc 2008;22:1131–4.
132. Roviaro GC, Rebuffat C, Varoli F, et al. Videoendoscopic pulmonary lobectomy for cancer. Surg Laparosc Endosc 1992;2:244–7.
133. Kirby TJ, Mack MJ, Landreneau RJ, et al. Initial experience with video-assisted thoracoscopic lobectomy. Ann Thorac Surg 1993;56:1248–53.
134. McKenna RJ, Houck W, Fuller CB. Video-assisted thoracic surgery lobectomy: experience with 1,100 cases. Ann Thorac Surg 2006;81:421–6.
135. Onaitis MW, Peterson RP, Bladerson SS, et al. Thoracoscopic lobectomy is a safe and versatile procedure: experience with 500 consecutive patients. Ann Surg 2006;244:420–5.
136. Swanson SJ, Herndon JE, D'Amico TA, et al. Video-assisted thoracic surgery lobectomy: report of Calgb 39802—a prospective, multiinstitution feasibility study. J Clin Oncol 2007;28:4993–7.
137. Roviaro G, Varoli F, Vergani C, et al. Long-term survival after videothoracoscopic lobectomy for stage 1 lung cancer. Chest 2004;126:725–32.
138. Suguira H, Morikawa T, Kaji M, et al. Long-term benefits for the quality of life after video-assisted thoracoscopic lobectomy in patients with lung cancer. Surg Laparosc Endosc 1999;9:403–10.

139. Guidicelli R, Thomas P, Lonjon T, et al. Video-assisted minithoracotomy versus muscle-sparing thoracotomy for performing lobectomy. Ann Thorac Surg 1994;58(3):712–7.
140. Landrenaeau RJ, Hazelrigg SR, Mack MJ, et al. Postoperative pain-related morbidity: video-assisted thoracic surgery versus thoracotomy. Ann Thorac Surg 1993;56:1285–9.
141. Sugi K, Kaneda Y, Esato K. Video-assisted thoracoscopic lobectomy achieves a satisfactory long-term prognosis in patients with clinical stage IA lung cancer. World J Surg 2000;24:27–31.
142. Yim AP, Wan S, Lee TW, et al. VATS lobectomy reduces cytokine responses to conventional surgery. Ann Thorac Surg 2000;70:243–7.
143. Nagashiro I, Andou A, Aoe M, et al. Pulmonary function, postoperative pain, and serum cytokine level after lobectomy: a comparison of VATS and conventional procedure. Ann Thorac Surg 2001;72:362–5.

Multidisciplinary Approach to Esophageal and Gastric Cancer

Roderick M. Quiros, MD[a],*, Courtney L. Bui, MD[b]

KEYWORDS

- Esophageal cancer • Gastric cancer • Surgery
- Chemotherapy • Radiation therapy • Neoadjuvant • Adjuvant

Cancers of the esophagus and stomach are a worldwide problem, constituting the eighth and fourth most common malignancies respectively.[1] These cancers tend to be diagnosed late and typically are advanced at presentation. Surgery traditionally has been the mainstay of treatment, although because of the high rate of locoregional and systemic recurrence with surgery alone, chemotherapy and radiation therapy have become integrated into the management of these cancers. Although exact treatment regimens may vary on a regional level, data suggest that the multimodal approach affords the best hope for improved outcomes in patients who have esophagogastric cancers.

ESOPHAGEAL CANCER

Esophageal cancer (EC) is fairly rare in the United States, with an estimated 16,500 new cases and 14,300 deaths in 2008.[2] Squamous cell carcinoma (SCC) and adenocarcinoma (AC) comprise the two major histologic subtypes of EC. SCC has a predilection for the proximal and midesophagus, and is more common in endemic parts of the world. SCC is associated with smoking and alcohol abuse. AC tends to occur in the distal esophagus and gastroesophageal (GE) junction, particularly in the setting of gastroesophageal reflux disease (GERD), obesity, or Barrett's esophagus.[3–5]

Clinically, patients with EC often present with dysphagia on ingestion of solids, often progressing to difficulty with liquids. Retrosternal pain may be noted. Decreased parenteral intake results, followed by weight loss. Tumor invasion into surrounding structures, such as the laryngeal nerves or tracheobronchial tree, may lead to

[a] Surgical Oncology, Cancer Care Associates, St. Luke's Hospital & Health Network, 801 Ostrum Street, Bethlehem, PA 18015, USA
[b] Radiation Oncology, Cancer Care Associates, St. Luke's Hospital & Health Network, 801 Ostrum Street, Bethlehem, PA 18015, USA
* Corresponding author.
E-mail address: quirosr@slhn.org (R.M. Quiros).

Surg Clin N Am 89 (2009) 79–96
doi:10.1016/j.suc.2008.09.019   surgical.theclinics.com
0039-6109/08/$ – see front matter © 2009 Elsevier Inc. All rights reserved.

hoarseness or severe coughing spells upon eating that interfere with breathing. Aspiration pneumonia can develop from fluid breathed into the lungs.

An esophagogram is usually the first diagnostic test performed in the work-up of suspected malignancy, and may help differentiate functional causes of symptoms from mass or mechanical causes, such as tumor. Alternatively, esophagogastroduo-denoscopy (EGD) may be performed first. This permits direct observation of the tumor and allows for biopsy and brushings to be obtained. Additionally, evaluation of tumor depth and regional nodes can be performed with endoscopic ultrasound (EUS) to stage the tumor and help determine the next course of treatment.[6,7]

Additional work-up includes CT of the chest with positron emission tomography using radiolabeled fluorodeoxyglucose (CT-PET). This allows for detection of distant metastases with an accuracy of greater than 90%.[8,9] It also may allow for the assessment of tumor response to preoperative therapy based on changes in detectable metabolic activity within the tumor.[10,11] Based on radiographic and histologic studies, EC can be considered localized or metastatic, with treatment based on extent of disease.

Surgery

Two surgical approaches are employed commonly in the United States. The Ivor-Lewis esophagectomy (ILE) uses a right-sided thoracotomy and a laparotomy. It allows for visible dissection of the intrathoracic esophagus and surrounding nodal tissue, although it is associated with a higher rate of pulmonary complications.[12] Moreover, because the final anastomosis is in the chest, a postoperative leak can impart a great degree of morbidity. Transhiatal esophagectomy (THE), which involves a laparotomy and a cervical incision and avoids a thoracotomy, is the other commonly used approach to esophageal resection. The esophagus is bluntly dissected from the surrounding mediastinal structures, and the anastomosis ultimately is created in the neck. The largest study on THE recently was published by Orringer and colleagues,[13] who reported a major complication rate of less than 3% in over 2000 operated patients over a 30-year period. Comparisons between the two techniques show that outcomes are ultimately similar in experienced centers,[12,14] with a direct correlation to both hospital volume and the number of esophagectomies performed annually.[15]

Minimally invasive esophagectomy (MIE) has been proposed as an alternative to ILE or THE. Luketich and colleagues[16] reported their experience with 222 patients who underwent the procedure using thoracoscopic mobilization of the esophagus. In their study, MIE offered results as good as or better than open operation; the authors observed a lower mortality rate (1.4%) and shorter hospital stay (7 days) than most open series. Given these results, a new intergroup trial (ECOG 2202) to assess MIE in a multicenter setting is underway.

Endoscopic mucosal resection (EMR) is a minimally invasive approach to early SCC that is used commonly in Japan.[17] It is applicable in particular to well-differentiated or moderately differentiated SCC confined to the lamina propria. Although there are no large randomized controlled trials evaluating its use in patients who have EC, smaller studies have shown that it may have some applicability to Western populations,[18] even in patients who have AC of the esophagus.[19]

Definitive, Nonsurgical Treatment

The use of radiation therapy as definitive treatment for EC has been evaluated in older series, with varying degrees of success.[20–23] Ultimately, radiation alone in EC yields few survivors.[24] Presently, the use of radiation alone has been relegated largely to patients who are either not surgical candidates or who are in need of palliation.

Additionally, patients who have cervical esophageal tumors that would require total pharyngolaryngectomy to resect, or with extensive mediastinal involvement, may derive some benefit from radiation therapy.

Chemoradiotherapy without surgery has the ability to cure a percentage of patients who have EC, although these tend to be patients who have SCC rather than AC. The landmark RTOG 85-01 study compared radiation alone (64 Gy) versus chemoradiotherapy (50 Gy given with concurrent and adjuvant cisplatin and fluorouracil [5-FU]) in patients who had T1-3N0-1M0 EC.[25] Eighty-two percent of patients had SCC carcinoma; the remainder had AC. Combined modality treatment yielded 5- and 8-year overall survival rates of 26% and 22% respectively; there were no survivors at 5 years in the radiation-alone arm. Distant metastases were reduced from 30% to 16% at 5 years with combined modality treatment. Of note, locally persistent or recurrent disease was the most common cause of treatment failure in both groups, and was seen in 38% of the combined modality arm. In the EST-1282 trial, another study comparing radiation alone with radiation plus chemotherapy, investigators demonstrated an improvement in median survival for those patients receiving both radiation and chemotherapy (14.8 versus 9.2 months).[26] Pattern of recurrence was not reported in this study.

Given the low overall survival and high local recurrence rate even in patients treated with chemoradiation, efforts have been made to increase the radiation dose or intensity of chemotherapy, with the goal of improving rates of local recurrence and distant metastases. Intergroup 0122 increased the radiation dose and added neoadjuvant chemotherapy to concurrent chemoradiation, but was unsuccessful because of treatment toxicity.[27] Intergroup 0123 used the same chemotherapy as the RTOG 85-01 trial, but increased the radiation dose from 50.4 Gy to 64.8 Gy.[28] There was no difference outcome, and there were more treatment related deaths in the high-dose arm. At this time, for patients who have inoperable tumors or in tumors of the cervical esophagus, definitive chemoradiotherapy is administered as per RTOG 85-01, until further studies show improvement in patient outcomes.

Combined Approaches Including Surgery

Because EC is characterized by locoregional and systemic recurrence even after resection, investigators have concentrated on treating EC with a bi- or trimodal approach, employing chemotherapy or chemoradiotherapy in addition to surgery, either before or after esophagectomy.

Induction chemotherapy followed by surgery has been compared with surgery alone in the treatment of EC. The American Intergroup 0113 trial was a multi-institutional randomized trial comparing 213 patients who received preoperative chemotherapy followed by surgery with 227 patients who underwent surgery alone for local and operable EC.[29] Preoperative chemotherapy included three cycles of cisplatin and 5-FU. Surgery was performed within 4 weeks after completion of the third cycle. Patients also received two additional cycles of chemotherapy after the operation. Patients assigned to surgery alone underwent the same operations as those patients who received preoperative chemotherapy. After a median follow-up of 55.4 months, there were no significant differences between the two groups in median survival: 14.9 months for the patients who received preoperative chemotherapy and 16.1 months for those who underwent immediate surgery (P = .53). The lack of a significant difference between treatment arms continued for the 2 years after initiation of treatment. With the addition of chemotherapy, there was no change in the rate of recurrence at locoregional or distant sites. A recent update on these patients has showed that while there was no difference in overall survival between patients receiving perioperative chemotherapy compared with the surgery-only group, a few patients who underwent a complete (R0) resection and who had objective tumor regression after preoperative chemotherapy did have improved survival.[30]

Another randomized controlled study on preoperative chemotherapy in patients who had EC was conducted by the Medical Research Council (MRC).[31] In contrast to the Intergroup 0113 study, overall survival was better in patients who received two cycles of preoperative cisplatin and 5-FU compared with those who had surgery alone (P = .004). Median survival was 16.8 months in the former group compared with 13.3 months in the surgery-alone group, with 2-year survival rates of 43% and 34%, respectively. Another trial conducted by the MRC used perioperative epirubicin, cisplatin, and 5-FU for patients who had resectable esophagogastric cancers (MRC Adjuvant Gastric Cancer Infusional Therapy/MAGIC trial).[32] Patients who had resectable adenocarcinoma of the stomach, esophagogastric junction, or lower esophagus were assigned to receive either perioperative chemotherapy and surgery or surgery alone. After a median follow-up of 4 years, the perioperative chemotherapy group had a higher likelihood of overall survival (P = .009), with a 5-year survival rate of 36% versus 23% in the surgery-alone group. Additionally, resected patients who received the perioperative regimen were found to have a decrease in both tumor size and stage. Although these results suggest that preoperative chemotherapy had some benefit with regards to overall survival, only 15% of patients in this study had true lower esophageal tumors.

Malthaner and colleagues[33] published a meta-analysis of patients with potentially resectable carcinomas of the esophagus who were randomized to having either chemotherapy or no chemotherapy before surgery, with the primary outcome being survival. Eight trials, including a total of 1729 patients, were included in the meta-analysis. There was some evidence to suggest that preoperative chemotherapy improves survival. Interestingly, there was no evidence that tumor recurrence differed in patients who received preoperative chemotherapy compared with surgery alone. The authors concluded that preoperative chemotherapy plus surgery may offer a survival advantage compared with surgery alone for resectable EC.

Historically, surgical resection has been the primary form of treatment for patients who have EC, with a 3-year overall survival rate after surgery alone ranging from 6% to 37%.[34–37] In patients undergoing R0 resection, 3-year overall survival remains only 39%,[30] with up to 29% of patients experiencing locoregional failure.[30] Distant metastases occur in up to 50% of patients undergoing curative resection.[29] Preoperative radiation alone has not been shown to significantly improve survival.[38] Several studies have evaluated the role of a brief course of concurrent chemoradiation followed by resection, to help achieve a more adequate surgical resection and sterilize micrometastatic disease. A selection of studies on neoadjuvant therapy in EC is presented in **Table 1**. Three trials studied patients with SCC only, and none showed a benefit to neoadjuvant therapy.[34,39,40] Two of these studies used sequential chemotherapy and radiation, which may be inferior to concurrent therapy; moreover, the radiation dose and fractionation in these studies were not considered standard in the United States.[34,39] The Chinese University Research Group for Esophageal Cancer (CURE) trial used more standard chemotherapy and radiation dose, but had very short median follow-up at 16.9 months.[40]

The remainder of the studies in **Table 1** includes both SCC and AC, with the exception of Walsh and colleagues.[36] Probably the most widely quoted study for neoadjuvant therapy, the study used preoperative radiation to 40 Gy with 5-FU and cisplatin during weeks 1 and 6, followed by surgery, compared with surgery alone. The authors found a difference in 3-year overall survival of 32% with preoperative

Table 1
Randomized trials of surgery with or without neoadjuvant chemotherapy and radiation in esophageal cancer

Trial	Year	Number of Patients	Histology	CRT Arm	3-Year Overall Survival		Comments
					Surgery	CRT	
Le Prise	1994	86	Squamous	Sequential to 20 Gy	14	19	Sequential low RT dose (20 Gy), underpowered
Walsh	1996	113	Adenocarcinoma	CTRT to 40Gy	6	32[d]	Lower than expected OS in surgery alone arm
Bosset	1997	297	Squamous	Sequential to 37 Gy	37	39	Sequential, altered RT fractionation
Urba	2001	100	75% adenocarcinoma	CTRT to 45 Gy	16	30	Underpowered
Burmeister	2005	256	62% adenocarcinoma	CTRT to 35 Gy	19.3 mo	22.2 mo[a]	One cycle of chemotherapy, low RT dose
Chiu	2005	81	Squamous	CTRT to 50–60Gy	54.5	58.3[b]	Limited follow-up (16.9 months)
Tepper	2008	56	75% adenocarcinoma	CTRT to 50.4 Gy	16	39[c,e]	Closed early due to slow accrual

Abbreviations: CRT, chemotherapy and radiation; CTRT, chemoradiation; RT, radiation therapy.

[a] Median survival.
[b] 2-year overall survival.
[c] 5-year overall survival.
[d] Statistically significant.
[e] Significance of 3-year overall survival not reported.

therapy versus 6% with surgery alone. Despite the results, however, he study has been criticized because of the very low survival rates of patients in the surgery-alone arm compared with other contemporary series.

Urba and colleagues[35] included both SCC and AC in a study using preoperative 5-FU and cisplatin with 45 Gy of concurrent radiation and found a difference in 3-year overall survival of 30% with neoadjuvant therapy versus 16% with surgery alone. Unfortunately, this study was not powered to detect this difference, and thus the finding, while promising, was not statistically significant. More recently, investigators in the Cancer And Leukemia Group B (CALGB) attempted a study of neoadjuvant 5-FU and cisplatin with radiation to 50.4 Gy, the regimen found to be effective in RTOG 85-01, and compared this with surgery alone.[37] The study closed prematurely because of slow accrual however, because practitioners were unwilling to randomize to a surgery alone at the time the study was performed. Only 56 of 475 planned patients were enrolled. Results were presented after 6 years of follow-up in 2008, with the median survival of patients in the neoadjuvant arm 4.5 years, compared with 1.8 years in the surgery-alone group.

Although a consistent benefit to neoadjuvant chemoradiation has not been demonstrated repeatedly in individual trials, several meta-analyses point to an improvement in survival. Gebski and colleagues[41] found an absolute survival difference of 13% at 2 years, favoring preoperative chemoradiation. In another meta-analysis, Fiorica and colleagues[42] calculated an odds ratio for mortality at 3 years after treatment of 0.53, favoring chemoradiation. In most of these studies involving neoadjuvant chemoradiation, pathologic response has been found to be an important endpoint, because patients found to have a complete response at the time of surgery consistently have shown an improved progression-free and overall survival.[43,44]

Given the findings of the previously mentioned studies, neoadjuvant chemotherapy and radiation followed by surgical resection are preferred treatments for EC in the United States. 5-FU and cisplatin, given concurrently with 45-50 Gy as in the CALGB study, is preferred over a shortened radiation course or altered fractionation, as these techniques may increase operative mortality or long-term morbidity.[34]

Is Surgery Required After Chemoradiation?

The results of definitive chemoradiation in RTOG 85-01 rival those studies of trimodality therapy. Subsequently, determining which patients actually will benefit from surgery following neoadjuvant treatment has emerged as an important issue. Two recent studies compared definitive chemoradiation to neoadjuvant therapy followed by surgery. A French study evaluated 444 patients with T3N0-1 tumors, 89% of whom had SCC of the esophagus.[45] All patients underwent initial therapy with two cycles of 5-FU and cisplatin given concurrently with 46 Gy of radiation. If patients responded to therapy, they randomly were assigned to surgical resection or to definitive chemoradiation. There was no significant difference in median survival (17.7 months with surgery versus 19.3 months with continued chemoradiation) or 2-year overall survival (34% with surgery versus 40% with continued chemoradiation). The surgery arm had fewer locoregional recurrences, but also experienced significantly higher 3-month mortality.

Stahl and colleagues[43] studied patients who had T3-4N0-1 SCC. Patients were randomized up front to neoadjuvant chemotherapy with 5-FU, leucovorin, etoposide, and cisplatin for three cycles followed by definitive chemoradiation with cisplatin and etoposide to 60 to 65 Gy, versus the same induction chemotherapy, then chemoradiation to 40 Gy, followed by surgery. Thirty-four percent of patients randomized to the surgery arm did not undergo resection, either because of patient refusal or development of metastatic disease. Of those patients who had surgery, 82% had complete tumor resection, and 35% had complete pathologic response. Overall survival at 2 years was similar, at 40% with surgery and 36% with continued chemoradiation. Median survival was also equivalent at 16.4 months in the surgery arm and 14.9 months with continued chemoradiation. Local progression-free survival was higher in the surgery arm, but treatment-related mortality was also significantly higher in the surgery group. On subgroup analysis of patients who responded to induction chemotherapy, 55% to 58% were alive at 3 years, while conversely, those who did not respond did poorly. In patients who responded poorly to induction chemotherapy who underwent R0 resection after chemoradiation, survival at 3 years was 32%, while the 3-year overall survival in the surgery arm for all nonresponders was 18%. Although numbers in this latter group were low, the results nevertheless suggest some benefit from surgery in patients who have minimal response to neoadjuvant therapy.

Results of studies evaluating definitive chemoradiation and neoadjuvant therapy followed by resection have produced surprisingly consistent results, with 3-year overall survival averaging 30% to 35%. Patients treated with chemoradiation alone still experience a high rate of locoregional recurrence, suggesting that surgery may be of benefit in these patients. Local recurrence in EC has profound effects on quality of life; thus surgery may be warranted even if overall survival is not prolonged. Patients who respond to neoadjuvant chemotherapy or chemoradiation fare particularly well, and may represent a subset of patients who may not benefit from surgery. Most patients in large studies of neoadjuvant chemoradiation followed by surgery versus definitive chemoradiation had SCC; conclusions regarding outcome of patients who have AC require further study. Regardless of tumor type, the difficulty in such studies lies in determining preoperatively whether a patient has a complete response to therapy, and therefore can avoid an operation. PET-CT has emerged as a potential indicator of response to induction therapy in EC,[46] and study of response-directed therapy in EC is warranted. The RTOG is evaluating a nonoperative regimen, adding cetuximab to paclitaxel, cisplatin, and radiation therapy, and this study is accruing.

GASTRIC CANCER

Gastric cancer (GC) is a fairly uncommon cancer in the United States, with 21,500 new cases and roughly 11,000 deaths expected in 2008.[2] Nevertheless, it is a serious health problem, as it is usually at an advanced stage at diagnosis. In Western countries, 5-year survival averages 20%. In Japan, where intense screening for GC is standard, tumors are found at an earlier stage, contributing to better overall survival.[1] Risk factors include *Helicobacter pylori* infection, high intake of salty or smoked foods, increased intake of nitrates, pernicious anemia, and smoking. Surgery is the mainstay of treatment, although because patients can recur both locally and distally, chemotherapy, radiation therapy, or combinations thereof have been used to help increase chance for cure.

Histologically, tumors are classified as intestinal-type or diffuse-type using the Lauren[47] classification system. Intestinal-type tumors often originate as metaplastic cells, which devolve into carcinoma. Diffuse-type tumors do not necessarily develop along a dysplastic pathway but can present because of genetic mutation, often appearing in younger patients. E-cadherin mutations are observed in roughly 25% of families who have predisposition to diffuse-type cancers, with an autosomal dominant inheritance pattern.[48]

Patients who have GC commonly present with epigastric pain, weight loss, and early satiety. Anemia caused by gastrointestinal bleeding may also be seen. Upper endoscopy is used to evaluate symptoms and obtain biopsies to confirm the diagnosis. Staging is done with a CT scan of the abdomen and pelvis, although diagnostic laparoscopy often is employed to help assess the possibility and extent of peritoneal involvement, given that small peritoneal nodules may be undetectable by CT scan. Treatment strategy is based on whether disease is found to be localized versus systemic.

Surgery

Although it is clear that surgery remains the primary treatment modality for GC, the actual extent of resection has been debated. Comparison between total and subtotal gastrectomy suggests that survival rates are comparable, with better quality of life and nutritional status in subtotal gastrectomy patients.[49] Extent of lymph node dissection is also a matter of controversy when evaluating studies on GC. The Japanese Research Society for the Study of Gastric Cancer has created a classification of lymph nodes based on location.[50] N1 nodes are perigastric lymph nodes along the lesser curvature (stations 1, 3, and 5) and greater curvature (stations 2, 4, and 6). N2 nodes are those found along the left gastric artery (station 7), common hepatic artery (station 8), celiac artery (station 9), and splenic artery (stations 10 and 11).

Classification of lymph node dissection is based on these stations. A D0 node dissection involves failure to remove N1 lymph nodes. A D1 dissection involves gastrectomy with the greater and lesser omenta along with N1 nodes. A D2 dissection involves gastrectomy along with removal of the omenta, the front leaf of the transverse mesocolon, and N2 nodes. Splenectomy and distal pancreatectomy are employed to allow removal of stations 10 and 11 for proximal tumors.

In Japan, D2 dissection has been advocated as the treatment of choice for patients who have GC.[50] Western investigators have attempted to perform extended lymphadenectomy in patients who have GC, but without significantly affecting overall survival. In a prospective study conducted by the MRC, 400 patients were randomized followed a staging laparotomy to undergo D1 or D2 resection.[51] After a median follow-up of 6.5 years, the 5-year survival rates were 35% for D1 resection and 33% for D2 resection. There was no difference in the overall 5-year survival between the two arms. Survival based on death from GC was similar in the D1 and D2 groups, as was recurrence-free survival. In a multivariate analysis, clinical stages 2 and 3, old age, male sex, and removal of spleen and pancreas were independently associated with poor survival. The MRC concluded that D2 resection offered no survival advantage over D1 surgery.

A Dutch group also evaluated the effect of extended lymph node dissection on GC patients.[52] Seven hundred eleven patients who had potentially curative resections were evaluated. In an effort to ensure quality control, a Japanese GC surgeon trained the participant surgeons in the study, with numbers and locations of lymph nodes detected at pathologic investigation graded in accordance to the guidelines of the Japanese Research Society for the Study of Gastric Cancer. Protocol adherence during the course of the trial and its impact on complications, hospital mortality, and survival were evaluated. Major noncompliance was noted in 15.3% of D1 and 25.9% of D2 patients. Intensification of quality control resulted in only a marginal improvement in protocol adherence and in the number of lymph nodes detected. The 5-year survival reported was 45% for D1 dissections and 47% for D2 dissections, suggesting that nonadherence to the protocol did not lead to increased hospital morbidity and mortality, but also had no impact on long-term survival. A follow-up after 11 years showed no difference in overall survival (30% and 35% for D1 and D2 dissections, respectively).[53] Risk for morbidity and mortality was higher in patients older than 70 years who underwent D2 dissections. Of all subgroups analyzed in the follow-up study, only patients who had metastases in 7 to 15 regional lymph nodes were found to have potential benefit from a D2 dissection, although the study admitted that it was difficult to preoperatively identify those patients who had that extent of disease.

Combined Approaches

Surgery alone leads to long-term survival of 77% to 90% for early, lymph node- negative lesions.[51,54] Because most of these patients recur locoregionally, and a significant portion develop distant metastases,[55] investigators have focused on developing pre- or postoperative therapies to improve outcome.

In the MAGIC study recently reported by Cunningham and colleagues at the MRC, the effects of perioperative epirubicin, cisplatin, and 5-FU (ECF) on patient outcome were compared with surgery alone in 503 patients who had resectable AC of the lower esophagus, GE junction, and stomach.[32] The primary endpoint was overall survival. In previous studies, ECF had been shown to achieve response rates in up to 56% of patients who received it,[56,57] and also had been shown to improve survival among patients who had incurable locally advanced or metastatic gastric adenocarcinoma.[56,58] Patients who had resectable tumors randomly were assigned to receive either perioperative chemotherapy and surgery or surgery alone. ECF was given as three preoperative and three postoperative cycles of intravenous epirubicin and cisplatin on day 1, and a continuous intravenous infusion of 5-FU for 21 days. Morbidity and mortality rates were similar between groups. The resected tumors were significantly smaller and less advanced in the patients who received perioperative ECF. Five-year survival rates for patients who received ECF versus those who did not were 36% and 23%, respectively. The perioperative chemotherapy group had a higher likelihood of overall ($P = .009$) and of progression-free survival ($P<.001$).

An Italian group recently reported the results after a 7-year follow-up of a study aimed at evaluating a different perioperative chemotherapy protocol in a group of patients who had locally advanced GC.[59] Twenty-four patients who had locally advanced GC underwent D2 gastrectomy after three preoperative cycles of chemotherapy (epidoxorubicin, etoposide, cisplatin). Three further cycles were planned after surgery. Of the 24 patients, 17 (71%) received postoperative treatment. Curative resection (R0) was achieved in 83.3% of patients. No pathologic complete responses were documented, but tumor downstaging was obtained in 10 of 24 patients (41.7%). Overall median survival was 40 months, and the 7-year survival rate was 46%. After univariate and multivariate analysis, R0 resection and tumor diameter were the most important prognostic factors. In this study, there was a clear benefit for patients treated by perioperative chemotherapy and D2-gastrectomy when compared with previously studied controls who had surgery with postoperative chemotherapy alone.

RTOG 99-04 is a phase 2 study that evaluated a neoadjuvant regimen of up to two cycles of 5-FU, cisplatin, and leucovorin followed by chemoradiation with 5-FU and weekly paclitaxel.[60] Forty nine patients who had stage 1b to 3 gastric cancer were entered. The R0 resection rate was 77%, and a complete pathologic response rate of 26% was observed. More patients who had a complete pathologic response were alive at 1 year than those with less response (82% versus 69%). The authors recommend further evaluation in a larger randomized trial, and this approach remains investigational.

Neoadjuvant chemoradiation may provide the benefit of tumor downstaging before surgery. Additionally, by administration before surgery, induction therapy increases the likelihood that patients receive a complete course of chemotherapy, given that some patients who are scheduled to receive therapy in the postoperative setting may not receive it because of postoperative complications. The risks of this strategy are that the tumor may progress during neoadjuvant therapy. Alternatively, surgery may be delayed or even abandoned because of treatment toxicity from chemotherapy or radiation, eliminating an opportunity for curative resection.

Historically, postoperative chemotherapy has yielded variable although mostly favorable effects on patient outcome, and it is considered standard therapy at most North American institutions. Liu and colleagues[61] recently published a meta-analysis on adjuvant chemotherapy for GC patients. Twenty-three trials including 4919 patients (2441 in the adjuvant chemotherapy arm, 2478 in the surgery-alone arm) were included. Nineteen studies reported survival rates at the end of follow-up; 60.6% were alive among 2286 patients in the adjuvant chemotherapy arm, while 53.4% were alive among 2313 patients in the surgery-alone arm. Additionally, the surgery-alone arm also had a shorter disease-free survival, and the adjuvant chemotherapy arm had a lower recurrence rate.

Other studies have not found such benefit to postoperative chemotherapy in GC patients. An Italian group conducted a randomized phase 3 trial on patients who had AC of the stomach (stages 1b, 2, 3a and b, or 4 [T4N2M0]) treated with potentially curative surgery, with half of patients randomly assigned to follow-up alone or to treatment with of 5-FU, epidoxorubicin, leucovorin, and cisplatin (PELF regimen).[62] After a median follow-up of 72.8 months, 49.6% of patients experienced recurrence, and 53.9% were dead of disease. Adjuvant chemotherapy did not increase disease-free survival or overall survival in this study. Another Italian group investigated the use of a weekly PELF as adjuvant treatment for high-risk radically resected GC patients.[63] Four hundred GC patients at high risk for recurrence (pT3 N0, or pT2/pT3 N1, N2, or N3) were enrolled. Two hundred one patients randomly were assigned to receive the PELF regimen, and 196 patients were assigned to a regimen consisting 5-FU and leucovorin. The 5-year survival rates were 52% in the PELF arm and 50% in the 5-FU/leukovorin arm. Compared with the 5-FU/leukovorin regimen, the PELF regimen did not reduce the risk of death or relapse. Moreover, only 9.4% of patients were able to complete the treatment in the PELF arm, while 43% of patients completed the treatment in the 5-FU/leukovorin arm, underscoring the unfavorable effect that treatment toxicity from an intensive weekly regimen had on patients' ability to receive treatment.

A Japanese study using adjuvant S-1 therapy after curatively resected GC was published recently.[64] S-1 is an oral fluoropyrimidine compound, comprised of the agents tegafur, 5-chloro-2,4-dihydroxypyridine, and oxonic acid. Patients with stage 2 or 3 gastric cancer who underwent gastrectomy with D2 lymph-node dissection randomly were assigned to undergo surgery followed by adjuvant therapy with S-1 or to undergo surgery alone. In the S-1 group, administration of S-1 was started within 6 weeks after surgery and continued for 1 year. There were 529 patients in the S-1 group and 530 patients in the surgery-alone group. The trial was stopped on the recommendation of the independent data and safety monitoring committee, because it was found that the S-1 group had a higher rate of overall survival than the surgery-only group at the 1-year interim analysis ($P = .002$). At 3 years after treatment, the overall survival rate was 80.1% in the S-1 group and 70.1% in the surgery-alone group. Another Japanese study showed that S-1 may have some applicability in GC patients initially deemed unresectable.[65] Patients receiving S-1 with cisplatin who showed a good clinical response underwent curative gastrectomy. A microscopically detailed examination of surgically obtained specimens showed the complete disappearance of malignant cells. These results are promising, although the study was small. The applicability of S-1 to a Western population remains uncertain, however.

Hallissey and colleagues[66] studied the use of postoperative radiation therapy alone in the treatment of patients who had GC. Their data, which failed to demonstrate an improvement in overall survival, did show a benefit toward reducing locoregional recurrence in patients who received radiation postoperatively. Given the persistence of distant relapse and potential benefit of chemotherapy, however, a trial evaluating radiation alone likely will not be repeated.

Intergroup 0116 evaluated the use of postoperative chemoradiation, and essentially changed the standard of care for gastric cancer in the United States.[67] In this study, 556 patients who had stage 1b to 4 M0 adenocarcinoma of the stomach or GE junction were randomized to surgery alone or to surgery followed by one cycle of 5FU/leucovorin, then chemoradiation with 5FU/leucovorin and radiation to 45 Gy, then a final two cycles of 5FU/leucovorin. Three-year overall survival rates were 50% and 41%, favoring adjuvant therapy. The median overall survival was 35 months with adjuvant therapy versus 26 months with surgery alone. Intergroup 0116 has been criticized because of its poor compliance rate with the recommended extent of lymph node dissection. Only 10% of patients underwent the recommended D2 dissection, with 36% having a D1 and 54% have a D0 dissection. The authors evaluated outcome according to dissection type, and all subsets seemed to benefit from adjuvant therapy. Intergroup 0116 was updated in 2004 after more than 6 years of follow-up.[68] Chemoradiation reduced the frequency of first relapse locally, but distant relapse remained a problem, emphasizing the need for more efficacious systemic therapy.

Intraperitoneal chemotherapy (IPC) has been used to treat appendiceal, colonic, peritoneal mesothelial, and ovarian cancers with varying degrees of success.[69–72] Some investigators have shown that the technique may have applicability to patients who have GC also.[73] A recent meta-analysis by Yan and colleagues[74] investigated the effectiveness and safety of adjuvant IPC for patients who had locally advanced resectable GC. Ten reports fit selection criteria and were included in the meta-analysis. A significant improvement in survival was associated with hyperthermic intraoperative intraperitoneal chemotherapy (HIIPC) alone or HIIPC combined with early postoperative IPC. There was a trend toward survival improvement with normothermic intraoperative IPC, but this was not significant with either early postoperative IPC alone or delayed postoperative IPC. IPC also was associated with higher risks of intra-abdominal abscess and neutropenia, confirming that the technique is not without risk.

Treatment for Advanced Malignancy of the Esophagus and Stomach

Numerous patients with EC or GC have unresectable, recurrent, or metastatic disease at diagnosis. Alternatively, there are patients with advanced but resectable EC or GC who would not tolerate surgery. Although surgery in such cases may not be possible, palliative interventions have an important role in managing these patients. The availability of newer cytotoxic agents has provided hope that current outcomes can be improved; indeed, several combinations have been shown to be effective and therefore good candidates for patients who have advanced disease.

The National Cancer Research Institute in the United Kingdom conducted a study of chemotherapy in 1002 patients who had advanced EC and GC.[75] The Randomized ECF for Advanced and Locally Advanced Esophagogastric Cancer 2 (REAL-2) Study evaluated capecitabine (an oral fluoropyrimidine) and oxaliplatin (a platinum compound) as alternatives to infused 5-FU and cisplatin, respectively, for untreated advanced esophagogastric cancer. Patients received triplet therapy with epirubicin and cisplatin plus either 5-FU (ECF) or capecitabine (ECX) or triplet therapy with epirubicin and oxaliplatin plus either 5-FU (EOF) or capecitabine (EOX). The primary endpoint was noninferiority in overall survival for the triplet therapies containing capecitabine as compared with 5-FU and for those containing oxaliplatin as compared with cisplatin. Median survival times in the ECF, ECX, EOF, and EOX groups ranged from 9 to 11 months, while survival rates at 1 year ranged from 38% to 47%. Progression-free survival and response rates did not differ significantly among the regimens. Compared with the regimens containing cisplatin, the regimens containing oxaliplatin were associated with a lower incidence of alopecia and renal toxicity. Other studies have confirmed an acceptable toxicity profile in oxaliplatin-containing regimens.[76–78] Additionally, alternative regimens containing other cytotoxic agents such as irinotecan may prove efficacious for patients who have advanced disease.[79,80]

The use of S-1 in conjunction with other chemotherapeutic agents is being studied. Japanese investigators have found some benefit to S-1 combined with cisplatin in patients who have advanced GC, with acceptable toxicity profiles.[81,82] Another group has initiated a prospective, multicenter, multinational, nonblinded, randomized phase 3 trial comparing S-1 alone versus an S-1/docetaxel combination (JACCRO GC-03 Study).[83] Six hundred twenty-eight patients who have advanced or recurrent gastric cancer (314 in each treatment arm) will be enrolled. The final results of this study are expected in 2010.

A randomized controlled trial has started in Japan and Korea to evaluate the role of gastrectomy for managing incurable advanced gastric cancer.[84] Patients diagnosed as having a single noncurable factor and who otherwise would tolerate surgery will be randomized to gastrectomy plus chemotherapy or chemotherapy alone. Three hundred thirty patients are to be recruited into the study. The primary endpoint will be overall survival, with secondary endpoints being progression-free survival and adverse events associated with either gastrectomy or chemotherapy.

New Treatment Approaches

Increased understanding of the molecular basis of cancer has led to the investigation of other treatments, often using biologic therapies to target malignancy. The addition of new agents to existing chemotherapeutic regimens has the potential to improve outcomes in patients who have malignancies of the esophagus, GE junction, and stomach.

GC has been shown to express varying amounts of epidermal growth factor receptors (EGFR), with high levels of EGFR associated with a shorter overall survival.[85] A recent phase 2 trial conducted by the Southwest Oncology Group (SWOG 0127 trial) studied erlotinib, an oral EGFR inhibitor, as a possible treatment for GE junction and distal gastric AC in patients who had no prior chemotherapy.[86] There was an overall response probability rate of 9%, all occurring in the subgroup with GE junction tumors; no responses were observed in group with distal GC. The median survival was 6.7 months in patients who had GE junction tumors and 3.5 months in the distal GC. Investigators concluded that erlotinib was active in patients who had GE AC, but inactive in GC. Another phase 2 trial evaluated gefitnib, another EGFR tyrosine kinase inhibitor, as adjuvant treatment for advanced, inoperable EC.[87] The primary endpoint was tumor response, with the effect of EGFR inhibition evaluated by gene expression analysis of tumor biopsies taken before gefitinib treatment and 28 days after. Out of 27 patients, three had a partial response, and seven had stable disease, giving a disease control rate of 37%. Microarray experiments on tumor biopsies showed that gefitinib also down-regulated oncogenes associated with tumor progression.

The use of bevacizumab, an angiogenesis inhibitor that targets and inhibits vascular endothelial growth factor (VEGF), has shown benefit in patients who have advanced colorectal,[88,89] lung,[90,91] and ovarian[92] cancers. Shah and colleagues[93] investigated its addition to irinotecan and cisplatin in patients who had metastatic or unresectable

AC of the GE junction and stomach. The primary endpoint was to demonstrate a 50% improvement in time to progression over historical values. With a median follow-up of 12.2 months, median time to progression was 8.3 months. In patients who had measurable disease, the overall response rate was 65%. Median survival was 12.3 months. The response rate and overall survival rates were encouraging, with time to progression improved over historical controls by 75%.

SUMMARY

Although surgery still plays a central role in the treatment paradigm for esophageal and gastric cancers, chemotherapy and radiation therapy have had increasingly important roles for treating these malignancies, such that their inclusion in treatment schema is now considered standard. Their use as pre- or peri-operative treatments in particular has been supported by several recent trials. As new drugs and biologic therapies are developed, and as the ability to assess tumor response to induction therapy continues to improve, strategies for managing these malignancies will continue to evolve.

REFERENCES

1. Kamangar F, Dores GM, Anderson WF. Patterns of cancer incidence, mortality, and prevalence across five continents: defining priorities to reduce cancer disparities in different geographic regions of the world. J Clin Oncol 2006; 24(14):2137–50.
2. Jemal A, Siegel R, Ward E, et al. Cancer statistics, 2008. CA Cancer J Clin 2008; 58(2):71–96.
3. Cameron AJ, Romero Y. Symptomatic gastro-oesophageal reflux as a risk factor for oesophageal adenocarcinoma. Gut 2000;46(6):754–5.
4. Gammon MD, Schoenberg JB, Ahsan H, et al. Tobacco, alcohol, and socioeconomic status and adenocarcinomas of the esophagus and gastric cardia. J Natl Cancer Inst 1997;89(17):1277–84.
5. Drewitz DJ, Sampliner RE, Garewal HS. The incidence of adenocarcinoma in Barrett's esophagus: a prospective study of 170 patients followed 4.8 years. Am J Gastroenterol 1997;92(2):212–5.
6. Vazquez-Sequeiros E, Norton ID, Clain JE, et al. Impact of EUS-guided fine-needle aspiration on lymph node staging in patients with esophageal carcinoma. Gastrointest Endosc 2001;53(7):751–7.
7. Brugge WR, Lee MJ, Carey RW, et al. Endoscopic ultrasound staging criteria for esophageal cancer. Gastrointest Endosc 1997;45(2):147–52.
8. Rankin SC, Taylor H, Cook GJ, et al. Computed tomography and positron emission tomography in the preoperative staging of oesophageal carcinoma. Clin Radiol 1998;53(9):659–65.
9. Wallace MB, Nietert PJ, Earle C, et al. An analysis of multiple staging management strategies for carcinoma of the esophagus: computed tomography, endoscopic ultrasound, positron emission tomography, and thoracoscopy/laparoscopy. Ann Thorac Surg 2002;74(4):1026–32.
10. Swisher SG, Maish M, Erasmus JJ, et al. Utility of PET, CT, and EUS to identify pathologic responders in esophageal cancer. Ann Thorac Surg 2004;78(4): 1152–60 [discussion: 1152–60].
11. Lordick F, Ott K, Krause BJ, et al. PET to assess early metabolic response and to guide treatment of adenocarcinoma of the oesophagogastric junction: the MUNICON phase II trial. Lancet Oncol 2007;8(9):797–805.

12. Hulscher JB, van Sandick JW, de Boer AG, et al. Extended transthoracic resection compared with limited transhiatal resection for adenocarcinoma of the esophagus. N Engl J Med 2002;347(21):1662–9.

13. Orringer MB, Marshall B, Chang AC, et al. Two thousand transhiatal esophagectomies: changing trends, lessons learned. Ann Surg 2007;246(3):363–72 [discussion: 372–4].

14. Chang AC, Ji H, Birkmeyer NJ, et al. Outcomes after transhiatal and transthoracic esophagectomy for cancer. Ann Thorac Surg 2008;85(2):424–9.

15. Birkmeyer JD, Siewers AE, Finlayson EV, et al. Hospital volume and surgical mortality in the United States. N Engl J Med 2002;346(15):1128–37.

16. Luketich JD, Alvelo-Rivera M, Buenaventura PO, et al. Minimally invasive esophagectomy: outcomes in 222 patients. Ann Surg 2003;238(4):486–94 [discussion: 494–5].

17. Soetikno R, Kaltenbach T, Yeh R, et al. Endoscopic mucosal resection for early cancers of the upper gastrointestinal tract. J Clin Oncol 2005;23(20):4490–8.

18. Pech O, Gossner L, May A, et al. Endoscopic resection of superficial esophageal squamous cell carcinomas: Western experience. Am J Gastroenterol 2004;99(7):1226–32.

19. Maish MS, DeMeester SR. Endoscopic mucosal resection as a staging technique to determine the depth of invasion of esophageal adenocarcinoma. Ann Thorac Surg 2004;78(5):1777–82.

20. Sykes AJ, Burt PA, Slevin NJ, et al. Radical radiotherapy for carcinoma of the oesophagus: an effective alternative to surgery. Radiother Oncol 1998;48(1):15–21.

21. Newaishy GA, Read GA, Duncan W, et al. Results of radical radiotherapy of squamous cell carcinoma of the oesophagus. Clin Radiol 1982;33(3):347–52.

22. Okawa T, Kita M, Tanaka M, et al. Results of radiotherapy for inoperable locally advanced esophageal cancer. Int J Radiat Oncol Biol Phys 1989;17(1):49–54.

23. Herskovic A, Martz K, al-Sarraf M, et al. Combined chemotherapy and radiotherapy compared with radiotherapy alone in patients with cancer of the esophagus. N Engl J Med 1992;326(24):1593–8.

24. Fok M, Sham JS, Choy D, et al. Postoperative radiotherapy for carcinoma of the esophagus: a prospective, randomized controlled study. Surgery 1993;113(2):138–47.

25. Cooper JS, Guo MD, Herskovic A, et al. Chemoradiotherapy of locally advanced esophageal cancer: long-term follow-up of a prospective randomized trial (RTOG 85-01). Radiation Therapy Oncology Group. JAMA 1999;281(17):1623–7.

26. Smith TJ, Ryan LM, Douglass HO Jr, et al. Combined chemoradiotherapy vs. radiotherapy alone for early stage squamous cell carcinoma of the esophagus: a study of the Eastern Cooperative Oncology Group. Int J Radiat Oncol Biol Phys 1998;42(2):269–76.

27. Minsky BD, Neuberg D, Kelsen DP, et al. Final report of intergroup trial 0122 (ECOG PE-289, RTOG 90-12): phase II trial of neoadjuvant chemotherapy plus concurrent chemotherapy and high-dose radiation for squamous cell carcinoma of the esophagus. Int J Radiat Oncol Biol Phys 1999;43(3):517–23.

28. Minsky BD, Pajak TF, Ginsberg RJ, et al. INT 0123 (Radiation Therapy Oncology Group 94-05) phase III trial of combined-modality therapy for esophageal cancer: high-dose versus standard-dose radiation therapy. J Clin Oncol 2002;20(5):1167–74.

29. Kelsen DP, Ginsberg R, Pajak TF, et al. Chemotherapy followed by surgery compared with surgery alone for localized esophageal cancer. N Engl J Med 1998;339(27):1979–84.

30. Kelsen DP, Winter KA, Gunderson LL, et al. Long-term results of RTOG trial 8911 (USA Intergroup 113): a random assignment trial comparison of chemotherapy followed by surgery compared with surgery alone for esophageal cancer. J Clin Oncol 2007;25(24):3719–25.

31. Medical Research Council Oesophageal Cancer Working Group. Surgical resection with or without preoperative chemotherapy in oesophageal cancer: a randomised controlled trial. Lancet 2002;359(9319):1727–33.

32. Cunningham D, Allum WH, Stenning SP, et al. Perioperative chemotherapy versus surgery alone for resectable gastroesophageal cancer. N Engl J Med 2006; 355(1):11–20.

33. Malthaner RA, Collin S, Fenlon D. Preoperative chemotherapy for resectable thoracic esophageal cancer. Cochrane Database Syst Rev 2006;(3):CD001556.

34. Bosset JF, Gignoux M, Triboulet JP, et al. Chemoradiotherapy followed by surgery compared with surgery alone in squamous-cell cancer of the esophagus. N Engl J Med 1997;337(3):161–7.

35. Urba SG, Orringer MB, Turrisi A, et al. Randomized trial of preoperative chemoradiation versus surgery alone in patients with locoregional esophageal carcinoma. J Clin Oncol 2001;19(2):305–13.

36. Walsh TN, Noonan N, Hollywood D, et al. A comparison of multimodal therapy and surgery for esophageal adenocarcinoma. N Engl J Med 1996;335(7):462–7.

37. Tepper J, Krasna MJ, Niedzwiecki D, et al. Phase III trial of trimodality therapy with cisplatin, fluorouracil, radiotherapy, and surgery compared with surgery alone for esophageal cancer: CALGB 9781. J Clin Oncol 2008;26(7):1086–92.

38. Arnott SJ, Duncan W, Gignoux M, et al. Preoperative radiotherapy for esophageal carcinoma. Cochrane Database Syst Rev 2005;(4):CD001799.

39. Le Prise E, Etienne PL, Meunier B, et al. A randomized study of chemotherapy, radiation therapy, and surgery versus surgery for localized squamous cell carcinoma of the esophagus. Cancer 1994;73(7):1779–84.

40. Chiu PW, Chan AC, Leung SF, et al. Multicenter prospective randomized trial comparing standard esophagectomy with chemoradiotherapy for treatment of squamous esophageal cancer: early results from the Chinese University Research Group for Esophageal Cancer (CURE). J Gastrointest Surg 2005;9(6):794–802.

41. Gebski V, Burmeister B, Smithers BM, et al. Survival benefits from neoadjuvant chemoradiotherapy or chemotherapy in oesophageal carcinoma: a meta-analysis. Lancet Oncol 2007;8(3):226–34.

42. Fiorica F, Di Bona D, Schepis F, et al. Preoperative chemoradiotherapy for oesophageal cancer: a systematic review and meta-analysis. Gut 2004;53(7):925–30.

43. Stahl M, Wilke H, Stuschke M, et al. Clinical response to induction chemotherapy predicts local control and long-term survival in multimodal treatment of patients with locally advanced esophageal cancer. J Cancer Res Clin Oncol 2005; 131(1):67–72.

44. Burmeister BH, Smithers BM, Gebski V, et al. Surgery alone versus chemoradiotherapy followed by surgery for resectable cancer of the oesophagus: a randomised controlled phase III trial. Lancet Oncol 2005;6(9):659–68.

45. Bedenne L, Michel P, Bouche O, et al. Chemoradiation followed by surgery compared with chemoradiation alone in squamous cancer of the esophagus: FFCD 9102. J Clin Oncol 2007;25(10):1160–8.

46. Wieder HA, Ott K, Lordick F, et al. Prediction of tumor response by FDG-PET: comparison of the accuracy of single and sequential studies in patients with adenocarcinomas of the esophagogastric junction. Eur J Nucl Med Mol Imaging 2007;34(12):1925–32.

47. Lauren P. The two histological main types of gastric carcinoma: diffuse and so-called intestinal-type carcinoma. An attempt at a histoclinical classification. Acta Pathol Microbiol Scand 1965;64:31–49.
48. Fitzgerald RC, Caldas C. Clinical implications of E-cadherin associated heredi-tary diffuse gastric cancer. Gut 2004;53(6):775–8.
49. Bozzetti F, Marubini E, Bonfanti G, et al. Subtotal versus total gastrectomy for gas-tric cancer: five-year survival rates in a multicenter randomized Italian trial. Italian Gastrointestinal Tumor Study Group. Ann Surg 1999;230(2):170–8.
50. Kajitani T. The general rules for the gastric cancer study in surgery and pathology. Part I. Clinical classification. Jpn J Surg 1981;11(2):127–39.
51. Cuschieri A, Weeden S, Fielding J, et al. Patient survival after D1 and D2 resec-tions for gastric cancer: long-term results of the MRC randomized surgical trial. Surgical Co-operative Group. Br J Cancer 1999;79(9–10):1522–30.
52. Bonenkamp JJ, Hermans J, Sasako M, et al. Quality control of lymph node dis-section in the Dutch randomized trial of D1 and D2 lymph node dissection for gastric cancer. Gastric Cancer 1998;1(2):152–9.
53. Hartgrink HH, van de Velde CJ, Putter H, et al. Extended lymph node dissection for gastric cancer: who may benefit? Final results of the randomized Dutch gas-tric cancer group trial. J Clin Oncol 2004;22(11):2069–77.
54. Abe S, Yoshimura H, Nagaoka S, et al. Long-term results of operation for carci-noma of the stomach in T1/T2 stages: critical evaluation of the concept of early carcinoma of the stomach. J Am Coll Surg 1995;181(5):389–96.
55. Gunderson LL, Sosin H. Adenocarcinoma of the stomach: areas of failure in a re-operation series (second or symptomatic look) clinicopathologic correlation and implications for adjuvant therapy. Int J Radiat Oncol Biol Phys 1982;8(1):1–11.
56. Webb A, Cunningham D, Scarffe JH, et al. Randomized trial comparing epirubi-cin, cisplatin, and fluorouracil versus fluorouracil, doxorubicin, and methotrexate in advanced esophagogastric cancer. J Clin Oncol 1997;15(1):261–7.
57. Ross P, Nicolson M, Cunningham D, et al. Prospective randomized trial compar-ing mitomycin, cisplatin, and protracted venous-infusion fluorouracil (PVI 5-FU) with epirubicin, cisplatin, and PVI 5-FU in advanced esophagogastric cancer. J Clin Oncol 2002;20(8):1996–2004.
58. Waters JS, Norman A, Cunningham D, et al. Long-term survival after epirubicin, cisplatin, and fluorouracil for gastric cancer: results of a randomized trial. Br J Cancer 1999;80(1–2):269–72.
59. Persiani R, Rausei S, Pozzo C, et al. 7-Year survival results of perioperative che-motherapy with epidoxorubicin, etoposide, and cisplatin (EEP) in locally ad-vanced resectable gastric cancer: up-to-date analysis of a phase II study. Ann Surg Oncol 2008;15(8):2146–52.
60. Ajani JA, Winter K, Okawara GS, et al. Phase II trial of preoperative chemoradiation in patients with localized gastric adenocarcinoma (RTOG 9904): quality of combined modality therapy and pathologic response. J Clin Oncol 2006;24(24):3953–8.
61. Liu TS, Wang Y, Chen SY, et al. An updated meta-analysis of adjuvant chemotherapy after curative resection for gastric cancer. Eur J Surg Oncol 2008;34:1208–16.
62. Di Costanzo F, Gasperoni S, Manzione L, et al. Adjuvant chemotherapy in com-pletely resected gastric cancer: a randomized phase III trial conducted by GOIRC. J Natl Cancer Inst 2008;100(6):388–98.
63. Cascinu S, Labianca R, Barone C, et al. Adjuvant treatment of high-risk, radically resected gastric cancer patients with 5-fluorouracil, leucovorin, cisplatin, and ep-idoxorubicin in a randomized controlled trial. J Natl Cancer Inst 2007;99(8): 601–7.

64. Sakuramoto S, Sasako M, Yamaguchi T, et al. Adjuvant chemotherapy for gastric cancer with S-1, an oral fluoropyrimidine. N Engl J Med 2007;357(18):1810–20.

65. Ina K, Kataoka T, Takeuchi Y, et al. Pathological complete response induced by the combination therapy of S-1 and 24-h infusion of cisplatin in two cases initially diagnosed as inoperable advanced gastric cancer. Oncol Rep 2008;20(2): 259–64.

66. Hallissey MT, Dunn JA, Ward LC, et al. The second British Stomach Cancer Group trial of adjuvant radiotherapy or chemotherapy in resectable gastric cancer: five-year follow-up. Lancet 1994;343(8909):1309–12.

67. Macdonald JS, Smalley SR, Benedetti J, et al. Chemoradiotherapy after surgery compared with surgery alone for adenocarcinoma of the stomach or gastro-esophageal junction. N Engl J Med 2001;345(10):725–30.

68. Macdonald JS, Smalley SR, Benedetti J, et al. Postoperative combined radiation and chemotherapy improves disease-free survival and overall survival in re-sected adenocarcinoma of the stomach and gastroesophageal junction: update of the results of Intergroup Study INT-116. Presented at: 2004 Gastrointestinal Cancers Symposium; January 22–24, 2004; San Francisco, CA.

69. Bijelic L, Yan TD, Sugarbaker PH. Failure analysis of recurrent disease following complete cytoreduction and perioperative intraperitoneal chemotherapy in patients with peritoneal carcinomatosis from colorectal cancer. Ann Surg Oncol 2007;14(8):2281–8.

70. Esquivel J, Sticca R, Sugarbaker P, et al. Cytoreductive surgery and hyperthermic intraperitoneal chemotherapy in the management of peritoneal surface malignancies of colonic origin: a consensus statement. Society of Surgical Oncology. Ann Surg Oncol 2007;14(1):128–33.

71. Yan TD, Sugarbaker PH. An evolving role of perioperative intraperitoneal chemotherapy after cytoreductive surgery for colorectal peritoneal carcinomatosis. Ann Surg Oncol 2007;14(7):2171–2.

72. Armstrong DK, Brady MF. Intraperitoneal therapy for ovarian cancer: a treatment ready for prime time. J Clin Oncol 2006;24(28):4531–3.

73. Scaringi S, Kianmanesh R, Sabate JM, et al. Advanced gastric cancer with or without peritoneal carcinomatosis treated with hyperthermic intraperitoneal chemotherapy: a single Western center experience. Eur J Surg Oncol 2008;34: 1246–52.

74. Yan TD, Black D, Sugarbaker PH, et al. A systematic review and meta-analysis of the randomized controlled trials on adjuvant intraperitoneal chemotherapy for resectable gastric cancer. Ann Surg Oncol 2007;14(10):2702–13.

75. Cunningham D, Starling N, Rao S, et al. Capecitabine and oxaliplatin for advanced esophagogastric cancer. N Engl J Med 2008;358(1):36–46.

76. Luo HY, Xu RH, Zhang L, et al. A pilot study of oxaliplatin, fluorouracil and folinic acid (FOLFOX-6) as first-line chemotherapy in advanced or recurrent gastric cancer. Chemotherapy 2008;54(3):228–35.

77. Liu ZF, Guo QS, Zhang XQ, et al. Biweekly oxaliplatin in combination with continuous infusional 5-fluorouracil and leucovorin (modified FOLFOX-4 regimen) as first-line chemotherapy for elderly patients with advanced gastric cancer. Am J Clin Oncol 2008;31(3):259–63.

78. Hwang WS, Chao TY, Lin SF, et al. Phase II study of oxaliplatin in combination with continuous infusion of 5-fluorouracil/leucovorin as first-line chemotherapy in patients with advanced gastric cancer. Anticancer Drugs 2008;19(3):283–8.

79. Muhr-Wilkenshoff F, Hinkelbein W, Ohnesorge I, et al. A pilot study of irinotecan (CPT-11) as single-agent therapy in patients with locally advanced or metastatic esophageal carcinoma. Int J Colorectal Dis 2003;18(4):330–4.

80. Park SH, Nam E, Park J, et al. Randomized phase II study of irinotecan, leucovorin and 5-fluorouracil (ILF) versus cisplatin plus ILF (PILF) combination chemotherapy for advanced gastric cancer. Ann Oncol 2008;19(4):729–33.
81. Koizumi W, Narahara H, Hara T, et al. S-1 plus cisplatin versus S-1 alone for first-line treatment of advanced gastric cancer (SPIRITS trial): a phase III trial. Lancet Oncol 2008;9(3):215–21.
82. Tsuji A, Shima Y, Morita S, et al. Combination chemotherapy of S-1 and low-dose twice-weekly cisplatin for advanced and recurrent gastric cancer in an outpatient setting: a retrospective study. Anticancer Res 2008;28(2B):1433–8.
83. Fujii M. Chemotherapy for advanced gastric cancer: ongoing phase III study of S-1 alone versus S-1 and docetaxel combination (JACCRO GC03 study). Int J Clin Oncol 2008;13(3):201–5.
84. Fujitani K, Yang HK, Kurokawa Y, et al. Randomized controlled trial comparing gastrectomy plus chemotherapy with chemotherapy alone in advanced gastric cancer with a single noncurable factor: Japan Clinical Oncology Group Study JCOG 0705 and Korea Gastric Cancer Association Study KGCA01. Jpn J Clin Oncol 2008;38(7):504–6.
85. Garcia I, Vizoso F, Martin A, et al. Clinical significance of the epidermal growth factor receptor and HER2 receptor in resectable gastric cancer. Ann Surg Oncol 2003;10(3):234–41.
86. Dragovich T, McCoy S, Fenoglio-Preiser CM, et al. Phase II trial of erlotinib in gastroesophageal junction and gastric adenocarcinomas: SWOG 0127. J Clin Oncol 2006;24(30):4922–7.
87. Ferry DR, Anderson M, Beddard K, et al. A phase II study of gefitinib monotherapy in advanced esophageal adenocarcinoma: evidence of gene expression, cellular, and clinical response. Clin Cancer Res 2007;13(19):5869–75.
88. McCormack PL, Keam SJ. Bevacizumab: a review of its use in metastatic colorectal cancer. Drugs 2008;68(4):487–506.
89. Hochster HS, Hart LL, Ramanathan RK, et al. Safety and efficacy of oxaliplatin and fluoropyrimidine regimens with or without bevacizumab as first-line treatment of metastatic colorectal cancer: results of the TREE Study. J Clin Oncol 2008; 26(21):3523–9.
90. Manegold C. Bevacizumab for the treatment of advanced nonsmall-cell lung cancer. Expert Rev Anticancer Ther 2008;8(5):689–99.
91. Di Costanzo F, Mazzoni F, Micol Mela M, et al. Bevacizumab in nonsmall cell lung cancer. Drugs 2008;68(6):737–46.
92. Garcia AA, Hirte H, Fleming G, et al. Phase II clinical trial of bevacizumab and low-dose metronomic oral cyclophosphamide in recurrent ovarian cancer: a trial of the California, Chicago, and Princess Margaret Hospital phase II consortia. J Clin Oncol 2008;26(1):76–82.
93. Shah MA, Ramanathan RK, Ilson DH, et al. Multicenter phase II study of irinotecan, cisplatin, and bevacizumab in patients with metastatic gastric or gastroesophageal junction adenocarcinoma. J Clin Oncol 2006;24(33):5201–6.

Liver-Directed Treatment Modalities for Primary and Secondary Hepatic Tumors

Brett Yamane, MD, Sharon Weber, MD*

KEYWORDS

- Liver-directed therapies • Hepatocellular carcinoma
- Colorectal metastases • Ablation • Radiotherapy
- Percutaneous ethanol injection • Embolization

Every year, approximately 150,000 new cases of colorectal cancer are diagnosed in the United States, with 10% to 25% of patients having hepatic metastases.[1,2] Hepatocellular carcinoma (HCC) claims 500,000 lives worldwide annually.[3,4] Although surgical resection is the gold standard for primary and secondary hepatic tumors, many patients are not surgical candidates because of inadequate liver functional reserve, extrahepatic disease, anatomic constraints of tumor, or medical comorbidities.[5] Therefore, other liver-directed therapies are used in the treatment of primary and secondary liver malignancies, including thermal ablative techniques (radiofrequency ablation [RFA], cryoablation, and microwave ablation [MWA]), directed radiotherapy, ethanol injection, and transcatheter arterial chemoembolization (TACE) and bland embolization. Although these therapies can be used alone or in combination, for various hepatic tumors, this article serves as a review of their usefulness as sole agents in the treatment of HCC and hepatic colorectal metastases.

EMBOLIZATION
Background

The liver obtains its blood supply from the portal system and the hepatic artery.[6] Various catheter-based therapies are used for liver tumors, exploiting the preferential blood flow to hepatic tumors by way of the hepatic arterial system.[7] TACE was introduced in the 1980s and delivers chemotherapeutics followed by either embolization or various materials to decrease intratumoral blood flow.[7] The reduction in blood flow to

University of Wisconsin, Department of Surgery, K4/764 Clinical Science Center, 600 Highland Avenue, Madison, WI 53792-7375, USA
* Corresponding author.
E-mail address: webers@surgery.wisc.edu (S. Weber).

Surg Clin N Am 89 (2009) 97–113
doi:10.1016/j.suc.2008.10.004
0039-6109/08/$ – see front matter © 2009 Elsevier Inc. All rights reserved.

surgical.theclinics.com

tumor leads to tumor ischemia and increased local concentrations of antitumor drug, thereby reducing systemic toxicity.[7]

Technique

TACE and bland embolization involve delivery of vascular occlusive agents to occlude tumor inflow by way of a temporary catheter placed in the hepatic artery.[8] The final position of the catheter tip in the hepatic arterial tree is directed under angiographic guidance, and is chosen according to the anatomy of the patient and the tumor. Ideally, the tip needs placement distally to avoid extrahepatic drug distribution, but not too distal to avoid arterial occlusion.[8] Chemotherapeutics may or may not be administered before embolization, marking the distinction between TACE and bland embolization. Embolization agents can be temporary (microspheres, degradable starch microspheres, collagen and gelatine sponge [Gelfoam]) or permanent (polyvinyl alcohol [Ivalon]).[8]

Specific to TACE, variations in protocols exist, including the chemotherapeutic used, the use of lipiodol, and the type of material used to decrease blood flow.[7] In the United States, doxorubicin, cisplatin, and mitomycin are the drugs used most often. Lipiodol is an iodinated ester from poppy-seed oil that is retained by liver tumors, and most protocols use this agent as a drug carrier and a tumor-seeking agent[7] because lipiodol has a microvascular occlusive effect and it is preferentially retained by hepatic tumor cells.[8] Some form of embolization with the agents mentioned above usually follows the administration of drug to reduce arterial blood flow, inducing tumor ischemia. However, it is important to maintain some flow to the tumor to repeat TACE treatments and to prevent hypoxia-induced up-regulation of stimulators of tumor metabolism, growth, and invasion-like vascular endothelial growth factor.[7]

Transcatheter Arterial Chemoembolization

Indications

The major tumor types for which TACE is indicated include HCC (as a bridge to transplantation and for unresectable tumors), neuroendocrine metastases, and metastatic sarcoma.[7] It can be used as a neoadjuvant therapy before surgery to reduce tumor size and vascularity, making lesions amenable to either surgery or ablation, in addition to its use in palliative indications and for symptomatic relief from tumors with invasion into Glisson capsule.[8]

Limitations

Limitations to TACE include extensive metastases involving both lobes of the liver, precluding treatment of all feeding vasculature at the expense of normally perfused tissue.[8]

Adverse effects/complications

Although TACE is usually well tolerated, the most common adverse effect is postembolization syndrome, consisting of right upper quadrant pain, nausea, vomiting, and fever with elevated liver enzymes.[7] This syndrome occurs in about 4% to 10% of patients undergoing this procedure, and is typically transient, with recovery within 7 to 10 days.[7] Serious complications such as tumor rupture, acute liver failure, liver abscess, and pulmonary lipiodol embolism are extremely rare.[7,8] Mechanical complications include catheter dislodgement, thrombosis and occlusion, site infection, mesenteric ischemia, and inadvertent infusion embolization of the hepatic artery.[8]

Outcomes

Transcatheter arterial chemoembolization

The Liver Cancer Study Group of Japan showed that TACE accounted for the most frequent treatment of HCC as initial therapy. Takayasu and colleagues[9] performed an 8-year prospective study with 8510 patients who had unresectable HCC treated with TACE, which found a median survival of 34 months (mean follow-up 19 months). The 5-year survivals, stratified by Tumor, Nodes, Metastases stage (I, II, III, and IV), were 47%, 32%, 20%, and 10%, respectively ($P = .001$), which demonstrates that the lower the stage, the better the survival rate after TACE therapy.

Combination transcatheter arterial chemoembolization + radiofrequency ablation

One limitation of TACE alone is tumor size.[9] Therefore, chemoembolization is often combined with other ablative modalities, and a recent randomized trial evaluated TACE combined with RFA versus TACE alone versus RFA alone in patients who had large HCC (>3 cm).[10] Overall survival was improved in patients undergoing TACE-RFA compared with either treatment alone, with a median survival of 24 months following TACE, 22 months following RFA, and 37 months following combination treatment ($P<.001$ for TACE versus the combination, $P\leq.001$ for TACE versus RFA). Prior to randomization, patients were stratified according to nodularity (uninodular versus multinodular). TACE-RFA demonstrated improved survival over RFA alone in patients who had either uninodular ($P = .001$) or multinodular HCC ($P<.001$). When subgroup analysis was performed according to lesion size, combination treatment increased survival over TACE ($P = .008$) and RFA ($P = .001$) in patients who had lesions between 3–5 cm in size. For lesions over 5 cm, survival was highest in the combination group ($P<.001$ TACE-RFA versus RFA, TACE-RFA versus TACE).

In addition, combination therapy with TACE-RFA was associated with a higher rate of complete responses on follow-up imaging (55% versus 5% for TACE [$P<.001$] and 37% for RFA [$P = .02$]). The same trend was noted when looking for objective responses, which included complete and partial responses. At 6 months, objective responses were noted in 54% of the TACE-RFA group, 35% of TACE, and 36% of the RFA group ($P = .009$ combo versus TACE, $P = .01$ combo versus RFA). Therefore, it appears that combination treatment has defined benefits in terms of complete and partial responses compared with either treatment alone.

Transcatheter arterial chemoembolization versus transcatheter arterial embolization (bland embolization)

Multiple studies comparing TACE with transcatheter arterial embolization (TAE) have shown no difference in survival or symptom management in patients who have neuroendocrine hepatic metastases.[11–13] In the treatment of HCC, these two therapies have been compared and showed no difference in survival.[14] In a randomized study by Llovet[14] comparing TACE, TAE, and symptomatic treatment of unresectable HCC, 112 patients received embolization with Gelfoam, chemoembolization with Gelfoam and doxorubicin, and symptomatic treatment. Treatments were administered at baseline, 2 months, 6 months, and then every 6 months thereafter. Treatment response was assessed by CT scan at 6 months, and magnitude was defined by a complete response (no disease evident) or partial response. Objective responses included complete and partial responses lasting for at least 6 months. The primary end point was survival (mean follow-up 22 months embolization, 21 months chemoembolization, and 15 months control groups). Two-year survival was 50% for embolization, 63% for chemoembolization, and 27% for control ($P = .009$ control versus chemoembolization, not significant embolization versus chemoembolization). The conclusion of the study was that chemoembolization improves survival compared with conservative therapy, but not with bland embolization.[14] It is clear that the choice of bland versus chemoembolization is institution dependent because no real differences in long-term outcome have been demonstrated.

ABLATION

Ablative techniques improve the ability to treat patients who have unresectable primary and secondary hepatic tumors.[15] Ablative techniques are used to destroy tumor by way of a source that changes temperature to levels that are associated with cell death while causing minimal damage to adjacent, normal liver.[7] These techniques include RFA, cryoablation, and MWA. Margins of at least 0.5 to 1.0 cm are needed to decrease the likelihood of recurrence.

The choice of ablative technique is dependent on equipment availability and surgeon/radiologist preference. Many ablation features overlap, with no randomized prospective studies demonstrating superior outcomes among modalities. Thus, it is unclear which specific modality is best for a given application. Currently, the most commonly used modality in the United States is radiofrequency, whereas in Europe and Asia, experience with MWA is extensive.

ABLATION, RADIOFREQUENCY ABLATION
Mechanism

RFA is the most frequently used thermoablative technique.[7] RFA produces coagulative necrosis by way of an alternating high-frequency electric current in the radiofrequency range (460–500 kHz), delivered through an electrode placed in the center of a lesion.[7] Ionic movement within the tissue creates frictional heat as the ions try to follow this alternating current, with local tissue temperatures exceeding 100°C.[7] This ionic agitation leads to tissue destruction by way of tissue boiling and creation of water vapor. Once lethal temperatures (>60°C) are reached, protein denaturation, tissue coagulation, and vascular thrombosis result in a zone of complete ablation. A zone of partial tissue destruction up to 8 mm in diameter can be seen surrounding the zone of coagulation.[15] Heat-based ablation modalities cause profound vascular thrombosis, making bleeding an unusual complication of RFA.[15]

RFA may be delivered in three ways: percutaneous, laparoscopic, or open (laparotomy).[7,15] The decision of which mode to use is based on known advantages of each technique. Most procedures require general anesthesia because RFA can cause severe pain while being applied.[15] Therefore, although percutaneous ablation avoids a laparotomy, patients require an anesthetic. In addition, when percutaneous techniques are used, the abdomen cannot be assessed for extrahepatic disease, and no access exists for intraoperative ultrasound, which can detect additional hepatic disease in 40% to 55% of patients.[15–17] Open and laparoscopic ablation allow for concurrent resection (liver and colon); however, laparoscopic ablation is technically difficult in its limited ability to image the liver in multiple planes, limiting accurate probe placement. Because of these drawbacks, open ablation is preferred for patients able to tolerate it.[15]

Indications

For RFA, indications include unresectable primary liver tumors, and colorectal and neuroendocrine liver metastases, as bridges to liver transplant for HCC, and as substitutes for surgical resection in those who have medical contraindications to surgery.[7]

RFA is the favored modality for coagulopathic patients because of the intrinsic cautery effect decreasing bleeding complications.[15]

Outcomes

No randomized studies have compared RFA with resection. A retrospective study from MD Anderson compared RFA, resection, and RFA + resection in 418 patients who had colorectal carcinoma (CRC) metastases.[18] RFA was used in operable candidates unable to undergo complete resection. RFA was associated with the highest rate of most local recurrence (9% RFA versus 5% combo versus 2% resection, $P = .02$). Liver-only recurrence was significantly higher in the RFA alone group (44%) compared with the combination (28%) and resection groups (11%) ($P<.001$ RFA versus combo, and RFA versus resection). Overall survival was highest (58% at 5 years) after resection (median follow-up 21 months). No difference was found between curatively treated patients in recurrence-free survival. Thus, resection continues to be the standard of care for patients who have resectable CRC, but ablation expands our ability to treat patients who have bilobar metastases that would have been considered unresectable.

RFA has been evaluated in patients who had unresectable HCC. Curley and colleagues[19] evaluated 110 cirrhotics who had HCC (Child class A–C) treated with RFA (open, laparoscopic, or percutaneous). Local recurrence developed in 3.6% of patients (median follow-up 19 months). New liver tumors or extrahepatic metastases developed in 50 patients (45.5%). Twenty-eight patients (25.4%) died of recurrent HCC, and 26 patients who had recurrence were alive at study termination. Sixty-five patients had no radiographic evidence of HCC recurrence. This study demonstrates that hepatic RFA can be performed with low morbidity and mortality in appropriately selected patients, with comparable recurrence rates to published data evaluating other ablation modalities.

Historically, evaluation of overall survival has been limited because of the heterogeneous patient population studied in these retrospective series. However, more recent series evaluating survival by tumor type have made it possible to compare outcome with series evaluating other types of treatment (resection or chemotherapy) for these tumors. Overall survival for colorectal and hepatocellular cancer after ablation (RFA and cryoablation) is listed in **Tables 1** and **2**, respectively.[15]

Table 1
Overall survival after ablation of colorectal hepatic metastases

Investigator	Ablation Type	N	Median FU (mo)	Median Survival (mo)	3YS (%)
Siperstein 2007[52]	RF	235	24	27	20.2
Sorensen 2007[53]	RF	102	Not given	52	64.0
Park 2007[54]	RF	30	Not given	35	Not given
Berber 2005[55]	RF	135	Not given	29	35.0
Solbiati 2004[56]	RF	38	33	33	46.0
Abdalla 2004[18]	RF	57	21	Not given	37.0
Yan 2003[57]	Cryoablation	172	23	28	41.0
Ruers 2001[58]	Cryoablation	30	26	32	37.0
Seifert 1998[23]	Cryoablation	116	21	26	32.0
Weaver 1995[59]	Cryoablation	47	26	26	Not given

Abbreviations: FU, follow-up; RF, radiofrequency; 3YS, three years.

Table 2
Overall survival after ablation of hepatocellular carcinoma

Investigator	Ablation Type	N	Median FU	Median Survival	3YS
Lencioni 2005[60]	RF	187	Mean 24 mo	57 mo	67%
Tateishi 2005[61]	RF	319	2.3 y	Not given	78%
Lin 2004[56]	RF	52	25 mo	Not given	74%
Lam 2004[62]	RF	51	Not given	Not given	61% (at 18 mo)
Curley 2000[19]	RF	110	19 mo	Not given	Not given; actual survival 59% at 19 mo FU

Abbreviations: FU, follow-up; RF, radiofrequency; 3YS, three years.

Limitations/Complications

The main limitation of RFA is attaining destruction of enough tissue volume. It is also difficult to treat lesions in all locations of the liver, especially those in the perihilar areas or near large vascular structures. Complications occur in 8% to 35% of patients undergoing RFA, and include abscess formation and biliary injury.[7,15]

ABLATION, CRYOABLATION
Mechanism

Another ablation technique, cryoablation involves a freezing and thawing process destroying cell membranes and organelles because of the mechanical stresses associated with the phase change from ice formation, resulting in a well-defined zone of tissue destruction.[15,20] Cryoablation can be performed with multiple applicators, allowing the operator to sculpt a cryolesion for maximal tumor coverage with minimal collateral damage. Regardless of the approach (open, laparoscopic, percutaneous), one of the main advantages of cryoablation over the heat-based ablation modalities is the ability to visualize the developing cryolesion with ultrasound, CT, and MRI, and the excellent correlation between the location of the cryolesion and the zone of cell death (**Fig. 1**). This advantage is important because the success of ablation requires an ability to visualize the complete destruction of the targeted tumor.[20–22]

Complications

Cryoablation has been rarely associated with substantial hemorrhage during large-volume freezes performed at open laparotomy because it has no intrinsic hemostatic properties.[20,23,24] With smaller probe sizes for cryoablation (1.7 mm), this problem is not clinically significant, except when freezing results in cracking of the liver capsule during thawing. However, percutaneous cryoablation does not appear to result in a high bleeding rate, perhaps because, in contrast to laparotomy, percutaneous ablation does not have the cryolesion–air interface, it is not performed in a low-pressure environment, and it has the benefit of surrounding tissues for tamponade.[25–28]

Cryoablation has been associated with a systemic complication termed cryoshock, which can lead to disseminated intravascular coagulopathy and multisystem organ failure, and leads to increased quantity of systemic inflammatory mediators in the blood compared with RFA.[29,30] The quoted incidence of 1% after large-volume ablations has likely decreased by limiting the volume of tissue destroyed by freezing.[20]

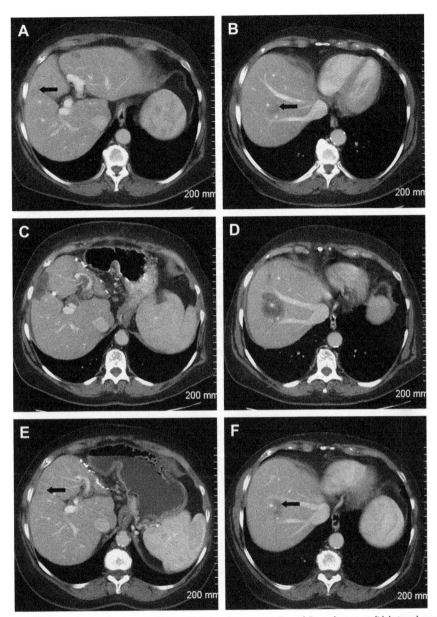

Fig. 1. Patient who had a large HCC in (L) lateral segment 2 and 3 underwent (L) lateral segmentectomy and cryoablation of two lesions in her (R) lobe. Ill-defined HCC in the R-hepatic lobe before cryoablation (*A, B*) (*arrows*), 1 month postablation (*C, D*), and 6 months postablation with resolving cryoablation lesion (*E, F*) (*arrows*). The patient has had no local recurrence noted at 18 months postablation. L, left; R, right; R-hepatic, right hepatic.

Outcomes

Although cryoablation has been found to be effective in causing cell death, concerns regarding increased local recurrence rates and higher complication rates have led to the decreased use of this technology.[25,26,31]

ABLATION, MICROWAVE ABLATION
Background

MWA is the newest of the ablation methods, and refers to all electromagnetic methods of inducing tumor destruction by using devices generating frequencies of a minimum of 900 MHz.[7,32] Under image guidance with CT, MRI, or ultrasonography, a microwave antenna is placed intratumorally. An electromagnetic wave is emitted from the microwave generator through the exposed, noninsulated portion of the antenna. This microwave transmission leads to agitation of water molecules in tumoral tissue, creating friction and heat, which leads ultimately to coagulative necrosis and cell death.[7,32]

Although MWA shares many advantages with the most commonly used ablative method, MWA has some theoretic advantages compared with RFA. Both offer flexible treatment approaches, consistent necrotic areas, and excellent patient tolerability. However, in MWA, transmission is not limited by tissue desiccation and charring (as in RFA, which relies on conduction of electricity), which allows intratumoral temperatures to be driven high, leading to a larger ablation zone, less treatment time, and more complete tumor killing.[32] MWA can be performed during laparoscopy or laparotomy, or percutaneously under ultrasound guidance, and it can be applied to multiple tumors, inducing necrosis within the tumor and in a margin of normal hepatic parenchyma.[7] Image findings indicative of tumor necrosis include echogenic change on ultrasonography, loss of contrast enhancement on CT, and decreased intensity on T2-weighted MRI.[33]

Indications

The indications for MWA include colorectal metastases,[33–35] unresectable HCC, HCC in anatomically difficult locations, and HCC patients unsuitable for surgery,[7,36] and it has been used in patients who have other metastatic tumors.[37]

Complications

Complications parallel those of RFA, including bile duct stenosis, intraperitoneal bleeding, liver abscess, colonic perforation, tumor seeding along the antennae track, and skin burns.[32] Because this technology has not yet been widely used in the United States, the morbidity and mortality data are still relatively unknown. Side effects associated with MWA include pain, postablative syndrome (fever/malaise), and asymptomatic pleural effusions that are self-limiting.[32,33]

Outcome

MWA for hepatocellular carcinoma

Liang and colleagues[36] evaluated prognostic factors for survival in 288 patients who had HCC. To be eligible, patients needed to have a single nodular HCC less than 8 cm, five or fewer lesions with diameters less than or equal to 6 cm, and absence of extrahepatic disease. One- and 5-year cumulative survival rates were 93% and 51% (mean follow-up 31 months). On multivariate analysis, patients who had a single nodule and tumors less than 4 cm had significantly improved survival rates. As expected, smaller tumors and less advanced disease demonstrated improved outcomes after therapy.

Resection versus MWA for colorectal metastases

In a randomized trial from Shibata and colleagues,[35] MWA was compared with resection in patients who had multiple colorectal metastases. Thirty patients who had multiple metastases who were potential surgical candidates were assigned to either hepatectomy or MWA. No statistical difference existed between the groups in regards to mean survival (MWA, 27 months versus surgery, 25 months, $P = .83$), postoperative complications, or death. Complications included one bile duct fistula and one hepatic abscess in the MWA group, and one patient each with bowel obstruction, bile duct fistula, and wound infection in the hepatectomy group. Clearly, the final conclusions of this study can only be made after longer follow-up.

MWA versus radiofrequency ablation for hepatocellular carcinoma

In 2002, a randomized study from Japan compared MWA with RFA in patients who had small HCC.[38] No difference existed in patient or tumor characteristics between the groups. Seventy-two patients who had 94 HCC lesions were randomly assigned to RFA or MWA with equivalent therapeutic effects, complication rates, and rates of residual foci observed between the two modalities.[38] After a mean follow-up of 18 months, no survival data were obtained, nor have follow-up studies been published to date.

Although the results of these studies are clearly limited by the small sample size, they represent the only prospective trials evaluating the efficacy of MWA. Based on these results and the results of other retrospective studies, the choice of ablative technique should be based on institutional and user experience and preference.

PERCUTANEOUS ETHANOL INJECTION
Background

Percutaneous ethanol injection (PEI) was first reported by Sugiura[39] in 1983.[39–41] PEI is an accepted treatment of patients who have small, unresectable HCC, given the limited indications for surgical resection in cirrhotic patients.[40]

Mechanism

Two to 8 mL of 95% ethanol is administered at a time, and PEI is performed under ultrasound guidance by way of a 21-gauge needle. Mechanistically, ethanol penetrates malignant cells promptly, inducing coagulative necrosis and thrombosis in the tumor microcirculation because of protein denaturation, platelet aggregation, and dehydration of parenchymal and surrounding endothelium.[41] With the different consistency between tumor tissue and the surrounding parenchyma, homogeneous distribution of ethanol occurs within the tumor nodule.[41] Although PEI offers the advantage of low cost and a favorable complication profile, most literature demonstrates the best results with small HCC (**Fig. 2**).[42,43] Complete tumor necrosis is correlated with tumor size, given that intratumoral fibrous septa limits the spread of ethanol, leading to irregular diffusion beyond the lesion and therefore not achieving an adequate margin in larger tumors.[42]

Indications

Given the size limitations associated with PEI, current indications often include HCC lesions less than 3 cm when used as a first-line therapy, and small HCC lesions recurring at distant sites after previous treatment.[40,43,44]

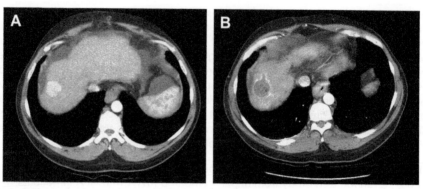

Fig. 2. Patient who has end-stage cirrhosis and ascites undergoing percutaneous ethanol injections for HCC. The liver tumor before (*A*) and after (*B*) PEI.

Outcome

Several studies have evaluated the effectiveness of PEI in HCC. Recently, randomized controlled studies comparing PEI with other ablative techniques or resection have been published (**Table 3**). In addition, some observational studies follow patients receiving PEI over the span of its use. The outcomes of patients who underwent PEI as first-line treatment of HCC in Japan since its development in the 1980s were evaluated in a recent observational study.[40] Indications for PEI in this study included HCC tumors less than or equal to 3 cm and a maximum of three tumors. Overall 5- and 10-year survival rates were 60% and 21%, respectively. The survival was best in Child class A patients who had a solitary HCC (2 cm or less), with 5-, and 10-year survival rates of 74%, and 31%, respectively. Results from a long-term follow-up of Korean patients demonstrate similar survival rates; their overall survival at 5 years was 39%, and 55% for patients who had tumors less than 2 cm in largest diameter.[44] Thus, long-term survival is possible after PEI alone for small HCC.

For the treated sites in Ebara's[40] study, 3-year local recurrence rate was 10%, whereas recurrence at untreated intrahepatic sites after PEI was 82%. Recurrence at other sites in the liver was lower in patients who had solitary lesions, serum alpha fetoprotein less than 20 ng/mL, and in tumors smaller than 2 cm.[40]

Depending on the study, when PEI is compared with surgical resection, PEI demonstrates conflicting survival profiles when used for small HCC lesions.[45–47] A recent randomized, controlled trial was performed to compare PEI with resection of HCC less than or equal to 3 cm in diameter, and less than or equal to two lesions.[43] All 38 patients in each group had hepatitis with or without cirrhosis. Patients who had cirrhosis were either Child class A or B without ascites or coagulopathy, with most having single tumors. Of the seventy-six patients who were randomized, the groups showed no statistical difference in either survival or recurrence. The 5-year tumor-free survival rates were 45% in the PEI group and 48% in the resection group. Higher recurrence rates were found in tumors greater than 2 cm and elevated alpha fetoprotein levels greater than 200 ng/mL. Although the number of treated patients was small, these results suggest that in these highly selected patients who had small, accessible HCC, PEI may have resulted in comparable outcome to resection.

PEI has also been compared with RFA and percutaneous acetic acid injection in a randomized study of patients who had Child class A/B cirrhosis and HCC less than or equal to 3 cm.[48] The primary end point was local recurrence, with overall and cancer-free survival as secondary end points. When comparing RFA to PEI,

Table 3
Summary of percutaneous ethanol injection trials for small hepatocellular carcinoma

				Results	
Investigator	N	Cohorts	Recurrence	FU	Survival (%)
Dettmer 2006[63]	101	PEI PEI + TACE	Not given	Not given	3-y survival PEI: 50 PEI + TACE: 52
Huang[a] 2005[43]	76	PEI Resection	Not given	Mean FU PEI: 38 mo Resection: 38 mo	3-y survival PEI: 97 Resection: 88
Lin[a] 2005[48]	187	PEI PAI RFA	3-y local PEI: 34% PAI: 31% RFA: 14%	Median FU 35 mo	3-y survival PEI: 51 PAI: 53 RFA: 74
Shiina[a] 2005[64]	232	PEI RFA	4-y overall PEI: 85% RFA: 70%	Median FU PEI: 3 y RFA: 3 y	4-y survival PEI: 57 RFA: 74
Lencioni[a] 2003[65]	102	PEI RFA	Not given	Not given	2-y survival PEI: 43 RFA: 64
Koda[a] 2001[66]	52	PEI TACE + PEI	Not given	Mean FU PEI: 31 mo TACE + PEI: 29 mo	3-y survival PEI: 66 TACE + PEI: 81
Yamamoto 2001[67]	97	PEI Resection	Study duration PEI: 85% Resection: 71%	Median FU PEI: 6 y Resection: 5 y	3-y survival PEI: 82 Resection: 84

Abbreviations: FU, follow-up; PAI, percutaneous acetic acid injection; PEI, percutaneous ethanol injection.
[a] Randomized controlled trial.

RFA was superior in terms of survival and local recurrence. The local recurrence rate was significantly worse in the PEI group, 35% versus 13% in the RFA group ($P = .012$). However, on subset analysis for tumors less than 2 cm, no difference in local recurrence existed among the three groups. Overall survival at 3 years was 74% in the RFA group and 51% in the PEI group ($P = .038$). In summary, in this study, RFA for HCC resulted in fewer local recurrences and longer overall survival.

Complications

In a 20-year observational study, complications after PEI treatment primarily included hyperthermia greater than 38°C (44%), elevated serum liver function tests (47.7%), and pain (14.4%).[40] Less common complications included seeding of HCC to body wall (1.9%), pleural effusion (1.5%), biliary stricture (3.3%), portal vein thrombosis (0.7%), and bleeding in the biliary tract (0.7%). Death and complications needing emergency treatment were not seen in any patients during the 20-year period. These results suggest that PEI can be used safely for the treatment of small HCC tumors, provided the dispersion area exceeds 1 to 2 cm of the maximal diameter of the tumor.[41]

Limitations

As shown by Lin and colleagues,[48] when comparing RFA to PEI, local recurrence rates increased in patients undergoing PEI with larger tumors. Larger tumors and multinodular tumors have a less uniform distribution of the ethanol because of intratumoral septae that prevent even distribution throughout the tumor, which may lead to recurrence at the peripheral aspect of the tumor.[41] Also, PEI usually requires multiple treatment sessions, increasing therapy time and potentially increasing the risk for tumor seeding.[41] No definitive criteria exist for the quantity and interval of ethanol injections; however, best results occur when dispersion exceeds 1 to 2 cm of the maximal tumor diameter to create a 1-cm ablation ring around the HCC nodule.[41] Because excessive ethanol increases side effects and unnecessary liver damage,[41] a delicate balance exists when PEI is considered for use in larger tumors or in patients who have severe hepatic dysfunction.

RADIOACTIVE PARTICLES
Background

The role of external beam irradiation for HCC is limited, given the radiosensitive nature of normal hepatic tissue.[4,6] Exposure to radiation in excess of 40 Gy can lead to radiation-induced liver disease (RILD), a clinical syndrome characterized by ascites, anicteric hepatomegaly, and elevated liver enzymes weeks to months after therapy.[4] RILD is the most prominent treatment-related complication in patients undergoing external beam hepatic irradiation.[4] Given this limitation and the need for higher doses to inflict lethal injury to malignant tissue, minimally invasive intra-arterial devices that deliver high doses of radiation internally to the tumor have emerged that use radioactive yttrium-90 microspheres to deliver high tumoricidal doses while limiting the development of RILD.[4]

Technique

Yttrium-90 intra-arterial radiotherapy, also known as radioembolization, is a minimally invasive catheter-based therapy delivering internal radiation by way of the arterial vessels feeding tumors. Treatment is selective because hepatic tumors derive their blood supply primarily from the hepatic artery, and normal liver parenchymal tissue is supplied primarily by the portal system.[49] Embolic particles are loaded with radionuclide containing the pure beta emitter, yttrium 90. The microspheres lodge in malignant microvasculature, delivering high doses of ionizing radiation to the tumor compartment while maintaining low radiation exposure of the normal liver. Two yttrium-90 microsphere devices are commercially available: TheraSphere (MDS Nordion, Ottawa, Ontario) (made of glass) and selective internal radiation (SIR) spheres (Sirtex Medical, Sydney, Australia) (made of resin).[4,49–51] SIRspheres are used primarily for hepatic colorectal metastases, and Theraspheres for HCC.

Contraindications

Absolute contraindications include a pretreatment technetium-99m macro-aggregated albumin scan demonstrating significant hepatopulmonary shunting (which results in >30 Gy being delivered to the lungs with a single infusion), and the inability to prevent deposition of microspheres to the gastrointestinal tract with modern catheter techniques. Relative contraindications include noncompromised pulmonary function, adequate liver reserve, serum creatinine less than 2.0 mg/dL, and a platelet count greater than $75 \times 10^9/L$.[4]

Morbidity

The most common clinical toxicity is a mild postembolic syndrome that includes fatigue, vague abdominal discomfort, pain, and fever. Other toxicities occurring as a result of nontarget radiation include cholecystitis, gastric ulceration, gastroduodenitis, pancreatitis, radiation pneumonitis, and RILD. Most of these toxicities can be limited with proper planning. Lymphopenia occurs in the immediate postprocedural period given the sensitivity of lymphocytes to radiation; however, no infectious complications have been documented.[4]

Outcomes (SIRspheres)

In a prospective study of SIRspheres in 46 patients who had unresectable primary and secondary liver malignancies, SIRspheres demonstrated activity primarily in patients who had CRC.[6] In this multi-institutional trial, patients were included if they had liver metastases with histologic confirmation of their primary tumor, and histologically confirmed HCC or radiologic evidence of a liver tumor consistent with hepatoma with elevated alpha-fetoprotein levels higher than 500. Complete responses were defined as a disappearance of all target lesions, and partial responses were defined as more than a 30% decrease in the sum of the longest dimension of the target lesion at 2 months. Of 32 patients who had metastatic CRC, 10 patients demonstrated partial responses, with a median duration of response of 9 months. In patients who had HCC, one partial response (20%) occurred, and the single gastrointestinal stromal tumor patient also had a partial response. This study had a few complications, including peptic ulceration, esophageal variceal bleed, and radiation hepatitis that resolved with conservative management.

In another prospective study by the same investigator, 30 patients who had failed 5-fluorouracil therapy were administered SIRsphere therapy for inoperative colorectal liver metastases (median follow-up 18 months).[49] Twenty-one patients underwent SIRsphere therapy and concomitant 5-fluorouracil. Ten partial responses occurred, with a median duration of 8 months. One patient achieved a complete response at 6 months. All responses were seen in patients who had disease limited to their liver. For all patients, the median time to progression was 5 months; however, for those achieving partial response, this time extended to 9 months.

Outcomes (TheraSpheres)

TheraSpheres are used for HCC, and in a recent prospective study looking at safety, tumor response, and survival, patients were stratified according to method of treatment, risk, Okuda classification, and Child class.[50] Patients were treated by liver segment or lobe, with the number of treatments dependent on tumor distribution, hepatic function, and vascular flow dynamics. The patients were divided into groups, including segmentally treated, lobar treated/low risk, and lobar treated/high-risk. High-risk classification was designated if patients presented with ascites, diffuse disease, greater than 70% tumor replacement of liver, aspartate aminotransferase or alanine aminotransferase levels more than five times the upper limit of normal, or total serum bilirubin greater than 2mg/dL. All patients treated in a lobar fashion with none of the above criteria were classified as being in the lobar, low-risk group. Forty-three patients were followed, and no difference existed among groups in terms of tumor response. Fifty-one percent of lesions demonstrated greater than 50% reduction in tumor size. Seventy-nine percent of patients were determined to have a tumor response when percent reduction or tumor necrosis was used as a measure.

Median overall survival was 47 months for the group undergoing segmental treatment, 17 months for those undergoing low-risk lobar treatment, and 11 months for those in the high-risk lobar group ($P<.0001$). In non–high-risk patients, median survival was 21 months compared with 11 months for high-risk patients ($P<.0001$). Based on Okuda classification, stage I patients had median survivals of 24 months, and stage II patients, 13 months ($P<.0001$). Child class A patients had improved survival, with median survivals of 21 months versus 14 months in class B/C patients ($P = .0061$). Based on these results, despite similar tumor response rates, patients who have better underlying liver function and less tumor burden have improved survival after directed radiotherapy for HCC.

Because this technology is new, its optimal efficacy remains to be determined. Further prospective studies are needed to compare other standard treatments with directed radiotherapy.

SUMMARY

Given the fact that most patients are inoperable at the time of their diagnosis with either HCC or metastatic colorectal cancer, other liver-directed therapies are needed. Currently, the most commonly used techniques include embolization, thermal ablation (RFA and MWA), PEI, and directed radiotherapy. These therapies can be administered alone but can also be effective when used in combination, or with other chemotherapeutic regimens. More randomized studies will be needed to better address which modalities are superior for each tumor type and the specific clinical scenario.

REFERENCES

1. Jemal A, Murray T, Ward E, et al. Cancer statistics, 2005. CA Cancer J Clin 2005; 55(1):10–30.
2. Cummins ER, Vick K, Poole GV. Incurable colorectal carcinoma: the role of surgical palliation. Am Surg 2004;70(5):433–7.
3. El-Serag HB. Hepatocellular carcinoma: an epidemiologic view. J Clin Gastroenterol 2002;35:72–8.
4. Ibrahim SM, Lewandowski RJ, Sato KT, et al. Radioembolization for the treatment of unresectable hepatocellular carcinoma: a clinical review. World J Gastroenterol 2008;14(11):1664–9.
5. Garrean S, Hering J, Saied A, et al. Radiofrequency ablation of primary and metastatic liver tumors: a critical review of the literature. Am J Surg 2008;195:508–20.
6. Lim L, Gibbs P, Yip D, et al. Prospective study of treatment with selective internal radiation therapy spheres in patients with unresectable primary or secondary hepatic malignancies. Intern Med J 2005;35(4):222–7.
7. Liapi E, Geschwind JF. Transcatheter and ablative therapeutic approaches for solid malignancies. J Clin Oncol 2007;25:978–86.
8. Vogl TJ, Zangos S, Eichler K, et al. Colorectal liver metastases: regional chemotherapy via transarterial chemoembolization (TACE) and hepatic chemoperfusion: an update. Eur Radiol 2007;17(4):1025–34.
9. Takayasu K, Arii S, Ikai I, et al. Liver cancer study group of Japan. Prospective cohort study of transarterial chemoembolization for unresectable hepatocellular carcinoma in 8510 patients. Gastroenterology 2006;131(2):461–9.
10. Cheng BQ, Jia CQ, Liu CT, et al. Chemoembolization combined with radiofrequency ablation for patients with hepatocellular carcinoma larger than 3 cm: a randomized controlled trial. J Am Med Assoc 2008;299(14):1669–77.
11. Pitt SC, Knuth J, Keily JM, et al. Hepatic neuroendocrine metastases: chemo- or bland embolization? J Gastrointest Surg 2008;12:1951–60.
12. Gupta S, Johnson MM, Murthy R, et al. Hepatic arterial embolization and chemoembolization for the treatment of patients with metastatic neuroendocrine tumors: variables affecting response rate and survival. Cancer 2005;104:1590–602.
13. Ruutiainen AT, Soulen M, Tuite CM, et al. Chemoembolization and bland embolization of neuroendocrine tumor metastases to the liver. J Vasc Interv Radiol 2005; 16:955–61, 2007;18:847–55.

14. Llovet JM, Real MI, Montaña X, et al. Barcelona Liver Cancer Group. Arterial embolisation or chemoembolisation versus symptomatic treatment in patients with unresectable hepatocellular carcinoma: a randomised controlled trial. Lancet 2002;349(9319):1734–9.

15. Weber SM, Lee FT Jr. Expanded treatment of hepatic tumors with radiofrequency ablation and cryoablation. Oncology 2005;19(11 Suppl 4):27–32.

16. Wallace JR, Christians KK, Quiroz FA, et al. Ablation of liver metastasis: is preoperative imaging sufficiently accurate? J Gastrointest Surg 2001;5:98–107.

17. Cervone A, Sardi A, Conaway GL. Intraoperative ultrasound (IOUS) is essential in the management of metastatic colorectal liver lesions. Am Surg 2000;66:611–5.

18. Abdalla EK, Vauthey J, Ellis LM, et al. Recurrence and outcomes following hepatic resection, radiofrequency ablation, and combined resection/ablation for colorectal liver metastases. Ann Surg 2004;239(6):818–25.

19. Curley SA, Izzo F, Ellis LM, et al. Radiofrequency ablation of hepatocellular cancer in 110 patients with cirrhosis. Ann Surg 2000;232:381–91.

20. Weber SM, Lee FT Jr. In: Diagnostic Imaging. New York; CMP Media, LLC; 2005. p. 3–6.

21. Steed J, Saliken J, Donnelly BJ, et al. Correlation between thermosensor temperature and transrectal ultrasonography during prostate cryoablation. Can Assoc Radiol J 1997;48:186–90.

22. Onik G, Gilbert J, Hoddick W, et al. Sonographic monitoring of hepatic cryosurgery in an experimental animal-model. AJR Am J Roentgenol 1985;144:1043–7.

23. Seifert JK, Morris DL. Prognostic factors after cryotherapy for hepatic metastases from colorectal cancer. Ann Surg 1998;228:201–8.

24. Seifert JK, Morris DL. World survey on the complications of hepatic and prostate cryotherapy. World J Surg 1999;23:109–13.

25. Adam R, Akpinar E, Johann M, et al. Place of cryosurgery in the treatment of malignant liver tumors. Ann Surg 1997;225:39–50.

26. Adam R, Hagopian EJ, Linhares M, et al. A comparison of percutaneous cryosurgery and percutaneous radiofrequency for unresectable hepatic malignancies. Arch Surg 2002;137:1332–9.

27. Harada J, Dohi M, Mogami T, et al. Initial experience of percutaneous renal cryosurgery under the guidance of a horizontal open MRI system. Radiat Med 2001; 19:291–6.

28. Lee Ft Jr, Chosy SG, Littrup PJ, et al. CT-monitored percutaneous cryoablation in a pig liver model: pilot study. Radiology 1999;211:687–92.

29. Seifert JK, France MP, Zhao J, et al. Large volume hepatic freezing: association with significant release of the cytokines interleukin-6 and tumor necrosis factor a in a rat model. World J Surg 2002;26:1333–41.

30. Ng KK, Lam CM, Poon RT, et al. Comparison of systemic responses of radiofrequency ablation, cryotherapy, and surgical resection in a porcine liver model. Ann Surg Oncol 2004;11:650–7.

31. Pearson AS, Izzo F, Fleming RY, et al. Intraoperative radiofrequency ablation or cryoablation for hepatic malignancies. Am J Surg 1999;178:592–9.

32. Liang P, Wang Y. Microwave ablation of hepatocellular carcinoma. Oncology 2007;72(1):124–31.

33. Seki T, Wakabayashi M, Nakagawa T, et al. Ultrasonically guided percutaneous microwave coagulation therapy for small hepatocellular carcinoma. Cancer 1994;74:817–25.

34. Fahy BN, Jarnagin W. Evolving techniques in the treatment of liver colorectal metastases: role of laparoscopy, radiofrequency ablation, microwave coagulation, hepatic

arterial chemotherapy, indications and contraindications for resection, role of transplantation, and timing of chemotherapy. Surg Clin North Am 2006;86(4):1005–22.

35. Shibata T, Niinobu T, Ogata N, et al. Microwave coagulation therapy for multiple hepatic metastases from colorectal carcinoma. Cancer 2000;89(2):276–84.

36. Liang P, Dong B, Yu X, et al. Prognostic factors for survival in patients with hepatocellular carcinoma after percutaneous microwave ablation. Radiology 2005; 235(1):299–307.

37. Martin RC, Scoggins CR, McMasters KM. Microwave hepatic ablation: initial experience of safety and efficacy. J Surg Oncol 2007;86(6):481–6.

38. Shibata T, Iimuro Y, Yamamoto Y, et al. Small hepatocellular carcinoma: comparison of radio-frequency ablation and percutaneous microwave coagulation therapy. Radiology 2002;223(2):331–7.

39. Sugiura N, Takara K, Ohto M, et al. Ultrasound-guided ethanol injection for the treatment of small hepatocellular carcinoma. Acta Hepatol Jpn 1983;21:920–3.

40. Ebara M, Okabe S, Kita K, et al. Percutaneous ethanol injection for small hepatocellular carcinoma: therapeutic efficacy based on 20-year observation. J Hepatol 2005;43(3):458–64.

41. Lin X-D, La L-W. Local injection therapy for hepatocellular carcinoma. Hepatobiliary Pancreat Dis Int 2006;5:16–21.

42. Guan YS, Liu Y. Interventional treatments for hepatocellular carcinoma. Hepatobiliary Pancreat Dis Int 2006;5:495–500.

43. Huang GT, Lee PH, Tsang YM, et al. Percutaneous ethanol injection versus surgical resection for the treatment of small hepatocellular carcinoma: a prospective study. Ann Surg 2005;242:36–42.

44. Sung YM, Choi D, Lim HK, et al. Long-term results of percutaneous ethanol injection for the treatment of hepatocellular carcinoma in Korea. Korean J Radiol 2006;7(3):187–92.

45. Cho YB, Lee KU, Suh KS, et al. Hepatic resection compared to percutaneous ethanol injection for small hepatocellular carcinoma using propensity score matching. J Gastroenterol Hepatol 2007;22(10):1643–9, 2007;22(10):1643–9.

46. Gournay J, Tchuenbou J, Richou C, et al. Percutaneous ethanol injection vs. resection in patients with small single hepatocellular carcinoma: a retrospective case-control study with cost analysis. Aliment Pharmacol Ther 2002;16(8):1529–38.

47. Daniele B, De Sio I, Izzo F, et al. Hepatic resection and percutaneous ethanol injection as treatments of small hepatocellular carcinoma. J Clin Gastroenterol 2003;36(1):63–7.

48. Lin SM, Lin CJ, Lin CC, et al. Randomised controlled trial comparing percutaneous radiofrequency thermal ablation, percutaneous ethanol injection, and percutaneous acetic acid injection to treat hepatocellular carcinoma of 3 cm or less. Gut 2005;54:1151–6.

49. Lim L, Gibbs P, Yip D, et al. A prospective evaluation of treatment with selective internal radiation therapy (SIR-spheres) in patients with unresectable liver metastases from colorectal cancer previously treated with 5-FU based chemotherapy. BMC Cancer 2005;5:1–6.

50. Salem R, Lewandowski RJ, Atassi B, et al. Treatment of unresectable hepatocellular carcinoma with use of 90Y microspheres (TheraSphere): safety, tumor response, and survival. J Vasc Interv Radiol 2005;16:1627–39.

51. Sharma RA, Van Hazel GA, Morgan B, et al. Radioembolization of liver metastases from colorectal cancer using yttrium-90 microspheres with concomitant systemic oxaliplatin, fluorouracil, and leucovorin chemotherapy. J Clin Oncol 2007; 25:1099–106.

52. Siperstein AE, Berber E, Ballem N, et al. Survival after radiofrequency ablation of colorectal liver metastases: 10-year experience. Ann Surg 2007;246:559–67.
53. Sorensen SM, Mortensen FV, Nielsen DT. Radiofrequency ablation of colorectal liver metastases: long-term survival. Acta Radiol 2007;48(3):253–8.
54. Park IJ, Kim HC, Yu CS, et al. Radiofrequency ablation for metachronous liver metastasis from colorectal cancer after curative surgery. Ann Surg Oncol 2007; 15(1):227–32.
55. Berber E, Pelley R, Siperstein AE. Predictors of survival after radiofrequency thermal ablation of colorectal cancer metastases to the liver: a prospective study. J Clin Oncol 2005;23:1358–64.
56. Solbiati L. Ablation for liver colorectal metastases: is it possible to equal the 5-year survival rates of surgery? Radiological Society of North America scientific assembly and annual meeting: Chicago (IL): November 28-December 3, 2004.
57. Yan DB, Clingan P, Morris DL. Hepatic cryotherapy and regional chemotherapy with or without resection for liver metastases from colorectal carcinoma - how many are too many? Cancer 2003;98:320–30.
58. Ruers TJ, Joosten J, Jager GJ, et al. Long-term results of treating hepatic colorectal metastases with cryosurgery. Br J Surg 2001;88:844–9.
59. Weaver ML, Atkinson D, Zemel R. Hepatic cryosurgery in treating colorectal metastases. Cancer 1995;76:210–4.
60. Lencioni R, Cioni D, Crocetti L, et al. Early-stage hepatocellular carcinoma in patients with cirrhosis: long-term results of percutaneous image-guided radiofrequency ablation. Radiology 2005;234:961–7.
61. Tateishi R, Shiina S, Teratani T, et al. Percutaneous radiofrequency ablation for hepatocellular carcinoma. An analysis of 1000 cases. Cancer 2005;103:1201–9.
62. Lam CM, Ng KK, Poon RT, et al. Impact of radiofrequency ablation on the management of patients with hepatocellular carcinoma in a specialized centre. Br J Surg 2004;91:334–8.
63. Dettmer A, Kirchhoff TD, Gebel M, et al. Combination of repeated single-session percutaneous ethanol injection and transarterial chemoembolisation compared to repeated single-session percutaneous ethanol injection in patients with non-resectable hepatocellular carcinoma. World J Gastroenterol 2006;12(23):3707–15.
64. Shiina S, Teratani T, Obi S, et al. A randomized controlled trial of radiofrequency ablation with ethanol injection for small hepatocellular carcinoma. Gastroenterology 2005;129(1):122–30.
65. Lencioni RA, Allgaier HP, Cioni D, et al. Small hepatocellular carcinoma in cirrhosis: randomized comparison of radio-frequency thermal ablation versus percutaneous ethanol injection. Radiology 2003;228(1):235–40.
66. Koda M, Murawaki Y, Mitsuda A, et al. Combination therapy with transcatheter arterial chemoembolization and percutaneous ethanol injection compared with percutaneous ethanol injection alone for patients with small hepatocellular carcinoma: a randomized control study. Cancer 2001;92(6):1516–24.
67. Yamamoto J, Okada S, Shimada K, et al. Treatment strategy for small hepatocellular carcinoma: comparison of long-term results after percutaneous ethanol injection therapy and surgical resection. Hepatology 2001;34:707–13.

Multidisciplinary Approach to Tumors of the Pancreas and Biliary Tree

Kimberly M. Brown, MD[a,b],*

KEYWORDS

• Pancreas • Pancreatic cancer • Pancreatic cyst
• Gallbladder cancer • Cholangiocarcinoma

Much of the progress made against pancreatic cancer in the last several decades has been in the areas of decreased morbidity and mortality from surgical resection, and improved quality of imaging studies, thus allowing for better selection of patients most likely to benefit from surgical therapy. Unfortunately, surgical resection, although the only hope of long-term disease control, does not result in a cure for most patients. Although the introduction of gemcitabine as an active agent in pancreatic cancer initially offered hope for improved outcomes, the dismal median and 5-year survivals of patients undergoing multimodal therapy demonstrate that there remains significant need for more effective chemotherapeutic and targeted therapies in this disease.

Cystic tumors of the pancreas represent a spectrum of diseases, from benign to frankly malignant. The ability to predict an individual lesion's risk of being malignant has improved with the advancement of cross-sectional imaging techniques and the introduction of endoscopic ultrasound (EUS) with aspiration of cyst contents for analysis, although diagnostic uncertainty still may be present in many cases. This may allow for the application of surgical resection in patients most likely to derive benefit.

Methods of early detection and effective systemic therapies are lacking for cholangiocarcinoma and gallbladder cancer and pancreatic cancer. Surgical resection offers the best hope of extended disease control, but is not possible in many cases because of the advanced stage of disease on presentation. A multidisciplinary approach to these challenging tumors can help expedite work-up and tailor available therapies to an individual patient's needs.

a Surgical Oncology, Saint Luke's Hospital of Kansas City, 4320 Wornall Road, Suite 420, Kansas City, MO 64111, USA
b Department of Surgery, Truman Medical Center, 2301 Holmes Street, Kansas City, MO 64108, USA
* 4320 Wornall Road, Suite 240, Kansas City, MO 64111.
E-mail address: kbrown4@saint-lukes.org

Surg Clin N Am 89 (2009) 115–131
doi:10.1016/j.suc.2008.09.022
0039-6109/08/$ – see front matter © 2009 Elsevier Inc. All rights reserved.
surgical.theclinics.com

CYSTIC LESIONS OF THE PANCREAS

Cystic lesions of the pancreas are encountered more and more frequently in clinical practice as higher-quality cross-sectional imaging studies are used for various related or nonrelated indications. These lesions encompass a spectrum of histopathologic entities, from benign with no metastatic potential to frankly malignant. Although there is no single test or combination of studies that definitively identify the malignant potential of cystic lesions of the pancreas, a rational approach to the work-up of such lesions can attempt to direct surgical therapy to those patients most likely to derive benefit.

The initial step in this process is a thorough history and physical examination, seeking to elicit current or past symptoms of pancreatitis, trauma, pancreatic insufficiency, or constitutional symptoms suggestive of malignancy. High-quality cross-sectional imaging is essential to the proper diagnostic algorithm, and may include multislice helical CT with intravenous contrast and fine cuts through the pancreas (less than or equal to 3 mm) or MRI with pre- and postgadolinium images. A comparison with prior studies, if possible, can help determine the rate of change of these lesions.

Some investigators have examined the use of 18-fluorodeoxyglucose positron emission tomography (18-FDG-PET) scanning in the work-up of cystic lesions of the pancreas. In a prospective study of 50 patients who had cystic lesions of the pancreas, Sperti and colleagues[1] found that 16 of 17 patients (94%) who had malignant cystic neoplasms displayed increased 18-FDG uptake with standard uptake values (SUV) greater than 2.5. Of the 33 patients with benign tumors, two had increased 18-FDG uptake, for an overall specificity and accuracy of 94%. The ability of PET to distinguish benign from malignant cystic tumors of the pancreas was better than that of CT, which had a sensitivity of 65%, specificity of 88%, and overall accuracy of 80%.[1] These findings were not corroborated by a retrospective study at Memorial Sloan-Kettering Cancer Center.[2] In this study, 79 patients who underwent PET imaging for cystic lesions of the pancreas were reviewed. Twenty-one patients underwent resection, and 47 were followed with imaging. Increased 18-FDG uptake was seen in four of seven patients (57%) who underwent resection of a malignant cystic tumor, and in 2 of 14 (14%) of patients who had a benign tumor, for a sensitivity of 57% and a specificity of 85%. Cross-sectional imaging revealed evidence of malignancy in all patients who had malignant tumors. Thus, 18-FDG PET imaging should not be considered a routine part of the work-up for cystic lesions of the pancreas, but in a patient who has equivocal findings on cross-sectional imaging, PET may help with operative decision making. The use of the National Oncologic PET Registry established by the Centers for Medicare and Medicaid is highly encouraged.[3]

EUS with aspiration of cyst contents has emerged as a possibly useful tool in the work-up of a cystic lesion of the pancreas. Although morphologic features seen with EUS may not allow for differentiation between benign and malignant lesions beyond that seen with standard cross-sectional imaging,[4] analysis of cyst fluid obtained by means of fine-needle aspiration of the cyst contents may help in the decision-making process, as will be discussed.[5]

Non-neoplastic cystic lesions of the pancreas primarily include pseudocysts, although parasitic cysts and cysts associated with congenital disease such as cystic fibrosis also may be seen. Pseudocysts may be diagnosed by history, although a history of pancreatitis does not exclude a cystic neoplasm. Further support of this diagnosis may come from serum and cystic fluid tumor markers such as carcinoembryonic antigen (CEA) and CA 19-9, which are normal in a pseudocyst. Furthermore, pseudocyst fluid is usually high in amylase and negative for tumor markers (**Table 1**).

Table 1
Clinical characteristics of the more common cystic lesions of the pancreas

	Pseudocyst	Serous Cystic Neoplasm	Mucinous Cystic Neoplasm	Intraductal Papillary Mucinous Neoplasm
Age	Any	60–80 y	30–50 y	60–80 y
Gender	Equal distribution	Female > male	Female >> male	Equal distribution
Location	Evenly distributed	Body/tail > head	Body/tail >> head	Head > body/tail
Appearance on imaging	Single cyst or multiloculated macrocystic; may have findings of chronic pancreatitis	Honey-combed microcystic; may have central scar; may have dominant cyst	Macrocystic, single or multi-loculated; thick, smooth wall; no connection to main duct	Polycystic lesion with dilation of pancreatic duct
Cyst fluid carcinoembryonic antigen	Low	Low	High	High
Cyst fluid amylase	High	Low	Low	Low
Cyst fluid mucin	Low	Low	High	High
Natural history	No malignant potential; resection indicated for diagnostic uncertainty, internal drainage for persistent symptoms	Invasive/metastatic disease extremely rare; resection for symptomatic or enlarging lesions, and is curative	Potential for invasive disease at diagnosis or with observation; resection recommended, is curative, although recurrence in 50% of patients with invasive component	Potential for invasive disease at diagnosis or with observation; resection recommended for main duct intraductal papillary mucinous neoplasm or branch duct >3 cm; recurrence in >50% of patients with invasive disease

Data from Brugge WR, Lauwers GY, Sahani D, et al. Cystic neoplasms of the pancreas. N Engl J Med 2004;351(12):1220. Katz MH, Mortenson MM, Wang H, et al. Diagnosis and management of cystic neoplasms of the pancreas: an evidence-based approach. J Am Coll Surg 2008;207(1):108.

The more common neoplastic cystic lesions of the pancreas include serous cystic neoplasms, mucinous cystic neoplasms (MCN), and intraductal papillary mucinous neoplasms (IPMN). Serous cystic neoplasms affect women more often than men at a ratio of approximately 3:1 to 4:1, and their incidence increases with age. Most of these tumors are benign, with a serous cystadenocarcinoma being a reportable event. Cross-sectional imaging findings consistent with serous cystic neoplasm include a central stellate scar, a honeycombed appearance, or a pattern sunburst calcification. When aspirated, the cyst contents demonstrate scant cellularity, a low CEA, and low CA 19-9 levels.[6] An asymptomatic serous cyst may be observed safely. In the symptomatic patient who is a good operative candidate, resection may be indicated. Lesions larger than 4 cm or that are rapidly growing or changing in appearance also may be considered for resection. Nonstandard pancreatic resections such as enucleation, central pancreatectomy, or spleen-preserving distal pancreatectomy may be considered for serous lesions.[7] In all cases of resected disease, patients are considered definitively treated, and further surveillance is not necessary.

Mucinous cystic neoplasms most frequently are found in middle-aged women. Cross-sectional imaging shows a macrocystic lesion, which may be multiloculated and typically has a thick wall. There is no communication with the main pancreatic duct. A lesion size greater than 3 cm, the presence of mural nodules, a solid component, and calcifications are indications of malignant disease.[8,9] EUS with cyst aspiration typically demonstrates viscous fluid with elevated mucin and CEA levels.[5] Elevated serum CEA or CA 19-9 suggests malignant or invasive disease, although sensitivity is low.[10,11] There is no reliable way to distinguish benign from malignant MCN, to detect malignant transformation, or to predict which lesions will go on to become malignant. Therefore, the diagnosis of MCN is an indication for resection, and a standard anatomic resection is preferred, although some authors advocate that low-risk MCNs may be treated with a less-extensive procedure.[9] When final pathologic analysis reveals noninvasive disease, long-term disease-free survival is expected. Invasive MCN may recur in up to 50% of patients, and as such, these patients should be followed with imaging.[6]

IMPNs, initially described in 1982,[12] are distributed equally between men and women, and increase in incidence with increasing age. The two variants are main duct and branch duct, and the histology can range from benign adenomas to invasive disease. Any portion of the pancreas or even the entire pancreas may be affected.[13] Cross-sectional imaging shows a polycystic lesion, with pancreatic ductal dilation in the main duct variant. Mural nodules, solid component, calcifications, and significant ductal dilation suggest malignant disease.[6] As with MCN, there is no reliable means to discriminate between invasive and noninvasive disease, or to detect transformation. Asymptomatic branch duct lesions less than 3 cm may be followed safely with serial imaging, while all symptomatic lesions, lesions greater than 3 cm and main duct lesions should be removed with a standard anatomic resection.[14] Intraoperative frozen section of the pancreatic duct margin should be examined with the goal of achieving a margin free of invasive disease or dysplastic epithelium. Some authors support achieving a margin free of invasive disease only;[15] in a retrospective review of patients undergoing resection for IPMN, eight patients with noninvasive IPMN at the final surgical margin had no recurrences, with a median follow-up of 34 months.[15] The prognosis following resection depends on the presence of invasive disease, with a 77% to 100% 5-year survival in the absence of invasive disease (median 85 months), and 5-year median survival as low as 36% with invasive disease (median 23 months).[15–17] Postoperative surveillance is tailored to the risk of recurrence, with more aggressive follow-up for patients who have invasive disease. An algorithm depicting the work-up and treatment of cystic lesions of the pancreas is presented in **Fig. 1.**

In summary, cystic lesions of the pancreas remain diagnostic challenges. Although data from demographics, cross-sectional imaging, serum tumor markers, and cyst fluid analysis may be helpful in determining the potential of a given lesion to harbor a malignancy, there are many cases in which these data are equivocal. In such cases, the age and comorbidities of the patient may influence the surgeon's decision to recommend excision versus observation. The patient's wishes may play a role in preoperative decision making also. Finally, the availability of minimally invasive techniques may alter the risk/benefit profile in favor of resection for patients in whom a preoperative diagnosis cannot be reached with certainty.

PANCREATIC DUCTAL ADENOCARCINOMA

Pancreatic ductal adenocarcinoma remains a formidable challenge from the standpoint of a lack of early diagnostic tests and effective therapies. Although ranking tenth in incidence of malignancies in the United States, it is the fourth most common cause of cancer-related deaths in men and women, with an estimated 37,680 new cases and 34,290 deaths expected in 2008.[18] Complete surgical resection offers the best hope for long-term control of disease, although only approximately 30% of patients present with potentially resectable disease by imaging studies, and less than 20% of all patients ultimately undergo resection.[19,20] A recent analysis of data from the National Cancer database revealed that among patients who had clinical stage 1 pancreatic cancer (T1-2N0M0), 38.2% of patients were not offered surgery, with an additional 15.5% of patients excluded for age or comorbidities. Additionally, increasing evidence shows that patients treated in high-volume centers, which largely incorporate a multidisciplinary evaluation and treatment approach, experience superior outcomes than those patients seen in lower-volume centers.[21,22]

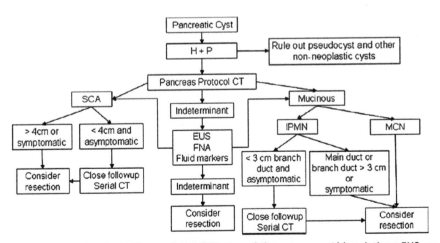

Fig. 1. Algorithm for the work-up of a cystic lesion of the pancreas. *Abbreviations:* EUS, endoscopic ultrasound; FNA, fine-needle aspiration; H&P, history and physical; IPMN, intraductal papillary mucinous neoplasm; MCN, mucinous cystic neoplasm; SCA, serous cystadenoma. (*From* Katz MH, Mortenson MM, Wang H, et al. Diagnosis and management of cystic neoplasms of the pancreas: an evidence-based approach. J Am Coll Surg 2008;207(1):116; with permission.)

Pancreatic cancer often remains asymptomatic until reaching an advanced stage. A cost-effective screening program has not been developed for the average-risk patient. Cigarette smoking, increased body mass index, high dietary fat, and exposure to beta-naphthlamine or benzidine have been associated with an increased risk of pancreatic cancer.[23] A small subset of pancreatic cancer has a familial predilection, including kindreds with a p16 germline mutation or the BRCA-2 gene mutation. In these high-risk individuals, EUS may be used as a screening modality to detect early stage tumors.[24]

DIAGNOSIS AND WORK-UP

Triphasic dynamic-phase helical or spiral CT scanning with fine cuts through the pancreas is the recommended method for evaluating known or suspected pancreatic lesions.[23] Approximately 70% to 85% of tumors will be resectable at the time of laparotomy if CT imaging demonstrates no evidence of extrapancreatic disease, no obstruction of the superior mesenteric vein (SMV)-portal vein (PV) confluence, and no tumor extension to the celiac trunk or superior mesenteric artery (SMA).[25]

PET has been investigated for diagnosis and staging of pancreatic malignancies. Earlier reports describe CT-PET as superior to CT in diagnosing pancreatic carcinoma (sensitivity and specificity 92% and 85% versus 65% and 62%),[26] but advances in the quality of CT and MRI imaging, and the increasing use of preoperative chemotherapy or chemoradiotherapy, which mandate tissue confirmation, leave open the question as to how PET or CT-PET contribute to the work-up of a patient who has suspected pancreatic cancer.

A study of PET for staging in a series of 42 patients who had untreated pancreatic cancer found that FDG-PET imaging detected metastatic disease in 13 of 16 patients (81% sensitivity), and identified eight metastatic sites in seven patients that were not seen on CT.[27] Overall, PET scanning changed the clinical staging in 5 of 42 patients (11.9%). The use of PET or CT-PET should be reserved for those patients in whom conventional imaging studies are equivocal, and it should be considered investigational. Again, the National Oncologic PET registry is recommended.[3]

EUS may be a useful tool in selected patients. For those patients suspected of having a pancreatic malignancy in whom no mass is seen on cross-sectional imaging, EUS may demonstrate a hypoechoic lesion consistent with a pancreatic tumor, with a sensitivity of 97% to 100%, including tumors smaller than 2 cm.[28,29] EUS with fine needle aspiration biopsy (FNAB) also allows for tissue confirmation. In addition, EUS can provide greater accuracy than other imaging modalities in assessing portal vein involvement or invasion by known pancreatic tumors, thus selecting patients who may require vessel resection or who may benefit from preoperative treatment.[30] EUS is the preferred method for obtaining tissue diagnosis in those patients who have unresectable disease or who will undergo preoperative treatment; however, biopsy of metastasis is appropriate in patients who have metastatic disease.[31]

In a patient with a clearly resectable pancreatic mass who is a good surgical candidate and is not being considered for preoperative treatment, endoscopic evaluation may not be necessary. The use of endoscopy for tissue diagnosis in this setting must be balanced with an understanding that a negative biopsy does not rule out a malignancy, and should not change the decision to proceed to surgery.[23]

The role of endoscopy for preoperative biliary decompression is controversial. Authors from Memorial Sloan-Kettering found an association between preoperative biliary decompression and increased risk of infections complications ($P = .022$) and death ($P = .021$) in patients undergoing biliary decompression before pancreaticoduodenectomy (PD).[32] Another retrospective review of 300 patients undergoing PD—172

(57%) with preoperative biliary decompression and 93 (31%) without—found no differ-ence in the incidence of complications, although the stent group had more wound in-fections $(P = .029)$.[33] Thus, patients who have symptomatic jaundice from an obstructing peri-ampullary tumor may undergo preoperative endoscopic stent place-ment, particularly if surgery is to be significantly delayed. Stenting, however, is indicated for obstructed patients with cholangitis, or those undergoing preoperative therapy. In these patients, temporary plastic stents are used most commonly; however, stent changes are necessary in 6 to 12 weeks because of stent obstruction. Some authors advocate the use of metallic, self-expanding stents, even in cases of patients planned for resection.[34]

Carbohydrate antigen 19-9 (CA 19-9) is a tumor marker associated with pancreatic adenocarcinoma. It is a derivative of the Lewis[a] blood group determinant, and as such is undetectable in patients who have a Lewis-negative blood group phenotype.[35] In addition, CA 19-9 often is elevated in patients who have biliary obstruction, even in the absence of malignancy.[36] Markedly elevated CA 19-9 in the nonjaundiced patient who had pancreatic cancer was found to be 84% to 88% predictive of unresectable disease in retrospective studies.[37,38] Although this laboratory value should not preclude a patient who has imaging studies consistent with resectable disease from receiving aggressive treatment, it may be a useful tool in selecting patients for addi-tional confirmatory studies or procedures to identify locally advanced or metastatic disease.[39] In addition, CA 19-9 response to treatment is a prognostic indicator, and its rise after treatment nadir is indicative of recurrent disease.[40]

Unrecognized occult metastatic disease may be found in as many as 25% of pa-tients brought to the operating room for planned resection, leading many surgeons to perform diagnostic laparoscopy before exploration. This procedure may be performed in the same setting as the planned resection, or in advance to allow for analysis of peritoneal cytology. The presence of malignant cells in peritoneal washings performed at resection has been found to correlate with a median survival of 8 months, compared with 16 months for patients who have negative cytology $(P<.001)$.[41] The survival pattern of patients who had positive cytology was comparable to those patients who had unresected metastatic disease (median survival 7 months, p = not significant). Although a staging laparoscopy is listed as a category 2B recom-mendation by the National Comprehensive Cancer Network (NCCN), patients most likely to benefit from its use include patients who have multiple comorbidities or those who have a high suspicion for vessel involvement or metastatic disease caused by markedly elevated CA 19-9 levels, large primaries or body/tail lesions.[23,39]

TREATMENT CONSIDERATIONS

Complete surgical resection, either by means of PD or distal pancreatectomy with splenectomy, is the only hope for long-term survival in patients who have pancreatic cancer. Short-term outcomes for these procedures have improved significantly over the past 20 years, and data suggest that surgical mortality and overall survival are improved when pancreatic resection is performed at a high-volume institution by a surgical team that performs at least 20 resections per year.[22,23] The goal of resection is complete removal of all gross and microscopic disease (R0 resection). Multiple technical aspects of PD have been studied, including extent of lymphadenectomy, method of pancreatic anastomosis, pylorus preservation, and vascular resection. A summary of these findings was presented in a prior issue of *Surgical Clinics of North America* and on the NCCN Web site.[23,42]

The antimetabolyte prodrug gemcitabine initially was found to have improved activity against pancreatic cancer compared with 5-FU in patients who have metastatic disease, and subsequently has been studied and incorporated into the adjuvant setting.[43] Patients who have metastatic disease are treated best by a gemcitabine-containing regimen, depending on performance status, and ideally should be treated on a clinical trial. Locally advanced, unresectable disease may be approached with chemotherapy or chemoradiation, with the role of radiation remaining controversial in both the adjuvant setting and in patients who have locally advanced, unresectable disease. Diagnostic laparoscopy may help confirm the absence of metastatic disease in patients being considered for chemoradiation, as 37% of patients who had locally advanced, unresectable tumors were found to have metastatic disease not detected by imaging studies when submitted to staging laparoscopy.[44]

The designation of borderline resectable tumors recently has emerged to describe a subpopulation of potentially resectable tumors with imaging features that indicate a higher likelihood of a margin-positive, or R1 resection. For tumors of the head or uncinate process, these criteria include SMV/PV impingement, SMA abutment, encasement of the gastroduodenal artery (GDA) up to its origin at the hepatic artery, limited inferior vena cava (IVC) involvement, short-segment SMV occlusion with patent vein proximally and distally, and colon or mesocolon invasion.[45] In addition, some authors include patients who have marginal performance status, or patients who have findings on imaging studies suspicious for but not clearly diagnostic of metastatic disease into the category of borderline resectable.[46]

Numerous studies have demonstrated the adverse impact of positive margins on survival, with median survivals ranging from 8 to 11 months in patients who had R1 or R2 resections, compared with 17 to 26 months for patients who had margin-negative (R0) resections.[47–49] The goal in the management of the borderline resectable patient is to maximize the chance of an R0 resection, which may be accomplished by delivering adjuvant treatment before surgery.[46,50] In addition to improving the rate of R0 resection, the use of preoperative treatment:

Allows for the identification of patients who develop rapidly progressive disease and likely would not benefit from surgical resection
Treats what is likely a systemic disease at diagnosis with a systemic treatment first
May allow for more patients to complete all modalities of treatment
May improve the efficacy of chemotherapy and radiation by delivering treatments to well-vascularized tissues
May render a subset of patients who have locally advanced unresectable disease amenable to surgical resection

Investigators at MD Anderson have demonstrated that the use of gemcitabine and cisplatin followed by gemcitabine-based chemoradiation delivered preoperatively was tolerated by 79 of 90 (88%) patients enrolled in a phase 2 trial. Fifty-two of the patients ultimately underwent PD, and the median survival for this subgroup was 31 months, compared with 10.5 months for patients who were not resected ($P<.001$). In a similar phase 2 trial employing preoperative chemoradiation with gemcitabine, 11 of 85 patients were deemed unresectable at restaging, because of medical comorbidity (three) or disease progression (eight). At surgery, another nine patients were found to have evidence of metastatic disease, for a total of 20/85 (23%) patients who progressed on preoperative treatment. Median overall survival for patients undergoing resection was 34 months compared with 7.1 months for patients who did not undergo PD (<0.001). Clearly a portion of the survival advantage of this treatment paradigm is derived from selecting out patients who likely would not have benefited from resection. In fact, to date, no randomized prospective trial has compared preoperative versus postoperative adjuvant treatment in resectable pancreatic cancer, so the true survival advantage to this regimen is unknown.

All patients who have undergone resection of a pancreatic adenocarcinoma should be considered for adjuvant treatment, as recurrence rates for surgery alone range from 50% to 80%.[51] In the United States, 5-FU based chemoradiotherapy has been the standard adjuvant treatment for resected pancreatic cancer, based on results from early phase 3 and single-institution studies demonstrating an improvement in median overall survival from 11 months to 20 months with the addition of 5-FU and concurrent radiation therapy.[52,53] A more recent phase 3 trial randomized 538 patients who had resected pancreatic cancer to gemcitabine followed by gemcitabine plus radiation or 5-FU followed by 5-FU plus radiation.[54] Median overall survival for the 388 patients who had pancreatic head tumors in the gemcitabine group was 20.5 months compared with 16.9 months in the 5-FU group, with 3-year survivals of 31% versus 22% ($P = .09$).

In Europe, radiation is not part of the standard treatment of pancreatic cancer. A phase 3 study from the European Study Group for Pancreatic Cancer (ESPAC) randomized 541 patients using a four-arm, 2×2 factorial design to compare the impact of chemotherapy, chemoradiation, chemoradiation plus chemotherapy, and observation on survival after resection.[55] Adjuvant chemoradiation was found to be associated with a lower median survival compared with regimens without chemoradiotherapy (17.9 months versus 15.9 months, $P = .05$). Patients receiving chemotherapy, however, had a median survival of 20.1 months compared with 15.5 months for those patients not receiving chemotherapy ($P = .009$).

More recently, the CONKO-001 (Charite Onkologie) trial reported phase 3 data on 368 patients who had resected pancreatic cancer randomized to either 6 months of gemcitabine or observation.[56,57] Disease-free survival at 3 and 5 years was 23.5% and 16% in the gemcitabine group, compared with 8.5% and 6.5% in the observation group ($P<.001$). Median overall survival was 22.8 months in the gemcitabine group compared with 20.2 months with observation ($P = .005$), with 3- and 5-year survivals of 36.5% and 21%, versus 19.5% and 9%.

Clearly the best hope for progress against pancreatic cancer remains the development of more efficacious systemic therapy. To date, targeted therapies have been largely unsuccessful in improving survival of patients who have pancreatic cancer. In a phase 3 trial, however, the epidermal growth factor receptor (EGFR) antagonist erlotinib demonstrated statistically significant improvement in overall survival in patients who had advanced or metastatic disease when given with gemcitabine, compared with gemcitabine alone (median survival 6.24 months versus 5.91 months, $P = .038$, 1-year survival 23% versus 17%, $P = .023$). The clinical significance of a 2-week improvement in overall survival remains to be clarified.

Pancreatic cancer is associated with symptoms such as pruritus from symptomatic biliary obstruction, nausea and vomiting from duodenal obstruction, and intractable pain from perineural tumor invasion. Various palliative treatments may be considered, including biliary stenting, operative biliary or gastric bypass, and celiac plexus neurolysis. In a review of 155 patients with locally advanced or metastatic disease who had been staged with laparoscopy and thus not submitted to prophylactic bypass procedures, 98% of the patients (152 of 155) did not require subsequent palliative procedures.[58] This suggests that laparotomy for prophylactic biliary or duodenal bypass is unnecessary. When possible, minimally invasive palliative treatments such as endoscopic biliary stenting, CT-guided celiac plexus neurolysis, or linear array EUS-guided chemical neurolysis should be employed over open surgical approaches.

BILIARY MALIGNANCIES

Tumors of the biliary tree include cholangiocarcinoma and gallbladder carcinoma. These cancers are less common than pancreatic cancer, with an estimated 9000 new cases of gallbladder and extrahepatic bile duct cancer in 2008,[18] but they present many of the same challenges, including advanced stage at presentation and a lack of effective systemic therapies. Like pancreatic tumors, surgery offers the best hope of cure for cholangiocarcinoma and gallbladder cancer. Long-term survival remains poor in these patients, with 5-year survivals in the range of 5%.

CHOLANGIOCARCINOMA

Cholangiocarcinoma is a relatively uncommon tumor, with an incidence that increases with age and a slight male predominance. Risk factors include cirrhosis, primary sclerosing cholangitis (PSC), chronic choledocholithiasis, bile duct adenoma, choledochal cyst, biliary papillomatosis, and parasitic or typhoid infection, although many patients who develop cholangiocarcinoma have no risk factors.[59] Cholangiocarcinoma can arise along any portion of the intra- or extrahepatic biliary tree. Tumors of the distal extrahepatic bile duct are managed in the same manner as pancreatic head cancers. Tumors of the intrahepatic bile ducts are approached in similar fashion to hepatocellular carcinoma, discussed elsewhere in this issue. The remainder of this article focuses on peri-hilar cholangiocarcinoma and cancer of the gallbladder.

The therapeutic goal of cholangiocarcinoma is a complete surgical resection with negative margins and adequate liver reserve, including inflow, outflow, and biliary drainage. As such, the preoperative work-up focuses on identifying the extent of disease within the bile ducts and the presence of metastases, which would preclude a curative resection.

Patients most commonly present with obstructive jaundice, with pain and constitutional symptoms typically occurring in more advanced disease. Physical examination may be unrevealing, or may demonstrate jaundice, right upper quadrant tenderness, or a palpable distended gallbladder, if the lesion is distal to the cystic duct. Laboratory studies are consistent with obstructive jaundice and may include a prolonged prothrombin time caused by malabsorption of fat-soluble vitamins. There are no sensitive and specific tumor markers for cholangiocarcinoma, with CA 19-9 being the most used test, in particular for screening patients who have PSC.

Ultrasonography is frequently the first test employed, and the pattern of ductal dilation may help identify the location of the obstructing tumor. Likewise, CT scanning may reveal a pattern of ductal dilation that suggests a location of an obstructing tumor; periportal, peripancreatic, celiac or mesenteric lymphadenopathy and intrahepatic metastases also may be visible on CT. MRI with magnetic resonance cholangiopancreatography using gadolinium contrast allows for more precise assessment of the location extent of intraductal tumor involvement, the relationship of tumor to the portal vein, and the presence of lymph node or distant metastases.

Cholangiography, either by means of percutaneous or endoscopic routes, is helpful in palliating symptomatic jaundice, obtaining brush cytology specimens for tissue diagnosis, and for assessing the extent of ductal involvement. Unfortunately, bile duct cytology may be nondiagnostic in up to 50% of patients who have a cholangiocarcinoma, highlighting the need for improved diagnostic techniques in these patients.[60]

The indications for surgical resection include a medically fit patient with no evidence of extrahepatic disease, including lymph node involvement beyond the porta hepatis, and no involvement of the contralateral bile duct beyond the secondary biliary radicals. The goal of resection is complete removal of all gross and microscopic disease (R0 resection), as this is associated with a prolonged disease-free survival.[61] For hilar cholangiocarcinoma, concomitant liver resection has been shown to decrease the incidence of local recurrence and should be considered in the preoperative planning.[61,62]

In patients who have unresectable disease, systemic treatment with 5-FU or gemcitabine-based chemotherapy may offer improvement in time to progression; however, no standard therapy has been established. Likewise, the role of adjuvant treatment is unproven and is approached best on a clinical trial. Liver-directed therapy, including transarterial chemoembolization (TACE), also may be used in patients who have unresectable or recurrent disease, and is discussed elsewhere in this issue.

Gallbladder Cancer

Gallbladder cancer remains a challenging clinical entity, both because of its insidious presentation (leading to diagnosis either at the time of cholecystectomy or upon pathologic review) and because of its relatively low incidence, approximately 5000 new cases in the United States per year.[59] Together, these make a prospective study very difficult.

Gallbladder cancer occurs approximately three times as often in women compared with men, and the incidence increases with age, with the peak incidence occurring in the seventh decade of life.[63] A history of gallstones, in particular larger gallstones, chronic cholecystitis, and a calcified gallbladder (porcelain gallbladder) may increase the risk of developing gallbladder cancer as much as eight times that of the general population.[64] Gallbladder polyps are thought to progress from adenomas to carcinomas, similar to colorectal cancer, with polyp size greater than 1 cm and broad-based, sessile polyps carrying the highest risk of malignancy in a retrospective review.[65]

The preoperative diagnosis of gallbladder cancer is made based on the appearance of a mass on imaging, which is usually ultrasonography. The sensitivity of ultrasound in detecting gallbladder cancer ranges from 50% to 85%, depending on how advanced the disease is at the time of imaging. This contributes to the high percentage of cases not recognized until the time of surgery or afterwards.[66] A suspicious mass on ultrasound should prompt further preoperative work-up or referral. Contrast-enhanced CT or MRI is appropriate for assessing the extent of local disease, vascular invasion, and lymphadenopathy. PET, chest radiograph, and diagnostic laparoscopy can be used to evaluate for the presence of metastases before definitive resection. ERCP, MRCP, or percutaneous cholangiography may be employed in those patients presenting with jaundice, for diagnostic or palliative purposes. Tissue biopsy is not required before proceeding with surgical resection for suspected gallbladder cancer.

In patients who have preoperatively known or suspected gallbladder cancer, surgery should be performed by a team with the training and resources to complete an oncologic resection in the same setting. The goal of surgical treatment is complete cholecystectomy to a negative bile duct margin with en bloc removal of the involved liver parenchyma and a periportal lymphadenectomy. Establishing the diagnosis intraoperatively entails the use of frozen section. A recent review of 31 patients with gallbladder cancer who underwent frozen section analysis found that one patient had a cancer that was missed on frozen section, as it was located away from the polypoid lesion, and two patients had tumors staged as pT1b on frozen section later reported as pT2.[67] The sensitivity for frozen section was 90% (28 of 31 patients), which is similar to previous studies,[68,69] although a lower accuracy in diagnosing depth of invasion was seen in earlier studies (70% of carcinoma cases had frozen section and permanent T stage agreement).[69]

For T1a tumors (invasion of lamina propria) found either incidentally on pathology review or at the time of cholecystectomy, no further surgery is required if the gallbladder was removed intact and the cystic duct margin is negative. For T1b lesions (invasion of muscle layer) or greater, patients should be considered for hepatic resection, lymphadenectomy, and re-excision of involved bile duct, if present.[23] Although a single procedure is the ideal scenario, a review of 410 patients evaluated for gallbladder cancer at Memorial Sloan-Kettering Cancer Center did not find previous surgery to be an independent predictor of outcome (44% 5-year survival for patients treated with a single operation versus 36% for those undergoing reresection, $P = .9$).[70] The group presenting without prior surgery, however, had a higher proportion of stage 4 patients and more patients presenting with jaundice, indicating more advanced disease. Thus, one cannot conclude that a staged operation is equivalent to a single procedure. Some authors recommend the excision of prior port sites, but this remains controversial.[71]

Long-term survival for patients who have unresectable disease remains dismal, with median survival between 5 and 8 months.[70] For those patients undergoing complete curative resection, 5-year overall survival ranges from 25% to 45%.[72] Patients who had T2 tumors experienced a 5-year survival of 59%, compared with 21% for patients who had T3 tumors. Likewise, the presence of nodal metastases reduced 5-year survival from 54% to 16%.[70,73]

Because of the relative rarity of this disease and the heterogeneity of the patient population, randomized prospective data on adjuvant treatments are scarce. A single phase 3 trial from Japan compared surgery alone with surgery plus adjuvant 5-FU/mitomycin and found an improvement in 5-year survival from 14.4% to 26% ($P = .04$).[74] A cohort of 21 patients treated at the Mayo Clinic with concurrent 5-FU and external beam radiation following potentially curative resection had an overall 5-year survival of 33%, with stage 1 to 3 patients having a 65% 5-year survival compared with 0% for stage 4 patients.[75] Patients undergoing potentially curative resection of any gallbladder cancer beyond a T1, N0 tumor should be considered for adjuvant chemoradiation.

Neoadjuvant therapy has been employed in an effort to select out patients most likely to benefit from surgical therapy, and to increase the chances of a complete surgical resection.[76,77] In a phase 2 study, 18 patients who had gallbladder cancer found on pathologic review underwent 5-FU based chemoradiotherapy before definitive operation. Seventeen patients completed treatment, and 13 patients ultimately underwent resection. Seven patients were alive at a median of 34 months follow-up, and none of those patients had residual disease at the time of definitive resection.[77]

Gemcitabine has been investigated in patients with metastatic or locally advanced unresectable gallbladder cancer with promising results. Its use in the adjuvant setting is under investigation.

SUMMARY

Tumors of the pancreas and biliary tree are approached best by a multidisciplinary team, to ensure optimal diagnostic imaging studies, expeditious staging, consideration for clinical trial participation, and tailored treatment, which may involve surgery, chemotherapy or radiation therapy. Interventional radiology and gastroenterology are essential disciplines in the multidisciplinary team, for diagnostic and therapeutic procedures such as biopsies, biliary stenting (endoscopic or percutaneous), and EUS. Gemcitabine-based chemotherapy is the most promising systemic treatment available, but still results in recurrence and disease progression in most patients treated in an adjuvant or palliative setting, respectively. Clinical trial participation is extremely important, so that newer, hopefully more promising therapies may be studied and incorporated into clinical care.

REFERENCES

1. Sperti C, Pasquali C, Decet G, et al. F-18-fluorodeoxyglucose positron emission tomography in differentiating malignant from benign pancreatic cysts: a prospective study. J Gastrointest Surg 2005;9(1):22–8 [discussion: 28–9].
2. Mansour JC, Schwartz L, Pandit-Taskar N, et al. The utility of F-18 fluorodeoxyglucose whole body PET imaging for determining malignancy in cystic lesions of the pancreas. J Gastrointest Surg 2006;10(10):1354–60.
3. Lindsay MJ, Siegel BA, Tunis SR, et al. The national oncologic PET registry: expanded medicare coverage for PET under coverage with evidence development. AJR Am J Roentgenol 2007;188(4):1109–13.
4. Ahmad NA, Kochman ML, Lewis JD, et al. Can EUS alone differentiate between malignant and benign cystic lesions of the pancreas? Am J Gastroenterol 2001; 96(12):3295–300.
5. Brugge WR, Lauwers GY, Sahani D, et al. Cystic neoplasms of the pancreas. N Engl J Med 2004;351(12):1218–26.
6. Katz MH, Mortenson MM, Wang H, et al. Diagnosis and management of cystic neoplasms of the pancreas: an evidence-based approach. J Am Coll Surg 2008;207(1):106–20.
7. Aranha GV, Shoup M. Nonstandard pancreatic resections for unusual lesions. Am J Surg 2005;189(2):223–8.
8. Allen PJ, D'Angelica M, Gonen M, et al. A selective approach to the resection of cystic lesions of the pancreas: results from 539 consecutive patients. Ann Surg 2006;244(4):572–82.
9. Crippa S, Salvia R, Warshaw AL, et al. Mucinous cystic neoplasm of the pancreas is not an aggressive entity: lessons from 163 resected patients. Ann Surg 2008; 247(4):571–9.
10. Bassi C, Salvia R, Gumbs AA, et al. The value of standard serum tumor markers in differentiating mucinous from serous cystic tumors of the pancreas: CEA, Ca 19-9, Ca 125, Ca 15-3. Langenbecks Arch Surg 2002; 387(7–8):281–5.
11. Fernandez-del Castillo C, Alsfasser G, Targarona J, et al. Serum CA 19-9 in the management of cystic lesions of the pancreas. Pancreas 2006;32(2):220.
12. Ohashi K, Murakami Y. Four cases of mucin-producing cancer of the pancreas on specific findings of papilla of vater. Prog Dig Endosc 1982;20:348–51.
13. Sarr MG, Murr M, Smyrk TC, et al. Primary cystic neoplasms of the pancreas. Neoplastic disorders of emerging importance—current state-of-the-art and unanswered questions. J Gastrointest Surg 2003;7(3):417–28.
14. Tanaka M, Chari S, Adsay V, et al. International consensus guidelines for management of intraductal papillary mucinous neoplasms and mucinous cystic neoplasms of the pancreas. Pancreatology 2006;6(1–2):17–32.
15. Raut CP, Cleary KR, Staerkel GA, et al. Intraductal papillary mucinous neoplasms of the pancreas: effect of invasion and pancreatic margin status on recurrence and survival. Ann Surg Oncol 2006;13(4):582–94.
16. Sohn TA, Yeo CJ, Cameron JL, et al. Intraductal papillary mucinous neoplasms of the pancreas: an updated experience. Ann Surg 2004;239(6):788–97.

17. D'Angelica M, Brennan MF, Suriawinata AA, et al. Intraductal papillary mucinous neoplasms of the pancreas: an analysis of clinicopathologic features and outcome. Ann Surg 2004;239(3):400–8.

18. Jemal A, Siegel R, Ward E, et al. Cancer statistics, 2008. CA Cancer J Clin 2008; 58(2):71–96.

19. Bilimoria KY, Bentrem DJ, Ko CY, et al. National failure to operate on early stage pancreatic cancer. Ann Surg 2007;246(2):173–80.

20. Li D, Xie K, Wolff R, et al. Pancreatic cancer. Lancet 2004;363(9414):1049–57.

21. Bilimoria KY, Bentrem DJ, Ko CY, et al. Multimodality therapy for pancreatic cancer in the U.S.: utilization, outcomes, and the effect of hospital volume. Cancer 2007;110(6):1227–34.

22. Birkmeyer JD, Stukel TA, Siewers AE, et al. Surgeon volume and operative mortality in the United States. N Engl J Med 2003;349(22):2117–27.

23. NCCN Clinical practice guidelines in oncology. Available at: www.nccn.org. Accessed November 8, 2008.

24. Canto MI, Goggins M, Yeo CJ, et al. Screening for pancreatic neoplasia in high-risk individuals: an EUS-based approach. Clin Gastroenterol Hepatol 2004;2(7):606–21.

25. Fuhrman GM, Charnsangavej C, Abbruzzese JL, et al. Thin-section contrast-enhanced computed tomography accurately predicts the resectability of malignant pancreatic neoplasms. Am J Surg 1994;167(1):104–11.

26. Rose DM, Delbeke D, Beauchamp RD, et al. 18Fluorodeoxyglucose-positron emission tomography in the management of patients with suspected pancreatic cancer. Ann Surg 1999;229(5):729–37.

27. Nishiyama Y, Yamamoto Y, Yokoe K, et al. Contribution of whole body FDG-PET to the detection of distant metastasis in pancreatic cancer. Ann Nucl Med 2005; 19(6):491–7.

28. Borbath I, Van Beers BE, Lonneux M, et al. Preoperative assessment of pancreatic tumors using magnetic resonance imaging, endoscopic ultrasonography, positron emission tomography, and laparoscopy. Pancreatology 2005;5(6):553–61.

29. Maguchi H. The roles of endoscopic ultrasonography in the diagnosis of pancreatic tumors. J Hepatobiliary Pancreat Surg 2004;11(1):1–3.

30. Brugge WR, Lee MJ, Kelsey PB, et al. The use of EUS to diagnose malignant portal venous system invasion by pancreatic cancer. Gastrointest Endosc 1996;43(6):561–7.

31. Micames C, Jowell PS, White R, et al. Lower frequency of peritoneal carcinomatosis in patients with pancreatic cancer diagnosed by EUS-guided FNA vs. percutaneous FNA. Gastrointest Endosc 2003;58(5):690–5.

32. Povoski SP, Karpeh MS Jr, Conlon KC, et al. Preoperative biliary drainage: impact on intraoperative bile cultures and infectious morbidity and mortality after pancreaticoduodenectomy. J Gastrointest Surg 1999;3(5):496–505.

33. Pisters PW, Hudec WA, Hess KR, et al. Effect of preoperative biliary decompression on pancreaticoduodenectomy-associated morbidity in 300 consecutive patients. Ann Surg 2001;234(1):47–55.

34. Mullen JT, Lee JH, Gomez HF, et al. Pancreaticoduodenectomy after placement of endobiliary metal stents. J Gastrointest Surg 2005;9(8):1094–104.

35. Magnani JL, Nilsson B, Brockhaus M, et al. A monoclonal antibody-defined antigen associated with gastrointestinal cancer is a ganglioside containing sialylated lacto-N-fucopentaose II. J Biol Chem 1982;257(23):14365–9.

36. Lamerz R. Role of tumour markers, cytogenetics. Ann Oncol 1999;10(Suppl 4): 145–9.

37. Schlieman MG, Ho HS, Bold RJ. Utility of tumor markers in determining resectability of pancreatic cancer. Arch Surg 2003;138(9):951–5.
38. Zhang S, Wang YM, Sun CD, et al. Clinical value of serum CA19-9 levels in evaluating resectability of pancreatic carcinoma. World J Gastroenterol 2008;14(23): 3750–3.
39. Karachristos A, Scarmeas N, Hoffman JP. CA 19-9 levels predict results of staging laparoscopy in pancreatic cancer. J Gastrointest Surg 2005;9(9):1286–92.
40. Sperti C, Pasquali C, Catalini S, et al. CA 19-9 as a prognostic index after resection for pancreatic cancer. J Surg Oncol 1993;52(3):137–41.
41. Ferrone CR, Haas B, Tang L, et al. The influence of positive peritoneal cytology on survival in patients with pancreatic adenocarcinoma. J Gastrointest Surg 2006; 10(10):1347–53.
42. Martin RF, Rossi RL. Multidisciplinary considerations for patients with cancer of the pancreas or biliary tract. Surg Clin North Am 2000;80(2):709–28.
43. Burris HA 3rd, Moore MJ, Andersen J, et al. Improvements in survival and clinical benefit with gemcitabine as first-line therapy for patients with advanced pancreas cancer: a randomized trial. J Clin Oncol 1997;15(6):2403–13.
44. Shoup M, Winston C, Brennan MF, et al. Is there a role for staging laparoscopy in patients with locally advanced, unresectable pancreatic adenocarcinoma? J Gastrointest Surg 2004;8(8):1068–71.
45. Varadhachary GR, Tamm EP, Abbruzzese JL, et al. Borderline resectable pancreatic cancer: definitions, management, and role of preoperative therapy. Ann Surg Oncol 2006;13(8):1035–46.
46. Katz MH, Pisters PW, Evans DB, et al. Borderline resectable pancreatic cancer: the importance of this emerging stage of disease. J Am Coll Surg 2008;206(5): 833–46.
47. Howard TJ, Krug JE, Yu J, et al. A margin-negative R0 resection accomplished with minimal postoperative complications is the surgeon's contribution to long-term survival in pancreatic cancer. J Gastrointest Surg 2006;10(10):1338–45.
48. Sohn TA, Yeo CJ, Cameron JL, et al. Resected adenocarcinoma of the pancreas-616 patients: results, outcomes, and prognostic indicators. J Gastrointest Surg 2000;4(6):567–79.
49. Benassai G, Mastrorilli M, Quarto G, et al. Factors influencing survival after resection for ductal adenocarcinoma of the head of the pancreas. J Surg Oncol 2000; 73(4):212–8.
50. Pingpank JF, Hoffman JP, Ross EA, et al. Effect of preoperative chemoradiotherapy on surgical margin status of resected adenocarcinoma of the head of the pancreas. J Gastrointest Surg 2001;5(2):121–30.
51. Griffin JF, Smalley SR, Jewell W, et al. Patterns of failure after curative resection of pancreatic carcinoma. Cancer 1990;66(1):56–61.
52. Klinkenbijl JH, Jeekel J, Sahmoud T, et al. Adjuvant radiotherapy and 5-fluorouracil after curative resection of cancer of the pancreas and periampullary region: phase III trial of the EORTC gastrointestinal tract cancer cooperative group. Ann Surg 1999;230(6):776–82.
53. Abrams RA, Yeo CJ. Combined modality adjuvant therapy for resected periampullary pancreatic and nonpancreatic adenocarcinoma: a review of studies and experience at The Johns Hopkins Hospital, 1991–2003. Surg Oncol Clin N Am 2004;13(4):621–38, ix.
54. Regine WF, Winter KA, Abrams RA, et al. Fluorouracil vs gemcitabine chemotherapy before and after fluorouracil-based chemoradiation following resection of

pancreatic adenocarcinoma: a randomized controlled trial. JAMA 2008;299(9): 1019–26.

55. Neoptolemos JP, Stocken DD, Friess H, et al. A randomized trial of chemoradiotherapy and chemotherapy after resection of pancreatic cancer. N Engl J Med 2004;350(12):1200–10.

56. Oettle H, Post S, Neuhaus P, et al. Adjuvant chemotherapy with gemcitabine vs observation in patients undergoing curative-intent resection of pancreatic cancer: a randomized controlled trial. JAMA 2007;297(3):267–77.

57. Neuhaus P, Riess H, Post S, et al. CONKO-001: final results of the randomized, prospective multicenter phase III trial of adjuvant chemotherapy with gemcitabine versus observation in patients with resected pancreatic cancer. J Clin Oncol 2008;26(May 20 suppl) [abstract LBA4504].

58. Espat NJ, Brennan MF, Conlon KC. Patients with laparoscopically staged unresectable pancreatic adenocarcinoma do not require subsequent surgical biliary or gastric bypass. J Am Coll Surg 1999;188(6):649–55.

59. de Groen PC, Gores GJ, LaRusso NF, et al. Biliary tract cancers. N Engl J Med 1999;341(18):1368–78.

60. Weber A, von Weyhern C, Fend F, et al. Endoscopic transpapillary brush cytology and forceps biopsy in patients with hilar cholangiocarcinoma. World J Gastroenterol 2008;14(7):1097–101.

61. Ito F, Agni R, Rettammel RJ, et al. Resection of hilar cholangiocarcinoma: concomitant liver resection decreases hepatic recurrence. Ann Surg 2008;248(2): 273–9.

62. Jarnagin WR, Fong Y, DeMatteo RP, et al. Staging, resectability, and outcome in 225 patients with hilar cholangiocarcinoma. Ann Surg 2001;234(4):507–17.

63. Maibenco DC, Smith JL, Nava HR, et al. Carcinoma of the gallbladder. Cancer Invest 1998;16(1):33–9.

64. Maringhini A, Moreau JA, Melton LJ 3rd, et al. Gallstones, gallbladder cancer, and other gastrointestinal malignancies. An epidemiologic study in Rochester, Minnesota. Ann Intern Med 1987;107(1):30–5.

65. Yeh CN, Jan YY, Chao TC, et al. Laparoscopic cholecystectomy for polypoid lesions of the gallbladder: a clinicopathologic study. Surg Laparosc Endosc Percutan Tech 2001;11(3):176–81.

66. Chattopadhyay D, Lochan R, Balupuri S, et al. Outcome of gall bladder polypoidal lesions detected by transabdominal ultrasound scanning: a nine year experience. World J Gastroenterol 2005;11(14):2171–3.

67. Kwon AH, Imamura A, Kitade H, et al. Unsuspected gallbladder cancer diagnosed during or after laparoscopic cholecystectomy. J Surg Oncol 2008;97(3):241–5.

68. Azuma T, Yoshikawa T, Araida T, et al. Intraoperative evaluation of the depth of invasion of gallbladder cancer. Am J Surg 1999;178(5):381–4.

69. Yamaguchi K, Chijiiwa K, Saiki S, et al. Reliability of frozen section diagnosis of gallbladder tumor for detecting carcinoma and depth of its invasion. J Surg Oncol 1997;65(2):132–6.

70. Fong Y, Jarnagin W, Blumgart LH. Gallbladder cancer: comparison of patients presenting initially for definitive operation with those presenting after prior noncurative intervention. Ann Surg 2000;232(4):557–69.

71. Steinert R, Nestler G, Sagynaliev E, et al. Laparoscopic cholecystectomy and gallbladder cancer. J Surg Oncol 2006;93(8):682–9.

72. Miller G, Jarnagin WR. Gallbladder carcinoma. Eur J Surg Oncol 2008;34(3): 306–12.

73. Chan SY, Poon RT, Lo CM, et al. Management of carcinoma of the gallbladder: a single-institution experience in 16 years. J Surg Oncol 2008;97(2):156–64.

74. Takada T, Amano H, Yasuda H, et al. Is postoperative adjuvant chemotherapy useful for gallbladder carcinoma? A phase III multicenter prospective randomized controlled trial in patients with resected pancreaticobiliary carcinoma. Cancer 2002;95(8):1685–95.

75. Kresl JJ, Schild SE, Henning GT, et al. Adjuvant external beam radiation therapy with concurrent chemotherapy in the management of gallbladder carcinoma. Int J Radiat Oncol Biol Phys 2002;52(1):167–75.

76. Sasson AR, Hoffman JP, Ross E, et al. Trimodality therapy for advanced gallbladder cancer. Am Surg 2001;67(3):277–83.

77. de Aretxabala X, Roa I, Burgos L, et al. Preoperative chemoradiotherapy in the treatment of gallbladder cancer. Am Surg 1999;65(3):241–6.

Multidisciplinary Care for Patients with Breast Cancer

Melissa C. Hulvat, MD[a,b,c], Nora M. Hansen, MD[a,b,c],
Jacqueline S. Jeruss, MD, PhD[a,b,c],*

KEYWORDS

- Breast cancer • Chemotherapy • Staging
- Neoadjuvant therapy • Radiation therapy
- Breast cancer surgery • Breast imaging

In 2007, the American Cancer Society estimated that there would be 180,500 new cases of breast cancer and 40,900 deaths from the disease.[1] Death rates for all cancers in women peaked in 1991 and have been steadily decreasing since then, largely because of a 7.5% absolute decrease in breast cancer deaths between 1991 and 2003. Despite these impressive gains, women in the United States can anticipate a 12.7% risk of being diagnosed with breast cancer during their lifetime.[2] The public and the medical community recognize breast cancer as a critical public health issue, and the dedication of public and private funding for the study and treatment of this disease continues to increase. Funding from the National Cancer Institute alone for breast cancer research increased from $522.6 million to $584.7 million between 2002 and 2006.[3] As advances are made and the treatment of breast cancer becomes ever more sophisticated, it simultaneously becomes more complex. Increasingly, women with breast cancer are seeking their care from comprehensive breast clinics staffed by breast surgeons, medical oncologists, radiation oncologists, plastic surgeons, genetic counselors, and other specialists. This article addresses the key components of multidisciplinary breast cancer care with a special emphasis on new and emerging approaches over the past 10 years in the fields of diagnostics, surgery, radiation, medical oncology, and plastic surgery.

PREOPERATIVE EVALUATION

The first step in appropriate treatment is an assessment of the extent of disease. Local, regional, and distant sites of disease all must be assessed to formulate the

ᵃ Northwestern University Feinberg School of Medicine, Department of Surgery, Chicago, IL 60611, USA
ᵇ Lynn Sage Comprehensive Breast Center, 250 E. Superior Street, Prentice 4-420, Chicago, IL 60611, USA
ᶜ Robert H. Lurie Comprehensive Cancer Center, Chicago, IL 60611, USA
* Corresponding author. Northwestern University Feinberg School of Medicine, Department of Surgery, 250 East Superior Street, Prentice, 4-420, Chicago, IL 60611.
E-mail address: j-jeruss@northwestern.edu (J.S. Jeruss).

Surg Clin N Am 89 (2009) 133–176
doi:10.1016/j.suc.2008.10.002
0039-6109/08/$ – see front matter © 2009 Elsevier Inc. All rights reserved.

surgical.theclinics.com

best treatment plan. All assessment must begin with a thorough history obtained from the patient. Along with an understanding of their overall health status, the history must focus on well-established risk factors for breast cancer, including age, ethnicity, family history of breast or ovarian cancer, age of menarche, age at menopause, age of first full-term pregnancy, personal history of breast biopsies and their results, and personal history of cancer. Several models use these and other risk factors to determine a woman's 5-year and lifetime risk of developing breast cancer. The Gail model is the most widely known, and the National Cancer Institute Breast Cancer Risk Assessment tool (**Table 1**) is based on this model with some additional variables.[4]

After the clinician obtains a comprehensive history, a clinical breast examination must be performed. The examination is crucial for diagnosing new or unsuspected abnormalities and clinically staging known malignancies. It also offers an opportunity to reinforce proper and consistent performance of breast self-examinations with patients.

Mammography

When discussing mammography, the distinction between screening and diagnostic mammography must be made clear. Mammography for screening purposes consists of two views (mediolateral oblique and craniocaudal) of each breast performed on an annual basis starting at age 40 for women without symptoms. The preponderance of the evidence is that screening mammography decreases breast cancer mortality for women aged 40 to 74. In one recent meta-analysis, the relative risk for screened women was 0.84 (95% CI, 0.77–0.91).[5] Diagnostic mammography is performed in response to a specific breast complaint (eg, a palpable mass, nipple discharge) and may contain additional views as necessary to evaluate for potential pathology. Magnification, compression, and computerized enhancement, used in conjunction with other imaging modalities, are available to image areas of abnormality and determine if these abnormalities are likely to be benign or malignant. Ability to identify the area

Table 1
Prognosis and risk assessment tools online

Tool	Use	Web Site
Van Zee nomogram	Risk of another positive node with a positive SLN	http://www.mskcc.org/mskcc/html/15,938.cfm
Memorial Sloan Kettering nomogram	Risk of having a positive SLN	http://www.mskcc.org/mskcc/html/15,938.cfm
Jeruss nomogram	Risk of another positive node with a positive SLN in a patient who had neoadjuvant chemotherapy	http://www.mdanderson.org/postchemoSLNnomogram
Neostaging worksheet	Prognosis after completion of neoadjuvant chemotherapy	http://www.mdanderson.org/postchemotherapystaging
Gail model	5-year and lifetime risk of breast cancer	http://www.cancer.gov/bcrisktool
Adjuvant online	Help determine risk and benefits of adjuvant chemotherapy	http://www.adjuvantonline.com

of interest on mammography makes tissue retrieval for pathologic inspection possible by stereotactic biopsy.

Recently, the question of traditional analog versus digital mammography was raised. The distinction between the modalities is in the way the image is processed and stored. Analog mammograms are radiographic images captured on film, whereas digital mammograms are radiographic images that have been digitized and stored in a computerized format that allows manipulation by the interpreting radiologist. Digital images can be magnified, and the contrast can be increased or decreased to allow better distinction between pathologic features and normal breast architecture. The Digital Mammography Imaging Screening Trial found that for women in general, digital and analog mammography were of similar accuracy, but digital mammography performed significantly better in women younger than age 50, women with dense breasts, and premenopausal or perimenopausal women.[6] This result was driven by the improved sensitivity of digital mammography compared with analog mammography without a difference in specificity. Subgroup analysis of the Digital Mammography Imaging Screening Trial continues to demonstrate an advantage for digital mammography in pre- or perimenopausal women younger than age 50 who had dense breasts, and it is reasonable to recommend this technology for that group of patients.[7]

Ultrasound

Of the more than 180,000 women in the United States who will be diagnosed with breast cancer this year, an estimated 16,150 will be under the age of 45.[8] The difficulty with assessing young women with dense breasts using standard mammography has prompted many to look for another modality to assess breast complaints in this population. Breast ultrasound is performed with a hand-held transducer of 10 to 15 mHz to achieve the proper resolution without sacrificing the necessary depth of penetration in most cases. It relies on an operator using the probe to image a point of interest from either another type of breast image (mammogram, MRI) or a palpable finding. One of the main criticisms of breast ultrasound is that the quality of the resulting images is based on the skill of the technician.

In patients younger than age 30, breast ultrasound can be the modality of choice for definitive diagnosis for a clinically palpable finding.[9] To date, breast ultrasound has been used and validated as an adjunctive tool for this type of patient, but not as a screening modality. Other patients who require breast ultrasound as the first choice for imaging are pregnant patients, juvenile or adolescent patients, and patients who have breast infections. In the first two groups, the main advantage of ultrasound is the lack of ionizing radiation exposure. For evaluation of breast infections, ultrasound is preferred over mammography because the necessary compression to perform mammography would not be tolerated. Ultrasonography can more accurately describe the dimensions of any abscess or fluid collection without the distortion caused by compression.

MRI

Another technology being increasingly applied to assessment of local, regional, and metastatic disease in patients who have breast cancer is MRI. Breast MRI interpretation is based on the presence of gadolinium-containing contrast media in the breast and its rate of uptake and washout. Smooth-, round-, or oval-shaped lesions are most often benign, whereas irregular or speculated lesions raise the suspicion of malignancy. It is generally accepted that MRI can detect lesions larger than 5 mm, whereas mammography does not have optimal sensitivity until lesions are 1 cm in size. The rate of uptake of contrast corresponds to the vascularity of the lesion in comparison to that of the surrounding breast and makes synchronous lesions in the breast more readily detectable.[10] Patients with proliferative breasts or a large amount of fibrocystic changes can have increased uptake throughout their mammary tissue, which makes distinction between normal and pathologic tissue more difficult.[11] Simultaneously, the rate of washout assists in distinguishing benign from malignant disease. Benign lesions progress in signal intensity over time, whereas malignant lesions wash out earlier.[12]

Of particular interest is the ability of MRI to delineate relative contraindications for breast conservation, such as nipple or chest wall invasion, larger than anticipated size causing an suboptimal lesion-to-breast size ratio, and the existence of multicentric disease.[13] MRI has an impact on the therapeutic approach in 15% to 27% of patients with biopsy-proven cancer, which generally results in a mastectomy instead of a breast-conserving approach. The advantage of finding additional, occult malignancy preoperatively is that the surgical approach can be modified as necessary to remove all malignancy from the breast. In one retrospective study, women who underwent preoperative breast MRI for staging had a 3-year recurrence rate of 1.2%, compared with a 6.8% rate in women who did not.[14] MRI is also useful for evaluation of the contralateral breast; in one large study, MRI detected clinically and mammographically occult breast cancer in the contralateral breast in 3.1% of patients.[15]

Because of the success in using MRI as a diagnostic tool, there is much interest and debate about the use of MRI as a screening modality. Currently, MRI is being used for screening young women at high risk for developing breast cancer: individuals with a known genetic mutation (including BRCA1 and BRCA2), strong family history, and personal history of lobular carcinoma in situ. The sensitivity of mammography for young women with a higher proportion of glandular tissue is poor. For women aged 40 to 50 years, the sensitivity of mammography is only 50% to 80% compared with 70% to 90% in woman older than 50.[16] Women with lobular carcinoma in situ develop invasive lobular carcinoma and invasive ductal carcinoma with the same incidence, but the sensitivity of mammography to detect invasive lobular carcinoma is lower than that for invasive ductal carcinoma.[17] Thus far, high-risk women have demonstrated the greatest screening benefit from MRI. A large study in 2004 examined the sensitivity of MRI in women with increased lifetime risk of breast cancer and women who were known BRCA1 and BRCA2 carriers. This work demonstrated a sensitivity rate of 40% for mammography and 71% for MRI to detect the presence of breast cancer.[18] The results of this study were confirmed by another group in 2005, which demonstrated a sensitivity rate of 40% for mammography and 77% for MRI, with the greatest benefit seen in the gene carrier group. Of note, the combined sensitivity of both modalities was 94%.[19] For BRCA1 and BRCA2 carriers specifically, the advantages of MRI for screening are even greater. For BRCA1 mutation carriers, adding MRI increases the sensitivity rate of annual screening from 35% to 85%, the proportion of axillary lymph-node negative cancers from 57% to 81%, and the false-positive rate from approximately 5% to only 25%. Overdiagnosis of invasive cancer is negligible. Outcomes for BRCA2 mutation carriers are similar.[20]

The benefits of increased detection with MRI must be weighed against the real risks of this procedure, however. The risks of harm associated with MRI include an increased cost (15 times the cost of a mammogram), anxiety caused by detection of small lesions of indeterminate importance, and the necessary recommendation for short-term follow-up studies and an increase in biopsies—many of which indicate that lesions are benign.

The most recent guidelines published by the American Cancer Society in March 2007 recommended MRI screening in addition to mammograms starting at the age of 30 for women who meet at least one of the following conditions: BRCA1 or

BRCA2 mutation; first-degree relative with a BRCA1 or BRCA2 mutation, even if they have yet to be tested themselves; lifetime risk of breast cancer of 20% to 25%; radiation to the chest between the ages of 10 and 30 years; or a diagnosis of Li-Fraumeni syndrome, Cowden syndrome, or Bannayan-Riley-Ruvalcaba syndrome.[21]

Positron Emission Tomography

Use of positron emission tomography (PET) scans with the glucose analog 2-[18F]fluoro-2-deoxy-D-glucose (FDG) is increasing for the staging of many types of human cancers, including breast cancer. The technique consists of determining a patient's baseline glucose level, injecting with FDG, and then scanning the body to determine the sites and intensity of uptake, which indicates glucose metabolism in these areas. Peak standardized uptake values are evaluated to determine the quantity of uptake of FDG in areas of interest. In theory, increased uptake of FDG indicates increased metabolism and a more aggressive tumor with a worse prognosis.[22]

Current reports of the sensitivity of whole-body PET for detecting primary breast tumors have been mixed. For large tumors, PET is up to 88% accurate and can provide additional information about the standardized uptake values intensity of a lesion.[23] For lesions smaller than 1 cm, the data are less encouraging. In the best of circumstances, the sensitivity of PET for these small tumors is 57%.[24,25] To overcome the limitations of whole-body PET in the detection of primary breast tumors, positron emission mammography was developed. This technology takes advantage of two planar FDG receptors used in conjunction with a conventional mammography system. The mammogram and FDG images are coregistered and read as a single image. The early data on these systems (between 2000 and 2006) revealed a sensitivity rate for detecting breast tumors of 50% to 90% and a specificity rate of 33% to 100%.[26] In the largest multi-institutional study to date on this technology by Tafra and colleagues,[27] positron emission mammography was useful in identifying extensive presence of ductal carcinoma in situ (DCIS) and was able to predict 75% of patients who would have failed breast conservation therapy (BCT) based on the extent of DCIS. If further studies validate the ability of positron emission mammography to reliably visualize DCIS, it could reduce the need for re-excisions after inadequate primary surgeries and would prove to be a valuable tool for preoperative assessment of the primary tumor.

PET scans also can be useful for determining the extent of locoregional disease in patients who have breast cancer. The use of PET to stage the axilla was evaluated in a prospective, multi-institutional trial by Wahl and colleagues.[28] PET with a threshold standardized uptake value of 1.8 yielded a 61% sensitivity and 80% specificity rate for detecting axillary metastasis in the 360 patients evaluated. This finding corresponded to a positive predictive value of only 62% and led the authors to recommend against PET for routine axillary staging. There is some evidence that uptake in the axilla of a higher standardized uptake value (2.3) can predict nodal positivity, but larger studies are needed before any definitive recommendations can be made.[29] Despite some promising developments, there is no current consensus that PET can replace other accepted modalities for axillary staging.[30]

Because of the low likelihood of metastatic disease in women with stage 1 breast cancer, no routine metastatic evaluation is recommended. In patients with stages 2 and 3 disease, further evaluation with a bone scan and CT are generally performed. PET scanning is useful for the assessment of patients with known stage 4 disease and patients with known or suspected recurrence. Recently, combined PET and CT systems (PET/CT) were applied to this specific situation. The CT portion of the study provided anatomic mapping of the PET images and, when merged, it produced high-quality fused images of activity and anatomy in the areas of interest.[31] PET/CT is particularly helpful in restaging cases of locally recurrent disease to confirm lack of unsuspected regional or distant sites of recurrence, because it may change patient management.[32] In a study of asymptomatic cancer patients with increasing tumor marker levels, PET/CT was 90% sensitive for diagnosing recurrence.[33] PET/CT also can be used to evaluate response to neoadjuvant chemotherapy. Initial data showed that the decrease in FDG uptake on PET/CT after the first course of neoadjuvant chemotherapy was significantly greater in patients who had a complete pathologic response than patients who did not.[34] This kind of early prognostic information on tumor response to therapy can be important in guiding the choice of future therapeutic strategies.

SURGERY
Lumpectomy

Multiple randomized trials with over a decade of follow-up have proved that BCT followed by radiation therapy is equally efficacious as mastectomy for treating breast cancer. Because the survival rate is equivalent, BCT has become the standard of care for women without contraindications to this approach.[35,36] BCT, as we refer to it in this article, goes by many different names, including lumpectomy, quadrantectomy, and segmental mastectomy. Regardless of the name, the principle is to remove the tumor with surrounding margins of negative breast tissue and preserve the breast with acceptable cosmesis for the patient.

Twenty-year data are available for National Surgical Adjuvant Breast and Bowel Project (NSABP) B-06, the landmark trial proving the equivalence of BCT to modified radical mastectomy in women with operative primary breast cancer. Between 1976 and 1984, more than 2000 women were randomized to receive modified radical mastectomy versus lumpectomy, axillary dissection and breast radiotherapy versus lumpectomy and axillary dissection. No significant differences were observed with respect to disease-free (DF) survival, distant DF survival, or overall survival (OS). The hazard ratio for death between the lumpectomy and axillary dissection alone and modified radical mastectomy groups was 1.05 (95% CI, 0.90–1.23; $P = .51$). The hazard ratio for death between the lumpectomy, axillary dissection and radiation group and the lumpectomy and axillary dissection alone group was 0.97 (95% CI, 0.83–1.14; $P = .74$). This finding supports equivalent survival with modified radical mastectomy and BCT.

Further, the data continue to support improved local control with the addition of breast radiotherapy to lumpectomy and control of the axilla. The incidence of recurrence in the same breast was 14.3% in women who underwent lumpectomy and breast radiotherapy, compared with 39.2% in women who underwent lumpectomy without irradiation ($P < .001$).[36] It must be noted that inherent to this concept of local control is adequate surgical resection to negative margins. In 30 of 34 studies on the topic of local recurrence after BCT, a persistent positive margin significantly increased the chance of a local recurrence regardless of any postsurgical adjuvant therapy.[37]

Recent studies show that achieving local control through adequate surgery and the inclusion of radiotherapy for all patients with an invasive cancer treated with less than a mastectomy not only decreases locoregional recurrence but also positively impacts survival. The Early Breast Cancer Trialists' Collaborative Group conducted a meta-analysis of 78 trials comparing more versus less surgery, radiotherapy versus no radiotherapy, and more surgery versus radiation. The analysis showed that avoidance of local recurrence in the conserved breast and avoidance of regional recurrence were of comparable relevance to the 15-year breast cancer mortality rate. Adequate local control avoided one breast cancer death over the 15-year period for every four local recurrences avoided, which reduced overall mortality.[38] Wapnir and colleagues[39] pooled data for node-positive women participating in five NSABP protocols (B-15, B-16, B-18, B-22, and B-25) to examine the effect of locoregional failure after BCT on the risk of distant disease and mortality. They found a hazard ratio for mortality associated with in-breast recurrence of 2.58 (95% CI, 2.11–3.15) and other local failure of 5.85 (95% CI, 4.80–7.13).

Mastectomy

Mastectomy is a procedure currently performed in two different subsets of women. It is an appropriate oncologic surgery for women with established breast cancers who are not candidates for BCT or who do not wish to undergo BCT. There is also a growing population of women who are identified as high risk for subsequent development of breast cancer because of more sophisticated methods of genetic testing. These women have no identified cancer but may seek prophylactic mastectomy as a means to modify their risk. These two groups are addressed separately.

Mastectomy for breast cancer

Approximately two thirds of women newly diagnosed with breast cancer are candidates for BCT. Absolute contraindications to BCT include inflammatory breast cancer, multicentric disease, and contraindications to radiotherapy, including previous mantle radiation and pregnancy. BCT is relatively contraindicated for tumors that comprise more than 20% to 25% of total breast volume. Some women who are candidates for BCT choose instead to have a mastectomy. Reasons include the greater peace of mind some women derive from having no breast tissue remaining after living through the diagnosis of a breast cancer. Some women do not want to participate in postoperative radiotherapy or do not have access to this treatment. Other women may opt for a mastectomy with immediate reconstruction, with or without a contralateral breast procedure, because of the possible cosmetic advantage. The modern mastectomy, in contrast to the Halstedian approach, seeks to leave as much of the normal architecture as possible while removing all the mammary tissue. The standard simple mastectomy excises the breast and skin envelope and leaves the pectoralis in place. The treatment of the axilla is discussed in a later section. The safety of the simple mastectomy in comparison to more radical approaches has been established over the past 25 years by several trials, including the landmark NSABP B-04 trial.[40] More recent advances in the performance of the simple mastectomy include the skin-sparing mastectomy (SSM), nipple-sparing mastectomy (NSM), and areola-sparing mastectomy.

The goal of the SSM is to remove all the mammary tissue, the nipple-areolar complex (NAC) and any biopsy scar and leave behind the breast skin envelope for reconstruction with either an implant or autologous tissue.[41] The primary concern with this procedure is ensuring comparable oncologic safety and equivalent rates of local recurrence non–skin-sparing mastectomy (NSSM), which has been addressed in multiple studies.[42] There is some debate over how often the skin is involved in patients with breast cancer. Two classic studies on this issue by Fisher and Wertheim[43,44] found rates of non-NAC skin involvement of 4.4% and 11.3%, respectively. In the most recent study on this topic by Ho and colleagues,[45] the rate of skin involvement outside of the NAC on serial sectioning of NSSM specimens was reported as 20%. In this study, skin involvement was clinically evident in half of the patients found to have pathologic involvement; the remaining half had T3 tumors. There is consensus that patients with clinically involved skin, including patients with inflammatory breast cancer, are not candidates for SSM. Based on these findings, care also should be taken when offering this procedure to women with large tumors.

The most important factor to consider when evaluating the oncologic safety of SSM is whether the procedure carries a higher risk of local recurrence than NSSM. Numerous studies have evaluated this issue. Chagpar[42] compiled a list of studies, and among the studies that compared SSM with control groups of NSSM, there was no significant difference in local recurrence.[46–51] The rate of local recurrence in these studies ranged from 3.2% to 9.5% in the NSSM group and 3.9% to 7.0% in the SSM group. In a further study by Carlson and colleagues[52] that compared the incidence of local recurrence to tumor size, T1, T2, and T3 lesions had recurrence rates of 3%, 10%, and 11%, respectively. An additional consideration for women with large T3 lesions who would not be ideal candidates for SSM is the use of neoadjuvant chemotherapy. With a good response, the tumor could shrink enough to facilitate performance of SSM in a breast that may otherwise have required NSSM.[53] Based on the available data, SSM seems to be equivalent to NSSM for prevention of local recurrence after mastectomy in properly selected patients.

With the success of SSM as an oncologically safe and cosmetically appealing approach to mastectomy, clinicians have taken it one step further and begun to argue that the NAC also might be preserved safely in selected patients. As with SSM, the most important question to ask when considering the option of NSM is whether it is oncologically safe. The nipple contains ductal tissue, and there is concern that preserving the NAC can leave behind tissue in which a new cancer can develop and/or leave behind tumor cells from the primary cancer. The risk of nipple involvement by direct extension of the primary tumor has been evaluated in numerous studies and has been reported as anywhere between 0% and 58%.[54]

In one study in which the NAC of mastectomy specimens were serially sectioned and examined, Laronga and colleagues[55] reported an incidence of NAC involvement by tumor of 5.6%. The only significant differences between the involved and uninvolved groups were a central location of the tumor and axillary nodal involvement. If these groups were excluded from analysis, the likelihood of NAC involvement with a node-negative peripheral tumor was only 2%. Numerous surgical incisions are described that can spare the NAC, including the "inverted teaspoon" incision over the top half of the NAC and with a lateral extension; a transareolar incision that is either transnipple or perinipple with lateral and medial extension; some variety of inframammary crease incision; and a mastopexy incision. The treatment of the actual nipple differs greatly among surgeons performing this procedure. Some surgeons evert the nipple and excise the ducts within, whereas some leave a small button of tissue under the nipple to preserve protrusion and lessen the chance of necrosis.[56]

At the European Institute of Oncology, Petit and colleagues[57] described leaving a 5-mm layer of retroareolar tissue after assessing for tumor involvement by frozen section then applying 16 Gy of intraoperative radiotherapy via their ELIOT delivery system to the remaining NAC. There is currently an inadequate level of data to recommend for or against NSM as an oncologically safe option for women with established breast cancers. Selection criteria have yet to be defined, and the follow-up period in trials assessing this technique is still too short. Even when potential candidates are limited to women with T1 lesions located 4 cm or more away from the NAC and without axillary involvement, frozen section analysis of the retroareolar tissue still precludes NSM in 16% to 46% of patients.[58,59] Currently, it seems that the subset of women with established malignancy who are appropriate candidates for NSM is small and ill-defined. More studies with longer follow-up periods are needed before this technique can be endorsed definitively.

A modification of NSM recently being explored is areola-sparing mastectomy. The assumption made with this method is that the areola is not different from the remainder of the breast skin and that all significant glandular tissue resides in the breast parenchyma and nipple proper. Simmons and colleagues[60] reported a less than 1% involvement of the areola in mastectomy specimens and noted that all tumors that involved the areola were located directly beneath it. Others have argued that the areola is not only pigmented skin with sebaceous elements but also contains ductal structures, such as the glands of Montgomery, that can connect to the underlying breast lobular units.[61] The largest experience with this technique was described by Simmons and colleagues,[62] whose study included 15 women undergoing 17 areola-sparing mastectomies and a 2-year follow-up. Patients were selected according to criteria similar to those used by others for NSM, and they reported no recurrences to date. Although no definitive recommendations regarding the oncologic safety of areola-sparing mastectomy can be made on the basis of these data, it does represent another intriguing avenue for ongoing research.

Prophylactic mastectomy

Any of the aforementioned approaches to mastectomy for cancer patients can be applied to prophylactic mastectomy in high-risk women. Individuals who are most likely to derive benefit from prophylactic surgery are women who are carriers of either BRCA1 or BRCA2 mutations.[63] According to estimates of lifetime risk, approximately 12.7% of women in the general population will develop breast cancer, compared with estimates of 36% to 85% of women with BRCA1 or BRCA2 genetic alterations.[64] Another group of women who may benefit from prophylactic mastectomy are individuals with a personal history of breast cancer. Follow-up studies of women with early-stage cancer in one breast show a cumulative risk of cancer in the contralateral breast of 17% at 20 years after diagnosis and up to 35% at 16 years in women with a strong family history.[65–67] These women may benefit from contralateral prophylactic mastectomy.

Bilateral prophylactic mastectomy for BRCA1 and BRCA2 carriers should intuitively offer a benefit. The Prevention and Observation of Surgical Endpoints study demonstrated a relative risk reduction for breast cancer of 95% in patients also undergoing prophylactic oophorectomy and 90% for women with intact ovaries, which is in line with previous observations on this subject.[68] Prophylactic mastectomy does not reduce this risk to zero, and no prospective clinical evidence proves an OS benefit. Theoretic modeling that takes into account the early age at diagnosis for breast cancer in BRCA1 and BRCA2 carriers predicts a 3.5-year survival advantage for genetic carriers who opt for bilateral prophylactic mastectomy, but actual data are needed to substantiate these claims.[69] Contralateral prophylactic mastectomy in BRCA1 and BRCA2 carriers who have already experienced an initial event has been shown to reduce the risk of a contralateral cancer by up to 97%.[70,71] As with bilateral prophylactic mastectomy, despite this impressive reduction in local events, an absolute survival benefit is still unproven for contralateral surgical prophylaxis.[63] Surgical technique for mastectomy in high-risk patients should follow the same general rules as in other patients who have breast cancer. Of paramount concern is removing all mammary tissue and providing the lowest risk for recurrence, which must be balanced with providing the optimal cosmetic outcome for these patients, who are often young women. It should be noted that the term "subcutaneous mastectomy" is historical and does not describe any of the currently advocated approaches to mastectomy.

Surgical prophylaxis must be considered along with other options for prevention, including surveillance and chemoprevention.[72] Clinical trials of tamoxifen given to women with an index estrogen receptor–positive breast cancer demonstrate a risk reduction of 50% for the contralateral breast. The same magnitude of risk reduction seems to apply to *BRCA1* and *BRCA2* carriers, with the risk of a contralateral event reduced by 30% to 40% with tamoxifen.[73] Breast MRI with an annual mammogram alternating at 6-month intervals provides additional screening for mutation carriers, and most experts agree that an annual MRI for these patients is appropriate.[72] As with surgical prophylaxis, more data are needed regarding chemoprevention and screening to decide which approach will yield the greatest benefit with the fewest adverse effects for this unique subset of women.

Staging and Treatment of the Axilla: Sentinel Lymph Node Biopsy and Axillary Dissection

The next step in the staging of breast cancer, after staging of the primary tumor, is determination of the axillary nodal status (**Table 2**). Lymph node metastases are the most significant prognostic indicator for patients who have breast cancer. Based on several trials and according to the American Society of Breast Surgeons, sentinel lymph node biopsy (SLNB) is the preferred method of axillary staging for patients with T1-3 invasive breast cancers that are clinically node negative, including multifocal/multicentric disease and prior breast surgery (**Table 3**).[74] Because approximately two thirds of patients are predicted to have a negative SLN result, these women can be spared an axillary dissection. Although SLNB still carries a risk of side effects, compared with axillary dissection, postoperative arm pain is decreased 3.2-fold, lymphedema is decreased 5-fold, and diminished arm strength is decreased 7.1-fold.[75] When performed correctly, SLNB is expected to have an identification rate of 95% and a false-negative result rate of 5% to 10%, as verified by complete axillary dissection.[76] The following discussion addresses the evolving roles of axillary dissection and SLNB in the treatment of patients who have breast cancer and the current controversies, including a discussion of therapy for isolated tumor cells (ITCs) N0(I+) and micrometastases N1(mi) and the use of SLNB in the setting of neoadjuvant chemotherapy.

The largest randomized trial to date evaluating treatment of the axilla in women with clinically node-negative breast cancers is the NSABP B-32 trial.[77] A total of 5611 women were randomized to either SLNB followed by axillary dissection or SLNB, with axillary dissection indicated only if the SLNB result was positive. Krag and colleagues[77] reported an identification rate of 97.2%, an accuracy rate of 97.1%,

Table 2	
Prognosis according to stage of breast cancer at diagnosis	
Stage	**5-Year Disease-Specific Survival Rate (%)**
0	100
I	100
IIa	92
IIb	81
IIIa	67
IIIb	35
IIIc	54
IV	20

Data from American College of Surgeons, Commission on Cancer: National Cancer Data Base. Available at: http://www.facs.org/cancer/ncdb/.

Table 3
Axillary recurrence after negative sentinel lymph node biopsy without axillary dissection

Study	Follow-up (mo)	# SLN-Negative Patients	# Recurrences (%)
Smidt[236]	26	401	2 (0.5)
Blanchard[228]	28	685	1 (0.1)
Chung[229]	26	208	3 (1.4)
Reisamer[233]	22	116	0
Schrenk[235]	22	83	0
Roumen[234]	24	100	1 (1.0)
Guiliano[230]	39	67	0
Jeruss[90]	28	611	2 (0.32)
Heuts[231]	43	344	3 (0.9)
Badgwell[227]	32	159	1 (0.6)
Palesty[232]	33	335	2 (0.6)

and a false-negative rate of 9.8%. These results were in line with previous findings, and some important caveats were identified. A nearly 20-fold variation in false-positive results was observed over a range of one to five SLNs removed, which led to the recommendation that all efforts should be made to remove several SLNs instead of only a single specimen. Previous excisional biopsies also doubled the false-negative rate, suggesting that clinicians must be aware that some alteration of the lymphatic drainage of the breast does occur in patients who have undergone reoperation. The data from the B-32 trial is not yet mature for analysis of differences in regional recurrence, OS, or DFS between the two groups.

The definition of a positive SLN has several caveats. The most recent American Joint Commission on Cancer staging manual (2002) and the International Union Against Cancer classified SLN metastases measuring 0.2 mm or smaller as ITCs and designated them pN0(i+).[78,79] SLN metastases between 0.2 mm and 2 mm are designated N1(mi) and are referred to as micrometastases. Metastatic deposits larger than 2 mm are N1 macrometastases. These distinctions have important ramifications for identification and treatment. The three standard methods of immediate, intraoperative identification of SLN metastasis are intraoperative frozen section, touch preparation, and cytologic smear. Overall, these methods have similar sensitivities (59% FS, 57% touch preparation, 59% cytologic smear), but each method was significantly better at detecting macrometastases (96% FS, 93% touch preparation, 93% cytologic smear) than micrometastases (27% FS, 27% touch preparation, 30% cytologic smear).[80] If a positive SLN is identified intraoperatively, standard of care is to perform an axillary dissection. In the case of a positive SLN identified at final pathology, the decision-making path is more complex and the standard of care continues to be debated. It is important to note that in approximately 60% of patients, tumor-positive SLNs are the only positive nodes and the risk of further non-SLN involvement increases with the size of the SLN metastasis.[81]

Of all positive SLNs, 40% are either ITCs or micrometastases.[82] It is imperative to understand the rationale for various treatment options for women with small-volume nodal disease. ITCs (SLN metastases measuring ≤ 0.2 mm) are designated N0(i+), and the recommendation for N0 disease is against complete axillary dissection. This designation is partly because of the unknown nature of ITCs. It is uncertain whether these ITCs are morphologically similar to true tumor cells or are artifacts or normal cells caught in transfer. Further questions about ITCs have to do with the reproducibility of this designation between independent pathologists and methods of histopathologic evaluation. ITCs identified on hematoxylin and eosin staining may have more prognostic significance than those seen by immunohistochemistry.[83] If an ITC is the only finding on SLNB, the risk of having another positive node on completion of axillary dissection is approximately 12%. This risk is compared with an 18% to 22% risk of additional positive nodes for micrometastases on SLNB and a 45% to 79% risk with macrometastatic disease.[76,84] Finding an ITC only in the SLN should not be an indication for further treatment of the axilla by either surgery or radiotherapy without another poor prognostic indicator, such as extensive invasive lobular component or lymphovascular invasion.

Micrometastatic disease (SLN metastases between 0.2 mm and 2 mm) is designated as N1(mi), node positive. For all N1 disease, the standard of care is a complete axillary dissection, but application of this standard to micrometastasis recently was called into question. The actual impact of micrometastasis on local or distant recurrence and on OS has not been well defined and is a subject of great interest that ultimately may impact therapy. Hansen and colleagues[85] prospectively examined the clinical impact of micrometastases in the SLNs of their patients at the John Wayne Cancer Institute with invasive breast cancer treated between 1992 and 1999. In this analysis, patients with micrometastatic tumor deposits, pN0 (i+) or pN1(mi) did not seem to have a worse 8-year DFS or OS compared with SLN-negative patients. As expected, there was a significant decrease in 8-year DFS and OS in patients with macrometastatic pN1 disease in the SLN.

This same issue was addressed by Chen and colleagues[86] using data from the Surveillance Epidemiology and End Results (SEER) database to evaluate the impact of N1(mi) disease in patients diagnosed with invasive breast cancer between 1992 and 2003, a time period over which the use of SLNB increased. The incidence of N1(mi) disease detection increased over this time period from 2.3% to 7% among 209,720 patients. On multivariate analysis, the presence of micrometastases in lymph nodes remained a significant prognostic indicator. Patients with micrometastases had a prognosis between N0(i-) and N1 disease even after adjusting for tumor and patient-related factors. This study, however, was limited by the use of a large retrospective database with no information as to the surgical technique or how the lymph nodes were evaluated. The heterogeneity of pathologic techniques and the experience of the pathologist may have led to some micrometastases being missed or overdiagnosed. The inability to determine which patients received adjuvant systemic therapy in this cohort also may have masked the true impact of the micrometastases. The question of whether women with N1(mi)-only disease must undergo complete axillary dissection is as yet unanswered.

American College of Surgeons Oncology Group Z0011 was a study designed to compare survival with SLNB without axillary dissection versus SLNB followed by axillary dissection in women with any positive SLN.[87] Unfortunately, this trial was closed prematurely because of slow accrual. We must continue to rely on smaller retrospective studies to address the question of whether axillary dissection can be omitted for certain women with a positive SLN, either N1(mi) or N1 (**Table 4**). The preponderance of the available evidence suggests that for women with small volume metastasis on SLNB who decline axillary dissection, the risk of an axillary recurrence is between 0 and 1.4%.[88–91] The number of patients evaluated in these studies with a positive SLNB result without axillary dissection was between 31 and 210. These studies were limited in their impact by short follow-up times (all ≤ 31 months). A possible confounding factor in these analyses was the use of either chemotherapy or axillary radiation as adjuvant therapy. More than 60% of patients in the cohort analyzed by Hwang

Table 4
Axillary recurrence after positive sentinel lymph node biopsy without axillary dissection

Study	Follow-up (mo)	# SLN-Positive Patients	# Recurrences
Jeruss[90]	28	73	0
Hwang[89]	29.5	196	0
Fant[88]	30	31	0
Naik[91]	46	210	3 (1.4%)

and colleagues[89] received some type of adjuvant therapy; the effect this may have on eliminating residual disease in the axilla is unknown. The use of axillary radiotherapy in place of axillary dissection is also unresolved. The European Organization for Research and Treatment of Cancer 10981 trial is currently enrolling patients to compare outcomes between axillary radiotherapy and axillary dissection with respect to local control and survival.

When deciding whether a patient will undergo complete axillary dissection after the identification of a positive SLN, an assessment of the risk of additional axillary metastasis can aid in the final decision-making process. The Van Zee/Memorial Sloan Kettering nomogram (see **Table 1**) uses patient, primary tumor, and SLNB information to estimate the risk for node positivity.[92,93] If the likelihood of an additional positive axillary node is low, an informed decision may be discussed to forgo axillary dissection if the calculated risk is acceptable to the patient and her oncology team.

The Van Zee nomogram is intended for women in whom surgical treatment is performed before any radiation or systemic therapy is administered, and the results may not be appropriately extrapolated to women who have received neoadjuvant systemic therapy.[94] For patients with clinically negative axillary nodes who have been treated with neoadjuvant chemotherapy before surgery, SLNB is also thought to be appropriate.[95] Jeruss and associates[96] at the MD Anderson Cancer Center developed a nomogram (see **Table 1**) for women treated in the neoadjuvant setting to predict the risk of harboring additional positive axillary lymph nodes. The Jeruss nomogram inputs five patient, primary tumor, and SLN variables to output the risk of an additional positive axillary lymph node. These five predictive variables are the presence of lymphovascular invasion, the method of SLN metastatic detection (hematoxylin and eosin vs immunohistochemistry), multicentric disease, presence of disease in a lymph node before systemic therapy, and pathologic tumor size. This nomogram was validated at the University of Michigan and provides a useful tool for counseling and decision making in this group of patients for whom the Van Zee nomogram may not accurately assess risk.

The following questions are important to ask when deciding whether an axillary dissection is warranted in an individual patient: What is the value is the information that will be obtained? Is there any potential benefit to the procedure itself? The current American Joint Commission on Cancer staging system for breast cancer does use the number of positive lymph nodes to define the categories of N1, N2, and N3, to establish the pathologic stage of the patient.[97] If finding additional positive lymph nodes and upstaging the patient potentially affect the adjuvant therapy regimen, such as the delivery or omission of chest wall radiotherapy for more than four positive nodes, then the risks of an axillary dissection may be justified. On the other hand, if the patient is likely to receive adjuvant treatments on the basis of her current diagnosis alone, identifying additional positive lymph nodes would expose her to the risks of the procedure with no change in her treatment plan. The second question, which asks whether clearance of all detectable regional disease confers an inherent survival benefit, is as yet unanswered. It seems intuitive that untreated nodal disease would act as a source of cells for distant metastasis and would worsen prognosis.[98] Some evidence indicates that clearance of the axilla can influence survival and locoregional control.[99] In one meta-analysis of randomized trials, a 5.4% survival benefit was associated with clearance of the axilla for clinically node-negative patients.[100] Others argue that the benefit of complete axillary dissection performed after positive SLNB is minimal.[101] Currently, the standard of care is complete axillary dissection for N1(mi) and N1 disease found by SLNB. Modification of this standard may be forthcoming, and as more mature data become available, the surgical treatment of the axilla may follow the trend seen in the surgical treatment of the breast: toward a more minimal approach for selected women.

Surgery on the Primary Tumor in Patients with Metastatic Disease

Identification of stage IV metastatic disease before performing surgery generally changes the extent, timing, and type of treatments offered to patients. The current recommendation regarding primary treatment modality for patients with metastatic breast cancer at the time of diagnosis is systemic therapy with surgical treatment of the primary tumor reserved for palliation of local symptoms. More recently, data emerged suggesting that resection of the primary breast tumor can prolong survival for women with stage IV disease.[102] This benefit seems to apply only to primary tumors that can be completely excised, because survival for women with positive margins of resection was equivalent to the group with no resection at all. Additional studies have supported this finding for either an OS advantage or a progression-free survival advantage.[103–105] All of these trials used review of National Cancer database records, SEER data, or retrospective review of institutional data. It is likely that significant bias exists regarding which patients were offered surgery, and further prospective randomized trials are needed in this area. Identifying metastatic disease before any intervention is important when contemplating a possible surgical plan, and all decisions regarding the care of patients who have stage IV breast cancer are best made by a multidisciplinary team on a case-by-case basis.

RADIATION THERAPY
Whole-Breast Radiotherapy

As mentioned in the previous discussion on BCT, a meta-analysis from the Early Breast Cancer Trialists' Collaborative Group in 2005 found that adequate locoregional control and a prevention of recurrence within the first 5 years after treatment translated into an absolute survival benefit.[38] For women opting for breast conservation, adequate local control is achieved with a combination of lumpectomy with negative margins and local radiotherapy. The standard method of delivering this radiation is via whole-breast radiation.

Two NSABP trials designed to assess the effect of whole-breast radiotherapy on outcomes for women treated with lumpectomy were NSABP B-06 and NSABP B-21. NSABP B-06 compared modified radical mastectomy to lumpectomy with axillary lymph node dissection with and without radiotherapy for women with tumors smaller than 4 cm. Among the findings was a difference between the lumpectomy groups with regard to in-breast recurrence. The lumpectomy-alone group experienced a 39.2% recurrence rate, whereas the lumpectomy plus radiation group had an in-breast recurrence rate of 14.3%.[106] The NSABP B-21 trial investigated whether women with node-negative invasive tumors smaller than 1 cm could avoid radiotherapy. Included were estrogen receptor–positive and –negative tumors. The cumulative incidence of in-breast recurrence was 16.5% with lumpectomy plus tamoxifen, 9.3%

with lumpectomy and radiation, and 2.8% with lumpectomy, radiation, and tamoxifen. Even in patients with favorable tumors, whole-breast radiation provided additional benefit in achieving local control.[107] Despite the advantages of whole-breast radiotherapy, it is not without its drawbacks. Whole-breast radiotherapy is typically administered 5 days per week for 6 to 7 consecutive weeks to a total of 50 Gy. This treatment course poses difficulty for some patients who find it difficult to comply with this plan because of mobility issues or travel concerns. In response to this concern, multiple ongoing investigations are determining which patients can have radiotherapy safely omitted from their treatment plans. Trials are currently examining alternative modalities to replace whole-breast radiotherapy and provide equivalent outcomes in less time for women who require this treatment.

In recent years, several trials have been designed to identify subsets of patients with early-stage breast cancer who could avoid radiation therapy after lumpectomy.[108] The Cancer and Leukemia Group B trial prospectively studied women aged 70 years and older with favorable tumors (< 2 cm, clinically lymph node-negative, hormone receptor-positive) who had lumpectomy for treatment of their primary tumors. In Cancer and Leukemia Group B 9343, they randomized these women to tamoxifen alone and tamoxifen with whole-breast radiotherapy. The addition of radiation did significantly lower the incidence of in-breast recurrence from 4% to 1%, but the absolute number of recurrences in both groups was low and there was no difference in OS.[109]

Another analysis with the same inclusion criteria was performed for women registered in the SEER database. Smith and colleagues[110] demonstrated a decreased risk of a second breast cancer event in the group treated with radiation therapy at 8 years (2.3% versus 8% in the no-radiotherapy group). In a further subgroup analysis, the authors found that radiation therapy was most likely to benefit patients aged 70 to 79 without comorbidities and was least likely to benefit patients aged 80 years or older with moderate to severe comorbidity. The suggestion of these trials—and others—is that radiotherapy lowers the risk of a second cancer event in the irradiated breast in all women, but the magnitude of this risk reduction differs according to patient and tumor characteristics. In some older women, a small increase in risk of recurrence may be acceptable if it avoids committing the patient to mastectomy because of inability or unwillingness to undergo radiotherapy, but this decision must be individualized and undertaken with caution. It seems most productive to continue to investigate modes of delivering adequate radiotherapy in less time and with less inconvenience to patients so that all women can derive the full benefit of this treatment modality.

Partial-Breast Irradiation

The biologic rationale for accelerated partial-breast irradiation (APBI) stems from the observation that most in-breast recurrences are found within the region of the previous lumpectomy site. More distant in-breast recurrences are much rarer, occurring only 3% of the time.[111–113] These findings have been consistent, despite the use of whole-breast radiotherapy, which that whole-breast irradiation may be overtreatment of the disease.[111] A major advantage of APBI lies in the shortened treatment time of 4 to 5 days as opposed to 5 to 6 weeks.[114] Thus far, techniques for delivering partial-breast irradiation include conformal external-beam radiotherapy, interstitial brachytherapy, balloon catheter-based brachytherapy, and high-dose intraoperative radiotherapy (**Box 1**).[115]

Three-dimensional conformal radiation therapy or intensity-modulated radiotherapy is a total external delivery system for APBI. This modality uses three-dimensional computer-based planning equipment to target the photon field directly at the lumpectomy cavity plus a 1- to 2-cm margin. The advantage is greater dose homogeneity in

> **Box 1**
> **Partial breast radiation modalities**
>
> Multicatheter interstitial brachytherapy
>
> MammoSite balloon catheter brachtherapy
>
> Three-dimensional conformal external-beam radiotherapy
>
> Intraoperative radiotherapy

the target field and less irradiation to surrounding breast and normal structures.[116] The Radiation Therapy Oncology Group 0319 trial, which closed in 2004, addressed the safety and efficacy of three-dimensional conformal radiation directed at the lumpectomy cavity (38.5 Gy total/10 fractions,2 fractions/d, given in 5 consecutive working days) versus standard 6-week radiation protocols.

Interstitial brachytherapy uses catheters placed into the tissue surrounding the lumpectomy cavity to deliver radiation to the cavity and adjacent tissue to a total of either 45 to 60 Gy over the course of 4 to 6 days or 32 to 37 Gy over the course of 4 to 5 days.[117] Compared with other APBI methods, interstitial brachytherapy offers the advantage of better tailoring of radiation dose to variations in the size and shape of the lumpectomy cavity.[118] Disadvantages of this technique are related to the relative complexity of delivery. The patient must be willing to tolerate the external portion of the catheters for the duration of the treatment, and the therapy must take place in a specially shielded facility. The difficulty of actualizing catheter-based brachytherapy, primarily as a consequence of technical intricacies, has limited the widespread use of this technique.[119] The use of alternative balloon catheter- based treatment, specifically MammoSite balloon brachytherapy, is also being implemented.[119]

Compared to interstitial brachytherapy, the MammoSite delivery system for intracavitary delivery of APBI is more standardized and easier to use. A single catheter and balloon unit is inserted either during the lumpectomy procedure or postoperatively under ultrasound guidance and inflated to conform to the size and shape of the lumpectomy cavity. Patients are dosed twice daily for 5 to 7 days, and the catheter is then deflated and removed.[116] Looking at patients with infiltrating ductal carcinoma, long-term follow-up data from several studies comparing high-dose catheter-based brachytherapy with standard whole-breast radiotherapy revealed similar outcomes with regard to local recurrence and cosmesis.[120] Keisch and colleagues[121] reported on MammoSite treatment outcomes for women with invasive ductal carcinomas smaller than 2 cm; cosmetic results were rated as good to excellent in 86% of the patients, and no local recurrences were reported in this study of 70 patients at 39 months of follow-up. There is evidence that the MammoSite radiotherapy delivery device is well tolerated and delivers a good cosmetic outcome with minimal toxicity, provided that it is placed 7 mm or deeper beneath the skin.[115]

The NSABP is currently enrolling to their B-39 trial (Radiation Therapy Oncology Group 0413), a randomized phase III study designed to determine whether APBI limited to the region of the tumor bed after lumpectomy provides equivalent local tumor control in the breast compared with conventional whole-breast irradiation in the local management of breast cancer in women with stages 0, I, and II disease. Acceptable modes of delivery of APBI for this trial are high-dose rate, multicatheter brachytherapy; high-dose rate, single catheter balloon brachytherapy (MammoSite); and three-dimensional conformal external beam radiation therapy based on patient choice and preferred technique of the treating facility.

Another form of APBI currently favored in Europe is high-dose intraoperative radiation therapy. This mode of radiation delivery uses a mobile linear accelerator unit to deliver a single dose of radiation with electrons to the involved quadrant of the breast in the operating room during the primary surgical procedure. Veronesi and others reported no significant increase in complications with this procedure and a low in-field rate of recurrence.[122] Their study of 1246 women treated with ELectron IntraOperative Therapy (ELIOT) at a single dose of 21 Gy demonstrated survival and local control equivalent to standard radiotherapy with increased patient satisfaction and excellent cosmetic results.[122] The obvious advantages of this approach are allowing the patient to completely avoid 6 weeks of daily postoperative radiation and expanded opportunities for immediate reconstruction. A potential downside to this approach is the delivery of radiation to the lumpectomy field without knowledge of the resection margin status or specifics of the tumor biology. Additional trials and longer follow-up are needed.

It is imperative to remember that for any form of APBI to be successful, reproducible treatment techniques must be available and the treatment target and patient selection criteria must be defined.[123] The American Society of Breast Surgeons' revised consensus statement from December 2005 set the inclusion criteria for APBI as 45 years of age or older, invasive ductal carcinoma or DCIS, total tumor size less than or equal to 3 cm, negative margins of excision and node-negative disease.[124] Any patient who may harbor disease that is a significant distance from the edge of the lumpectomy cavity as to fall outside of the expected clinical target volume and any patient with the potential for multifocal disease must be excluded.[125]

Postmastectomy Radiation

For some patients, even treatment with mastectomy and level I and II axillary lymph node dissection alone is not enough to gain local control. Patients with a high likelihood of microscopic disease beyond the boundaries of the surgical field likely benefit from postmastectomy radiation therapy (PMRT) to reduce the chance of a locoregional recurrence.[126] Evidence indicates that PMRT delivered to the appropriate patient population reduces local recurrence by as much as threefold, but the effect of this reduction on OS is debatable.[127] Because of the evolving nature of this topic, the American Society of Clinical Oncology published guidelines for the use of PMRT in 2001.[128] The group recommended PMRT for patients with four or more positive axillary nodes and patients with T3 tumors or stage III cancers. Radiation fields for this indication should include the chest wall and supraclavicular nodal bed. There is insufficient evidence to date to recommend axillary radiation for patients who already underwent a complete level I and II axillary dissection and for inclusion of the internal mammary nodes in the radiated field. In an update of earlier data, the 2005 Early Breast Cancer Trialists' Collaborative Group meta-analysis of trials involving node-positive women concluded that PMRT administration produces a moderate, but definite, reduction in long-term breast cancer mortality and improvement in local control.[38]

Many additional variables in the delivery of postmastectomy radiation still need to be defined. The question of whether patients with high-risk, node-negative disease or one to three positive nodes should receive PMRT remains an issue of debate.[129] The Southwest Oncology Group study 9927 entitled "A Randomized Trial of Post-Mastectomy Radiotherapy in Stage II Breast Cancer in Women with One to Three Positive Axillary Nodes" was designed to answer this question, but unfortunately it closed because of slower-than-anticipated enrollment. Another trial with the same goal, the Selective Use of Postoperative Radiotherapy after Mastectomy BIG 2-04 study, is currently accruing postmastectomy patients in this group of patients with one to three positive axillary lymph nodes. Several prognostic factors—patient related and tumor related—have been proposed to determine which subgroup of patients with one to three positive lymph nodes would benefit most from PMRT. These factors include age, lymphovascular invasion, tumor grade, percent positive axillary nodes, extracapsular extension of lymph node metastasis, hormone receptor status, gene expression profile, and margin status. Larger trials that focus on these particular groups of women and longer follow-up are needed to answer these questions.

Post-Neoadjuvant Radiotherapy

The indications for neoadjuvant therapy have expanded in recent years. The use of postsurgical radiation in the setting of mastectomy has been particularly difficult to address in patients treated with neoadjuvant therapy. The controversy about this issue stems primarily from the fact that decisions regarding postmastectomy radiation have been based on primary tumor size and the number of positive lymph nodes in an axillary dissection. Particularly if neoadjuvant therapy alters the information found at final pathology, how can decisions regarding patient selection criteria for postmastectomy radiation be accomplished? Buchholz and colleagues[130] examined the recurrence pattern for patients treated with neoadjuvant therapy and mastectomy. Their study confirmed that patients who presented with lesions larger than 5 cm, T4 disease, or bulky adenopathy had a high risk for locoregional recurrence. In the study, patients treated with neoadjuvant therapy and postmastectomy radiation were found to have a lower rate of locoregional recurrence than patients who did not receive radiation. For some high-risk groups, the use of radiation therapy also contributed to improved overall and disease-specific survival, which was found to be true for patients who presented with stage III disease and exhibited a complete pathologic response. Data from the NSABP B-18 and B-27 trials showed a higher locoregional recurrence rate for patients who had residual positive lymph nodes after neoadjuvant therapy.[131–133] Based on information available, postmastectomy radiation has been recommended for patients who present with T3 lesions or stage III disease. Postmastectomy radiation has been recommended for patients with four or more positive lymph nodes after neoadjuvant therapy. For patients with one to three positive residual nodes, treatment may be beneficial. Management questions remain for stage II patients who are found to be node negative at final pathology. The treatment of this patient population may be best addressed by a prospective trial.

The use of adjuvant radiation after neoadjuvant chemotherapy and breast conservation is more straightforward. All patients treated with this surgical modality after neoadjuvant chemotherapy require radiotherapy. Breast-conserving surgery should be limited to cases in which negative margins of resection can be achieved and the patient is able to receive standard postoperative radiotherapy.[134] It is imperative to mark the location of the primary tumor before chemotherapy is delivered to ensure that the tumor bed can be localized for excision should a complete pathologic response be achieved.

SYSTEMIC THERAPY

According to the most recent National Comprehensive Cancer Network guidelines, adjuvant chemotherapy is a part of the recommended treatment for more than 70% of all women with invasive breast cancer.[135] Selecting patients who are most likely to receive benefit that outweighs the risks inherent to treatment is of paramount importance. It is widely accepted that women with node-positive disease receive a survival benefit from systemic therapy, and it has been standard practice to offer patients with hormone receptor–negative disease or tumors larger than 1 cm some form of chemo-therapeutic regimen. Patients who fall outside of these recommendations have a more uncertain risk/benefit profile. Two new treatment decision technologies have emerged to offer assistance in these indeterminate cases: gene panels used to calculate recurrence scores and computer-based prognostic models.

Treatment Decision Tools

The most widely used gene panel in the United States is the Oncotype DX (Genomic Health, Inc., Redwood City, California) breast cancer assay. Quantitative expression analysis of 16 cancer genes and 5 reference genes is determined from analysis of the patient's tumor cells using paraffin-embedded tissue. The information obtained from this assay is used to calculate a recurrence score (low, medium, or high). This score predicts the likelihood of a distant recurrence at 10 years after diagnosis. The Oncotype DX technology is validated in women with stage I or II disease who are node negative and estrogen receptor positive.[136] An ECOG-sponsored trial is currently recruiting patients to evaluate the benefit of this technology in a multicenter prospective fashion. The Trial Assigning Individualized Options for Treatment (TAILORx) will examine whether genes identified by Oncotype DX that are frequently associated with risk of recurrence for women with early-stage breast cancer can be used to assign patients to the most appropriate and effective treatment plan. Expected accrual is 10,046 women at more than 900 sites in the United States and Canada; the trial has been ongoing since 2006. Other commercially available multigene assays are Mammoprint (Amsterdam Signature; Agendia), and GeneSearch (Rotterdam Signature; Veridex). These systems have the disadvantage of requiring fresh (as opposed to paraffin-embedded) tissue but analyze a greater number of genes. The European Organization for Research and Treatment of Cancer Microarray in Node-negative Disease may Avoid ChemoTherapy (MINDACT) trial is currently enrolling patients for risk stratification and outcome analysis based on clinicopathologic risk and the Mammoprint 70 gene panel profile.

The computer program Adjuvant! Online (http://www.adjuvantonline.com), based largely on estimates of prognosis from the SEER database, predicts 10-year breast cancer outcomes for patients with and without systemic therapy (see **Table 1**).[137] This program calculates outcome risk estimates for women with invasive cancer after definitive tumor resection and axillary staging but before any systemic therapy. Women with inflammatory cancer, unusual pathologic tumor subtypes, or metastatic disease require additional steps for analysis. Patient data, including patient age, menopausal status, comorbidities, estrogen receptor status, nodal status, and tumor size, are entered into the program at www.adjuvantonline.com. The prognostic factor impact calculator then uses a Bayesian approach to estimate the expected benefits of adjuvant treatment (hormonal, chemotherapeutic, and combination therapy). A confirmation study of this tool using the British Columbia Breast Cancer Outcomes Unit was performed by Olivotto and colleagues[138] in 2005. Adjuvant! Online predicted OS, disease-specific survival, and event-free survival to within 2% for most patients evaluated. Patients younger than 35 years and patients with lymphovascular invasion in their tumor specimens were the only two groups that required additional modification to the program to derive reliable predictions. Thus far, Adjuvant! Online is proving to be an important tool for assessing the benefit of adjuvant therapies in women with stages I and II breast cancer.

Systemic Regimens

Once the decision has been made to embark on adjuvant treatment with chemotherapeutic agents, several regimens are available. Polychemotherapy has proved superior to single-agent therapy by a preponderance of evidence (**Box 2**). Combined systemic therapy regimens for breast cancer have advanced from cyclophosphamide, methotrexate, and fluorouracil in the 1970s, to the introduction of anthracyclines in the 1980s, to the addition of taxanes in the 1990s, to modern targeted therapies, biologics, and alternate dosage and duration schemas.

The gold standard for polychemotherapy in breast cancer for many years was cyclophosphamide, methotrexate, and fluorouracil, which can be administered in either intravenous or oral formulations. In an Oxford meta-analysis that compared cyclophosphamide, methotrexate, and fluorouracil to anthracycline-containing regimens, the anthracyclines had a more than 5% increased DF and OS.[139] Cyclophosphamide, methotrexate, and fluorouracil therapy is no longer considered first line in the treatment of breast cancer. Currently, an anthracycline-based regimen, the most widely used being doxorubicin with cyclophosphamide (AC), shows the greatest

---

Box 2
Breast cancer therapeutic regimens

Chemotherapies

    For early-stage breast cancer

        AC (doxorubicin and cyclophosphamide)

        AC followed by T (doxorubicin and cyclophosphamide followed by paclitaxel)

        CAF (cyclophosphamide, doxorubicin, and 5-fluorouracil)

        Cyclophosphamide, methotrexate, and 5-fluorouracil

        TAC (docetaxel, doxorubicin, and cyclophosphamide)

    For metastatic disease

        Gemcitabine with paclitaxel

        Capecitabine with docetaxel

        Bisphosphonates (zoledronic acid and pamidronate)

Hormonal therapies

    Selective estrogen receptor modulators

        Tamoxifen

        Toremifene

        Fulvestrant

    Aromatase inhibitors (AIs)

        Anastrazole

        Exemestane

        Letrozole

Bioimmunotherapies

    Traztuzumab

    Bevacizumab

    Vaccines in trial

Tyrosine kinase inhibitors

    Lapatinib

benefit in younger age groups.[140] This benefit is lower for hormone receptor-positive patients when compared with patients who are hormone receptor negative and is significantly decreased for human epidermal growth factor receptor (HER-2)–positive patients.[141,142]

The absolute benefit of therapies that include taxanes can be hard to quantify because they are given either in combination or in series with anthracyclines in nearly all published trials. It is reasonable to assert that almost all patient groups respond to taxanes.[143] Four cycles of AC followed by paclitaxel provided a longer DF survival and OS in the Cancer and Leukemia Group B 9344 and NSABP B-28 trials.[144,145] Docetaxel also demonstrated benefit when combined with standard therapy in the BCIRG 001 trial, with the greatest survival benefit in node-positive patients.[146] Regarding appropriate taxane usage, Sparano and colleagues[147] presented an update of the ECOG 1199 trial evaluating AC chemotherapy followed by paclitaxel given either weekly or every 3 weeks or docetaxel given either weekly or every 3 weeks at the 2007 American Society of Clinical Oncologists meeting. This group found the greatest benefit to patients who received weekly paclitaxel, followed by patients who received docetaxel every 3 weeks. Upon subgroup analysis, hormone receptor–negative women had a higher recurrence-free survival rate when treated with paclitaxel, whereas hormone receptor–positive women derived a greater benefit from treatment with docetaxel. Overall, the greatest benefit in DF and OS was seen with weekly paclitaxel after standard adjuvant chemotherapy with AC.

One group of patients who have breast cancer who require special consideration when constructing an adjuvant treatment plan is patients with triple-negative (estrogen receptor/progesterone receptor (PR)-negative, HER-2–negative) disease. This phenotype is most often seen in African American women who are premenopausal and accounts for 15% of all breast cancer cases. This disease subtype carries a poor prognosis, with earlier local and distant recurrence than that seen in receptor-positive disease, and is commonly associated with BRCA1 mutations.[143] Because the BRCA1 gene mutation affects DNA repair, mitomycin-C and platinum agents such as cisplatin are expected to have increased activity in patients who have breast cancer who harbor this mutation. The mechanism of action for these agents is mitigated by DNA cross-linking and works by impairing DNA synthesis, transcription, and function.[148]

Neoadjuvant Therapy Indications

Neoadjuvant chemotherapy is the standard of care for women with inflammatory breast cancer and women with bulky disease that causes it to be inoperable. Recently, the indications for neoadjuvant therapy were expanded to include patients with large primary tumors interested in breast conservation or patients who might achieve a more cosmetic SSM with good tumor response to treatment. The delivery of maximal chemotherapy first provides an opportunity to study the clinical effectiveness of a particular chemotherapeutic regimen. NSABP B-18 was designed to evaluate the worth of neoadjuvant chemotherapy with AC for the treatment of stage I and II breast cancers. There was no difference in DF or OS in the neoadjuvant versus adjuvant treatment groups. The neoadjuvant group did experience other advantages. The rate of BCT in the neoadjuvant group versus the adjuvant group was 67.8% compared with 59.8%. All outcomes were better in women who experienced a pathologic complete response from chemotherapy before excision of their tumor, which allowed identification of women with this important prognostic factor.[149]

The addition of docetaxel to AC also in a neoadjuvant fashion increased the rate of clinical response in women who initially failed to respond to AC and resulted in a significantly greater complete pathologic response in women with anthracycline-sensitive tumors than that seen with AC alone.[150] Numerous subsequent trials echoed this result of improved clinical complete response and complete pathologic response when a taxane was added to AC in the neoadjuvant setting, making this the current standard of care.[151] The results of equivalent survival with a higher rate of successful BCT were demonstrated in subsequent meta-analyses of the available data.[152,153] If the cancer progresses during neoadjuvant therapy, the default should be to revert to surgery immediately with all subsequent chemotherapy given postoperatively. Staging of disease for patients treated in the neoadjuvant setting should include pretreatment clinical stage and postoperative pathologic stage (**Table 5**). To account for clinical and pathologic staging factors, a new mechanism for prognostic determination has been devised that assigns point values to the individual clinical and pathologic substages and includes biologic markers: estrogen receptor and tumor grade (see **Table 1**).[154,155] This scoring system currently provides the most refined distant metastasis free and disease specific survival data for patients treated with neoadjuvant therapy. Validation for this work is forthcoming.

HER-2 Disease Treatments

Expression of HER-2 traditionally was a negative prognostic factor for breast cancer patients. HER-2–positive patients tend to have more aggressive disease, which has a higher likelihood of being locally advanced and an increased resistance to endocrine therapy.[156] HER-2/*neu* (ErbB2) is one of a family of epidermal growth factors that encodes for the extracellular domain of HER-2 and is overexpressed in 20% to 30% of all

Table 5
Prognosis according to clinical pathologic scoring system after completion of neoadjuvant chemotherapy

Clinical Stage	Score	Pathologic Stage	Score	Tumor Marker	Score
I	0	0	0	ER negative	1
IIA	0	I	0	Nuclear grade 3	1
IIB	1	IIA	1		
IIIA	1	IIB	1		
IIIB	2	IIIA	1		
IIIC	2	IIIB	1		
		IIIC	2		

CPS total score	5-y DSS (%)	95% CI	CPS + EG total score	5-y DSS (%)	95% CI
0	99	96–100	0	100	
1	93	89–96	1	98	94–100
2	83	78–88	2	96	91–98
3	76	68–83	3	88	83–92
4	48	27–67	4	72	64–79
			5	57	42–70
			6	22	3–51

Abbreviations: CPS, clinical pathologic score; DSS, disease specific survival; EG, estrogen receptor grade.
Modified from Jeruss JS, Mittendorf EA, Tucker SL, et al. Staging of breast cancer in the neoadjuvant setting. Cancer Res 2008;68(16):6479; with permission.

breast cancers.[157] Therapies targeted to this protein have been a topic of intense research and development. The success of HER-2–targeted therapies turned this previously negative prognostic factor into an opportunity for exciting new treatment modalities that can decrease local recurrence and increase OS. The two HER-2–targeted therapies with the most evidence for their use are trastuzumab and lapatinib.

Trastuzumab (Herceptin, Genentech BioOncology) is a recombinant, humanized IgG monoclonal antibody that targets the extracellular domain of HER-2.[158] Trastuzumab interferes with multiple steps in the tumor cell cycle and sensitizes HER-2–positive cancers to other cytotoxic therapies.[159] The US Food and Drug Administration (FDA) first approved trastuzumab for use in patients with metastatic HER-2–positive breast cancer in combination with paclitaxel.[160] In response to findings of significantly greater time to progression and an improvement in median OS, the National Cancer Institute sponsored two trials of adjuvant treatment with trastuzumab, led by the NSABP and the North Central Cancer Treatment Group. Both trials compared standard chemotherapy (doxorubicin and cyclophosphamide followed by paclitaxel) with the same regimen plus trastuzumab administered after or concurrent with paclitaxel. The data from NSABP B-31 and North Central Cancer Treatment Group N-9831 were merged and the trials closed prematurely because of superiority in the groups treated with trastuzumab. Romond and colleagues[161] reported a 52% reduction in the risk of recurrence and a 33% reduction in the risk of death in the trastuzumab groups compared with patients who received standard regimens alone. Subsequent trials of trastuzumab in combination with other adjuvant and neoadjuvant chemotherapeutic regimens sought to answer questions regarding the optimal sequencing and duration of trastuzumab therapy.

Other phase III trials to evaluate the optimal patient population and timing of trastuzumab therapy are the Breast International Group HERceptin Adjuvant trial, the Breast Cancer International Research Group (BCIRG) 006 trial, and the FINland Herceptin trial (FINHer). In an interim analysis, the Breast International Group HERceptin Adjuvant trial (BIGHER), which is evaluating the use of trastuzumab after rather than concurrent with standard chemotherapy, showed a 46% risk reduction for new events.[162] BCIRG 006 compared docetaxel with carboplatin and trastuzumab (DCT; six cycles, with 1 year of trastuzumab) with adriamycin/cyclophosphamide (AC; four cycles) followed by docetaxel (four cycles) without (AC-D) and with (AC-DT) trastuzumab for 1 year in node-positive and high-risk node-negative HER-2–positive patients. Four-year data show superiority in DF survival for trastuzumab groups compared with the AC-D group. Trastuzumab/docetaxel after anthracycline provided a greater benefit than trastuzumab/docetaxel after carboplatin, with mortality rates also favoring AC-DT (1.9%) over AC-D (3.4%) and DCT (2.6%).[163] FINher evaluated docetaxel compared with vinorelbine and randomized the HER-2–positive patients to receive or not receive a shorter 9-week course of trastuzumab. The women who received this shorter course of trastuzumab enjoyed a similar improvement in DFS compared with the other studies mentioned, with less cardiotoxicity.[164]

A major limitation to the use of trastuzumab in all of these trials is its cardiotoxicity. Anthracyline-based chemotherapy also has known cardiotoxicity, with a rate of severe cardiac decline of 3.7%. The addition of trastuzumab therapy concurrent with adriamycin increased this rate to 16.1%, whereas the risk associated with administering trastuzumab after adriamycin treatment was only 2.2%. Of equal importance is the cardiac decline seen with sequential trastuzumab, which was more often reversible compared with the effects of trastuzumab given concurrent with anthracycline.[165] A shorter 9-week course of trastuzumab was not associated with cardiac risk above that conferred by anthracycline therapy in the data analysis thus far.

Resistance to trastuzumab eventually develops in most patients with metastatic breast cancer who initially respond to trastuzumab, and in the adjuvant setting, 15% of patients still experience relapse despite trastuzumab-based therapy.[166] There are multiple mechanisms by which HER-2–positive tumor cells become resistant to trastuzumab, and novel modalities are being explored to circumvent resistance by targeting other members of the epidermal growth factors family.[156] One such agent is lapatinib (Tykerb, GlaxoSmithKline). Lapatinib is an orally delivered dual tyrosine kinase inhibitor targeted against epidermal growth factor and HER-2. In vitro data demonstrate a synergistic effect activity of lapatinib in combination with trastuzumab.[167] Lapatinib was also shown to inhibit growth of HER-2–overexpressing breast cancer cells that were maintained long-term on trastuzumab and exhibited trastuzumab resistance.[168]

Nahta and colleagues[166] described lapatinib-induced apoptosis in trastuzumab-resistant cells as occurring to the same degree as that seen in parental, trastuzumab-sensitive cells. Also of importance was the observation that lapatinib may have better central nervous system penetration than trastuzumab and may be a potential agent to treat HER-2–positive brain metastases.[169] Currently, the data support an improvement in time to progression for lapatinib in combination with capecitabine in patients whose disease has progressed on trastuzumab.[170] Beyond these observations, how to integrate lapatinib into other established treatment plans is not currently known, and it should not be used in the adjuvant setting outside of clinical trials until further studies have been conducted.[171] The cardiotoxicity of HER-2–targeted treatments seen with trastuzumab use seems to be a class effect, but the degree of toxicity varies among agents. The rate of high-grade left ventricular ejection fraction decline for patients treated with lapatinib thus far is 1.3%, with 57% of cases either improving or resolving after cessation of treatment.[172] Other novel agents, such as pertuzumab (a monoclonal antibody against HER-2 and HER-3), erlotinib (an inhibitor of the tyrosine kinase activity of epidermal growth factor), and geldanamycin (a HER-2–destabilizing protein), are under investigation for the treatment of trastuzumab-resistant HER- 2–positive breast cancers. Trials comparing different combinations of therapeutic agents and alternative timing of treatment are also ongoing.

Hormonal Therapies: Tamoxifen and Aromatase Inhibitors

Hormonal therapy is recommended as adjuvant therapy for all women with estrogen receptor–positive breast cancers, regardless of patient age, lymph node involvement, HER-2 status, or menopausal status unless there is a compelling contraindication. Hormonal therapy falls into three categories. First is the blockade of estrogen activity. The gold standard for this type of therapy is tamoxifen, which competitively inhibits estrogen binding to estrogen receptors in the breast. Second is surgical or medical ovarian ablation, which definitively blocks estrogen synthesis in premenopausal women. This type of therapy is generally reserved for patients with known genetic predispositions to breast cancer, such as BRCA1 and BRCA2 carriers. Third, estrogen continues to be synthesized in postmenopausal women by the conversion of androgens to estrogens via the aromatase enzyme. Aromatase inhibitors (AIs) such as exemestane, letrozole and anastrozole block this pathway. Exemestane is a type I steroidal AI that irreversibly binds aromatase, whereas letrozole and anastrozole are type II nonsteroidal AIs that reversibly bind the aromatase enzyme. The best choice of hormonal agent and duration of therapy for the treatment of estrogen receptor–positive breast cancer has been the topic of intense study.

Tamoxifen is recommended for the treatment of women with estrogen receptor-positive tumors larger than 1 cm for a duration of 5 years. Such therapy is associated with a 47% reduction in the annual odds of recurrence and a 26% reduction in the annual odds of mortality, with the benefit seen for node-positive and node-negative disease.[173,174] The main risks associated with tamoxifen therapy are uterine cancers and venous thromboembolism. Because of its mechanism of action, tamoxifen is effective antihormonal therapy in premenopausal and postmenopausal women. AIs are also effective in postmenopausal women, and the question is which drug class is superior in this subset.

In the Arimidex, Tamoxifen, Alone or in Combination (ATAC) trial, anastrozole was compared with tamoxifen for 5 years in more than 9000 postmenopausal women with stage I and II breast cancer. Anastrozole significantly prolonged DFS (hazard ratio 0.87, $P = .01$) and time-to-recurrence (hazard ratio 0.79, $P = .0005$) and significantly reduced the incidence of distant metastases (hazard ratio 0.86, $P = .04$) and contralateral breast cancers (42% reduction, $P = .01$). There were also fewer side effects with anastrozole, but arthralgia and fractures were increased.[175] Coombes and colleagues[176] asked the question of whether postmenopausal women who had already begun treatment with tamoxifen should continue for the full 5 years or switch to therapy with an AI. Of the 4742 women enrolled in a study to address this question, 2362 were randomly assigned to change therapy from tamoxifen to exemestane after 2 to 3 years, for a total duration of 5 years of therapy. There was an absolute benefit in terms of DFS of 4.7% in the exemestane group ($P = .001$), although OS was not significantly affected. In postmenopausal women who have completed the full 5 years of therapy with tamoxifen, the addition of an AI can still confer additional benefit. Goss and colleagues[177] conducted a double-blind, placebo-controlled trial of 5 years of tamoxifen followed by either 5 years of letrazole or a placebo. The letrazole group had longer DFS (93% versus 87% at 4 years, $P = .001$) when compared with placebo without a statistically significant difference in OS. The preponderance of the evidence supports 5 years of therapy with an AI for postmenopausal women with hormone receptor–positive breast cancers.

Hormonal agents are used for more than adjuvant treatment of breast cancers. Tamoxifen therapy has been shown to confer a survival benefit to patients with DCIS and is used as chemoprevention for patients at an increased risk of developing breast cancer. Tamoxifen for chemoprevention was compared with raloxifene, another competitive inhibitor of estrogen binding also used to prevent osteoporosis in the Study of Tamoxifen and Raloxifene (STAR) trial. In that trial, both drugs reduced the risk of developing invasive breast cancer by approximately 50%. The raloxifene group also had 36% fewer uterine cancers and 29% fewer venous thromboembolic events than the women who were randomized to tamoxifen.[178] This study was unblinded, and women have been allowed to cross over from tamoxifen to raloxifene after 4 years of treatment. Further data accrued after crossover have yet to be published.

Antiangiogenic Agents

For tumors to grow and metastasize, they must be able to induce the formation of a vascular supply. This hypothesis was first expressed in 1971 by Folkman[179] when he proposed that without the ability to grow and recruit a blood supply, solid tumors could only grow to 2 to 3 mm and could not metastasize. Inhibition of this process of neoangiogenesis is an appealing strategy for the treatment of various malignancies, including breast cancers. Among the many angiogenic factors active in the human body, vascular endothelial growth factor (VEGF) plays a pivotal role in the formation of new blood vessels under physiologic and pathologic conditions and has been the most popular target for antiangiogenic therapies.[180] VEGF binds to cellular surface receptors and activates an intracellular tyrosine kinase-dependent signaling pathway that leads to cell proliferation, increased vascular permeability, inhibition of apoptosis, and neoangiogenesis.[181] Elevated levels of VEGF are found in breast cancers of ductal cell origin and at higher levels in estrogen receptor–positive tumors.[182] Increased VEGF expression and the intensity of this expression also seem to be strongly associated with a high microvessel density and poorer outcomes in breast cancer.[183]

The first chemotherapeutic agent to successfully block the action of VEGF and inhibit tumor neoangiogenesis was bevacizumab (Avastin, Genentec BioOncology). Bevacizumab is a humanized monoclonal antibody directed at the VEGF-A ligand; when it binds, bevacizumab disrupts the initiation signal through VEGF and the entire downsteam pathway.[184] Bevacizumab showed benefit in the treatment of metastatic colon and lung cancers and recently showed promise in the treatment of advanced breast cancer.[185] After some initially disappointing results, the Eastern Oncology Cooperative Group was able to show in a phase II randomized controlled trial (ECOG E2100) that combination therapy with paclitaxel plus bevacizumab significantly increased tumor response rates over paclitaxel alone (28.2% versus 14.2%) and an improved progression-free survival (11.4 versus 6.11 months). Unfortunately, this did not result in improved OS.[186] The side-effect profile of bevacizumab includes hypertension (23%), including hypertensive crisis and nephritic syndrome, thrombosis (including deep venous thrombosis), myocardial infarction, and cerebrovascular accident, congestive heart failure, bleeding, impaired wound healing and bowel perforation.[180]

Some controversy surrounded the FDA approval of bevacizumab for the treatment of metastatic breast cancer in February 2008, because an FDA advisory committee had voted 5 to 4 against approval. In the past, the FDA only approved chemotherapeutic drugs that extended a patient's lifespan, but bevacizumab slowed progression-free survival without an improvement in OS.[187] Questions also remain as to the proper duration and sequencing of therapy, possible synergistic effects with other cytotoxic chemotherapeutic agents, and how to select patients who are most likely to benefit from antiangiogenic therapy.[188] Data continue to be analyzed from E2100; E2104 will investigate adding bevacizumab to an AC-T regimen, and the Breast Cancer Intergroup E5103 trial will evaluate the efficacy of bevacizumab in the adjuvant setting. Other inhibitors of angiogenesis, such as sunitinib and sorafenib, have met with success in other tumor types and are being evaluated for the treatment of breast cancer, along with axitinib and pazopanib.[171]

Vaccines

The perfect treatment for any disease would be inexpensive, easy to administer, well tolerated, and specifically target only the disease entity and not the host. Vaccines have offered these features for treatment of many infectious diseases, and the idea of a vaccine directed against cancer is as exciting as it has proven evasive. Vaccine trials directed against various human cancers are ongoing and are fueled by an ever-growing understanding of tumor biology. A successful vaccine must have (1) a target antigen on the tumor cell to effect an immune response, (2) a delivery platform, and (3) necessary adjuvants to enhance immune response.[189] Early results of antitumor vaccines have been disappointing, with reported response rates of only 2.6%.[190] Some reasons for this have to do with the nature of tumor antigens. Tumor cells may only express low levels of any one particular antigen, they may change their antigenic profile as they grow and metastasize, and most tumor antigens are self-antigens and in the best case are only mildly immunogenic. Another likely reason for suboptimal results for cancer vaccines may be caused by the patients in advanced stages of disease who are recruited into phase I and II trials. In particular, large and metastatic tumors are less amenable to vaccination because the inoculum cannot reach cells on the inside of the tumor mass, and metastatic cancers can have an immunomodulatory effect on the host.[191] Investigators are currently embarked on numerous trials of novel agents and delivery methods for a breast cancer vaccine that can hopefully overcome these hurdles.

Myriad potential target antigens that can be recognized by human T lymphocytes on breast cancer cells have been identified. These antigens are expressed by normal cells but are either mutated or overexpressed by breast cancer cells and are ideal for eliciting a specific immune response against these cells.[189] Among them are mammoglobulin A, the membrane associated glycoprotein MUC-1, the adhesion molecule glycoprotein CEA, telomere reverse transcriptase hTERT and the epidermal growth factor receptor HER-2/*neu*, specifically the E75 peptide portion.

The next important element of a successful vaccine is an appropriate delivery system. DNA vaccines come in two varieties: those that use full-length cDNA molecules and those that present fragments of material from whole tumor cells to the host. For creating the full-length pieces of DNA, established recombinant DNA techniques permit rapid optimization of the DNA molecule to form the vaccine.[192] Once the molecule is created, it is cloned into a bacterial plasmid along with promoter/enhancer sequences and immunostimulatory factors. It is injected, and in vivo transfection of the DNA molecule into the target cells causes production of the encoded antigen and presentation by normal mechanisms.[191] One approach to using genomic fragments of whole tumor cells is transfer of these fragments into a fibroblast line for antigen presentation.[193] Creating a chimera of an antigen-presenting cell with a human tumor antigen is a delivery system designed to boost a tumor antigen's weak inherent immunogenicity.

Another such fusion being explored for multiple cancers is that of the tumor antigen with a dendritic cell. Dendritic cells and tumor cells are cocultured in polyethylene glycol to generate fusion cells, which do cause a measurable immune response, but it has not proved to be a sufficiently robust process to generate enough cells for multiple vaccinations.[194] Use of infectious vectors is another possible delivery platform for a breast cancer vaccine. Numerous different viral vectors and bacterial vectors, such as *Listeria monocytogenes* and *Escherichia coli,* are being produced to express highly immunogenic forms of cancer antigens for presentation to the immune system.[195–197] Peptide-based vaccines are another take on delivery strategies. These peptide vaccines use antigenic epitopes derived from tumor antigens to induce immune regulators that then recognize and lyse tumor cells that express the same immunogenic peptide on their surface. When combined with an immunoadjuvant, these peptides can be injected without an additional delivery system. Mittendorf and colleagues[198] are involved in phase II trials using an E75 HER2/*neu* peptide mixed with an immunoadjuvant to immunize node-positive and node-negative DF breast cancer patients. The vaccine has shown effect in stimulating clonal expansion of E75-specific CD8+ T cells and reduction in recurrence rate in inoculated patients trends toward significance.

There have been major advances in the understanding of tumor biology and its relation to therapeutic vaccination, but as of yet this has not translated into significant clinical benefit. Many of the currently available data deal with therapeutic vaccination, whereas a practical approach to prophylactic cancer vaccination has been elusive. Immunotherapy and vaccination for therapy and prevention of breast cancer continue to be an exciting topic for research in the years ahead.

RECONSTRUCTIVE SURGERY

The diagnosis of breast cancer poses many simultaneous concerns for a woman. She is likely focused on seeking a treatment plan that will give her the greatest chance of long-term survival, but she is probably also worried about what this treatment will mean for her self-image and sexuality. The emotional impact of losing a breast for patients who undergo mastectomy can be devastating, and it is the responsibility of the physicians who make up the care team to include a plastic surgery consultation in the initial phase of the treatment plan to inform the patient of all her reconstructive options. Data show the positive effects of breast reconstruction on the psychologic well-being of patients who have breast cancer.[199] When the primary surgeon has a discussion with the patient regarding options for reconstruction, this can significantly influence the patient's ultimate choice of whether to include reconstruction in her treatment plan.[200] The Federal Breast Reconstruction Law, passed in 1998, bars insurance companies from considering breast reconstruction after oncologic surgery as elective and requires coverage for reconstruction of the affected breast and contralateral symmetry procedures. Reconstruction is a vital part of comprehensive breast cancer therapy.

The timing and type of this reconstruction can vary. Immediate reconstruction can ease the sense of loss that accompanies mastectomy because the patient is never without a "breast" and it can accomplish two procedures with only one general anesthetic and recovery period. Delayed reconstruction can be necessary if no reconstructive surgeon is available at the time of the primary surgery or if the patient desires more time to consider her options. A third option, termed "delayed-immediate" reconstruction, entails placing an implant expander concurrent with mastectomy and then waiting until after radiation therapy is completed to replace it with a permanent implant. This approach allows the skin envelope to be preserved but negates the risk of capsular contraction around an implant during radiation therapy.[201]

The type of reconstruction that is most appropriate for an individual patient must take into account her medical comorbidities, body habitus, oncologic treatment plan, and preference. The general categories for reconstruction after mastectomy are implant based and autologous tissue based or a combination of the two modalities.

Implant Reconstruction

Breast reconstruction with a prosthetic implant can be accomplished in more than one way. The patient can receive either standard or adjustable implants at the initial surgery, which achieves a single-stage reconstruction. Alternately, the patient can have a two-stage approach, with a tissue expander initially and then a permanent implant at a later date.

Single-stage reconstruction is best suited to patients with small breasts who have undergone a SSM or a nipple-sparing prophylactic mastectomy.[202] These women can be fitted with a prefilled permanent implant made of either saline or silicon, or they can be fitted with an adjustable permanent implant and port that can be inflated postoperatively until desired volume is reached, after which the port removed. In women who started with a large breast or significant ptosis, this technique may not provide enough inferior volume to yield an acceptable result, or a contralateral breast reduction may be considered.[203] An adjunctive technique to single-step, implant-based reconstruction first published by Breuling[204] in 2005 is the use of acellular dermal grafts. Alloderm (LifeCell Corporation, Branchburg, New Jersey) is an acellular dermal matrix composed of cadaveric human skin. The ability of this substance to survive as a graft is attributed to its ability to encourage vascular ingrowth and incorporation. Instead of lifting the serratus muscle to form the inferolateral aspect of the subpectoral implant pocket, Alloderm is sewn to the pectoralis major muscle, chest wall, and inframammary fold to form an inferior sling for the implant and increase the total volume of the implant pocket. The advantage of this procedure is the ability to adequately fill out the mastectomy skin flaps immediately without need for expansion. The graft significantly reduces downward migration of the implant. Although there are limited long-term follow-up data regarding this approach, early excellent cosmetic results with minimal complications are encouraging.[205]

The most common way to achieve an implant-based reconstruction is via a two-step approach. At the time of mastectomy, an implant expander is placed in a subpectoral position. After the mastectomy incision has healed, the expander is filled in increments on an incremental basis until the desired volume is reached months later. The expander is then replaced with a permanent saline or silicon implant during a second outpatient surgical procedure. Of note, silicon gel implants were unavailable for patients outside of FDA trials between 1992 and 2005. In 2006, the FDA launched a Web site with statements concluding that the preponderance of available research has determined that silicon implants are safe and effective for general use.[206] Silicon implants offer a softer and more natural feel to the reconstructed breast and are a good option for most women who are not averse to receiving a silicon implant.[201]

Implant-based reconstructions have the clear advantage of being relatively minor procedures that require no donor tissue from other parts of the body to deliver an aesthetically pleasing result. One limitation of implant reconstruction is the way the reconstructed breast looks and feels without clothing because it does not have the same feel and contour as a native breast. This difference can be minimized by performing bilateral reconstruction so that the symmetric appearance of the breasts provides a more natural-looking result.[207] The most common and disfiguring late complication of implant insertion is capsular contraction, which may require additional surgical procedures to either release or excise the abnormally thickened capsule. The risk and severity of contracture increase with radiation therapy, and implant reconstruction may not be the most ideal reconstructive option for patients expected to receive postmastectomy radiation.[208]

Autologous Tissue-Based Reconstructions

When it is known preoperatively that a patient will likely need postmastectomy radiation, autologous reconstruction in a delayed fashion using the patient's own tissue is the preferred approach. The donor sites appropriate for tissue removal for autologous breast reconstruction are the abdomen, the gluteus, and the latissimus dorsi.

The most common of the reconstructions based on abdominal tissue is the transverse rectus abdominis muscle flap (TRAM). The skin, subcutaneous fat, and rectus abdominis muscle of the lower abdomen are used to reconstruct the breast mound. This procedure can be accomplished as a pedicled flap that relies on the superior epigastric vessels for its blood supply or as a free flap with a microvascular anastomosis. TRAM reconstruction can be offered to women with substantial abdominal tissue and is not a good choice for thin women. An additional benefit of TRAM reconstruction for many women who are candidates is that they essentially receive an abdominoplasty from the harvest of the abdominal flap. Abdominal tissue-based flaps are contraindicated for women who smoke, have medical comorbidities (including diabetes), are obese, have had previous liposuction to the donor area, and have multiple abdominal surgical scars, especially ones that would disrupt the epigastric vessels. The main risk of a TRAM, besides the risk of flap failure inherent to any autologous reconstruction, is the risk of abdominal wall hernias.

A newer reconstructive strategy that uses abdominal skin and subcutaneous tissue but preserves the rectus abdominis muscle involves the deep inferior epigastric perforator flap (DIEP). The inferior epigastric vessels are dissected down to their origin from the iliac and removed along with the flap, and the procedure requires microvascular anastomosis to the thoracodorsal or internal mammary vessels. The advantages of DIEP when compared with TRAMs are less deformity of the abdominal wall and better perfusion and improved flap survival.[209]

For women in whom abdominal flap reconstruction is contraindicated for anatomic reasons, other sites for donor tissue can be used. An alternate site for donor tissue is the gluteus either as a superior artery gluteal perforator flap or an inferior gluteal artery perforator flap. The perforating vessels for each are carefully dissected free from the surrounding gluteus maximus muscle, which is spread in the direction of the muscle fibers and safely preserved. The vascular pedicle is anastomosed to recipient vessels in the chest and the donor site is closed primarily.[210] The main disadvantage of the superior artery gluteal perforator flap is that harvest is from high on the buttock and can leave a noticeable deformity. Inferior gluteal artery perforator flap harvest is based lower on the buttock, and the donor site scar usually falls in or near the crease under the buttock, but it has a higher chance of producing discomfort upon sitting after the surgery. These techniques are promising alternatives but currently not widely used.

A third potential site for tissue useable for reconstruction of the breast is the latissimus dorsi. Flaps from this area are usually pedicled myocutaneous flaps based from the subscapular blood supply. Latissimus flaps have a low rate of graft loss and can be useful in salvage situations in irradiated tissue beds.[211] The disadvantage of a latissimus flap is that there is often not enough tissue to reconstruct the breast without need for additional volume provided by an implant. Another consideration when bringing the pedicle of a latissimus dorsi flap through the axilla is staging of the axillary lymph nodes. Final positive SLNB after negative intraoperative assessment subsequent to this type of reconstruction could risk loss of the graft, secondary to the need for complete axillary dissection. Special care must be taken to appropriately stage the axilla if this reconstructive approach is chosen. Assistance from a plastic surgeon is suggested if reoperative axillary surgery is necessary.

Oncoplastics

Women who are candidates for BCT are not immune from concerns about poor aesthetic outcome. As many as 20% to 30% of women treated with BCT require additional reconstructive surgical procedures to repair contour deformity, and an unknown number sustain poor cosmesis and do not seek additional surgery.[212] Poor cosmetic result is associated with patient- and treatment-related risk factors. Important patient-related risks are younger age, larger body habitus, larger tumor size, and tumor in the medial or inferior lateral position. Treatment-related risk factors for poor postoperative symmetry include the need for re-excision after initial lumpectomy, postoperative seroma, and subsequent radiation therapy.[213] When BCT necessitates an excision of more than 20% of breast volume, the final result is likely to be rated as poor by the patient and independent observers.[214] If an excision of this size or larger is anticipated, a breast reconstruction procedure should be considered if cosmetic outcome is to be enhanced.

The term "oncoplastics" was first used by Audretsch[215] in 1998 to describe the technique of avoiding mastectomy by using mastoplasty and other plastic surgical techniques to reconstruct the breast after wide local excision of the primary breast tumor. Oncoplastic surgery combines optimal oncologic resection with the best achievable aesthetic result, and it can provide equivalent oncologic outcomes when compared with BCT without reconstruction.[216] Depending on the volume of breast issue removed, the appropriate reconstructive technique may be local tissue rearrangement, rotational flaps, replacement of tissue with flaps from distant donor sites, or the use of a prosthetic implant.[205] Another important concept in an oncoplastic approach is the treatment of the contralateral breast. The timing for a symmetry procedure on the unaffected breast is somewhat controversial, with some surgeons advocating for accomplishing it in the same operative setting as the oncologic resection and some preferring to wait until it is known that there is no need for re-excision or mastectomy on the affected side.[217] No randomized trials have evaluated the safety and efficacy of the oncoplastic approach, but reports with up to 74 months of follow-up do not show inferiority to BCT without reconstruction.[218] The development of new techniques that fall under the umbrella of oncoplastic breast surgery are ongoing and offer exciting options for breast conservation with improved cosmetic results, as long as negative tumor margins are first obtained.

ONCOFERTILITY

A breast cancer diagnosis can be devastating for a woman of any age, but for women of reproductive age who have not completed their families, the diagnosis poses additional fertility issues. A successful strategy for fertility preservation must be made as part of the overall oncologic treatment plan, and it is important to address this topic with younger patients before treatment rather than after therapy for her cancer has begun. The threat to fertility is conferred by the need for systemic chemotherapy, and the decision to administer these treatments depends on the stage at diagnosis. Women with stage I disease (small tumors, no axillary involvement) and favorable tumor biology (estrogen receptor–positive, PR-positive, HER-2–negative tumors) are typically treated with surgery as the primary modality. Once surgical treatment is completed, subsequent antiestrogen therapy and radiation therapy may be necessary. Thus far, indirect evidence suggests that antiestrogen therapy can be delayed to allow for pregnancy after surgery and radiotherapy have been completed.[219,220] Pregnancy or harvesting of eggs for in vitro fertilization should not occur during treatment with radiotherapy, because internal scatter from standard radiation therapy can reach the pelvis and ovaries during treatment.[221]

Patients with tumors larger than 1 cm, metastases to regional lymph nodes, or estrogen receptor/PR–negative tumors probably need chemotherapy and face more serious threats to their future fertility. The impact of chemotherapy on fertility depends on the woman's baseline ovarian reserve, and the initial evaluation should include an assessment of ovarian function through blood testing or an ultrasound-guided antral follicle count or both.[222] Patients anticipating treatment with an alkylating agent, including cyclophosphamide, run a high risk of ovarian toxicity and menopause as a result of their treatment. The options for fertility preservation for these women are varied and must take each patient and her tumor biology into account. One option involves delay of treatment to undergo a cycle of hormone stimulation and retrieval of oocytes. This approach may be less favorable for women with hormonally sensitive estrogen receptor/PR–positive tumors. Recent data suggest that exogenous estrogens can have an indirect mitogenic effect on hormone receptor-negative tumors, potentially making hormone stimulation oncologically unfavorable for these women.[223]

Another fertility preservation technique that does not require exposure to exogenous hormones is ovarian tissue retrieval. Once the ovarian tissue is retrieved, oocytes can be aspirated from the ovary and cryopreserved, or ovarian cortical tissue strips can be preserved.[224] Ovarian cortical tissue can be used for subsequent retransplantation, but this procedure is considered suboptimal because it carries a risk of reintroducing cancer cells to the patient. Another option in which the patient is not exposed to whole pieces of retransplanted tissue is still an experimental procedure called "in follicle maturation." This procedure entails recovering immature follicles from cryopreserved ovarian tissue, growing and maturing the oocytes in vitro, and then using them for in vitro fertilization. This procedure has been successful in animal models and shows promise in human tissue studies.[225,226]

SUMMARY

As technology advances, our understanding of the complex mechanisms of breast cancer pathogenesis evolves. This improved understanding can translate directly into improved diagnostics and therapeutics. Several recent impactful changes have occurred in the management of breast cancer, including the implementation of SLNB and the use of trastuzumab. The future holds great promise for a less morbid approach to the treatment of disease with the implementation of gene arrays to refine treatment planning and simultaneously minimize systemic toxicity. A vaccine against HER-2–positive breast cancer also may be on the horizon. As clinical practice and scientific discovery continue to progress, there is just cause for optimism as we approach the next decade of breast cancer care.

REFERENCES

1. Jemal A, Siegel R, Ward E, et al. Cancer statistics 2007. CA Cancer J Clin 2007; 57(1):43–66.
2. National Cancer Institute Web site. Available at: http://www.cancer.gov. Accessed July 1, 2008.
3. National Institutes of Health Web site. Available at: http://www.nih.gov. Accessed July 1, 2008.
4. National Cancer Institute Breast Cancer Risk Assessment. Available at: http://www.cancer.gov/bcrisktool. Accessed July 1, 2008.
5. Humphrey LL, Helfand M, Chan BK, et al. Breast cancer screening: a summary of the evidence for the US Preventive Services Task Force. Ann Intern Med 2002; 137(5 Pt 1):347–60.
6. Pisano ED, Gatsonis C, Hendrick E, et al. Diagnostic performance of digital versus film mammography for breast-cancer screening. N Engl J Med 2005; 353(17):1773–83.
7. Pisano ED, Hendrick RE, Yaffe MJ, et al. Diagnostic accuracy of digital versus film mammography: exploratory analysis of selected population subgroups in DMIST. Radiology 2008;246(2):376–83.
8. American Cancer Society. Breast cancer facts & figures 2007–2008. Atlanta (GA): American Cancer Society, Inc.; 2007.
9. Yang W, Dempsey PJ. Diagnostic breast ultrasound: current status and future directions. Radiol Clin North Am 2007;45(5):845–61.
10. Blair S, McElroy M, Middleton MS, et al. The efficacy of breast MRI in predicting breast conservation therapy. J Surg Oncol 2006;94(3):220–5.
11. van den Bosch MA, Daniel BL, Mariano MN, et al. Magnetic resonance imaging characteristics of fibrocystic change of the breast. Invest Radiol 2005;40(7): 436–41.
12. Kuhl CK. MRI of breast tumors. Eur Radiol 2000;10(1):46–58.
13. Kuhl C, Kuhn W, Braun M, et al. Pre-operative staging of breast cancer with breast MRI: one step forward, two steps back? Breast 2007;16(Suppl 2):S34–44.
14. Fischer U, Zachariae O, Baum F, et al. The influence of preoperative MRI of the breasts on recurrence rate in patients with breast cancer. Eur Radiol 2004; 14(10):1725–31.

15. Lehman CD, Gatsonis C, Kuhl CK, et al. MRI evaluation of the contralateral breast in women with recently diagnosed breast cancer. N Engl J Med 2007; 356(13):1295–303.
16. Fletcher SW, Black W, Harris R, et al. Report of the international workshop on screening for breast cancer. J Natl Cancer Inst 1993;85(20):1644–56.
17. Boetes C, Veltman J, van Die L, et al. The role of MRI in invasive lobular carcinoma. Breast Cancer Res Treat 2004;86(1):31–7.
18. Kriege M, Brekelmans CT, Boetes C, et al. Efficacy of MRI and mammography for breast-cancer screening in women with a familial or genetic predisposition. N Engl J Med 2004;351(5):427–37.
19. Leach MO, Boggis CR, Dixon AK, et al. Screening with magnetic resonance imaging and mammography of a UK population at high familial risk of breast cancer: a prospective multicentre cohort study (MARIBS). Lancet 2005; 365(9473):1769–78.
20. Plevritis SK, Kurian AW, Sigal BM, et al. Cost-effectiveness of screening BRCA1/2 mutation carriers with breast magnetic resonance imaging. JAMA 2006;295(20): 2374–84.
21. Saslow D, Boetes C, Burke W, et al. American Cancer Society guidelines for breast screening with MRI as an adjunct to mammography. CA Cancer J Clin 2007;57(2):75–89.
22. Tafra L. Positron emission tomography (PET) and mammography (PEM) for breast cancer: importance to surgeons. Ann Surg Oncol 2007;14(1):3–13.
23. Samson DJ, Flamm CR, Pisano ED, et al. Should FDG PET be used to decide whether a patient with an abnormal mammogram or breast finding at physical examination should undergo biopsy? Acad Radiol 2002;9(7):773–83.
24. Eubank WB, Mankoff DA. Evolving role of positron emission tomography in breast cancer imaging. Semin Nucl Med 2005;35(2):84–99.
25. Kumar R, Chauhan A, Zhuang H, et al. Clinicopathologic factors associated with false negative FDG-PET in primary breast cancer. Breast Cancer Res Treat 2006;98(3):267–74.
26. Rosen EL, Eubank WB, Mankoff DA. FDG PET, PET/CT, and breast cancer imaging. Radiographics 2007;27(Suppl 1):S215–29.
27. Tafra L, Cheng Z, Uddo J, et al. Pilot clinical trial of 18F-fluorodeoxyglucose positron-emission mammography in the surgical management of breast cancer. Am J Surg 2005;190(4):628–32.
28. Wahl RL, Siegel BA, Coleman RE, et al. Prospective multicenter study of axillary nodal staging by positron emission tomography in breast cancer: a report of the staging breast cancer with PET study group. J Clin Oncol 2004;22(2):277–85.
29. Chung A, Liou D, Karlan S, et al. Preoperative FDG-PET for axillary metastases in patients with breast cancer. Arch Surg 2006;141(8):783–8 [discussion: 8–9].
30. Byrne AM, Hill AD, Skehan SJ, et al. Positron emission tomography in the staging and management of breast cancer. Br J Surg 2004;91(11):1398–409.
31. Tatsumi M, Cohade C, Mourtzikos KA, et al. Initial experience with FDG-PET/CT in the evaluation of breast cancer. Eur J Nucl Med Mol Imaging 2006;33(3):254–62.
32. Eubank WB, Mankoff DA. Current and future uses of positron emission tomography in breast cancer imaging. Semin Nucl Med 2004;34(3):224–40.
33. Radan L, Ben-Haim S, Bar-Shalom R, et al. The role of FDG-PET/CT in suspected recurrence of breast cancer. Cancer 2006;107(11):2545–51.
34. Berriolo-Riedinger A, Touzery C, Riedinger JM, et al. [18F]FDG-PET predicts complete pathological response of breast cancer to neoadjuvant chemotherapy. Eur J Nucl Med Mol Imaging 2007;34(12):1915–24.

35. Poggi MM, Danforth DN, Sciuto LC, et al. Eighteen-year results in the treatment of early breast carcinoma with mastectomy versus breast conservation therapy: the National Cancer Institute Randomized Trial. Cancer 2003;98(4):697–702.

36. Fisher B, Anderson S, Bryant J, et al. Twenty-year follow-up of a randomized trial comparing total mastectomy, lumpectomy, and lumpectomy plus irradiation for the treatment of invasive breast cancer. N Engl J Med 2002;347(16):1233–41.

37. Singletary SE. Surgical margins in patients with early-stage breast cancer treated with breast conservation therapy. Am J Surg 2002;184(5):383–93.

38. Clarke M, Collins R, Darby S, et al. Effects of radiotherapy and of differences in the extent of surgery for early breast cancer on local recurrence and 15-year survival: an overview of the randomised trials. Lancet 2005;366(9503):2087–106.

39. Wapnir IL, Anderson SJ, Mamounas EP, et al. Prognosis after ipsilateral breast tumor recurrence and locoregional recurrences in five National Surgical Adjuvant Breast and Bowel Project node-positive adjuvant breast cancer trials. J Clin Oncol 2006;24(13):2028–37.

40. Fisher B, Jeong JH, Anderson S, et al. Twenty-five-year follow-up of a randomized trial comparing radical mastectomy, total mastectomy, and total mastectomy followed by irradiation. N Engl J Med 2002;347(8):567–75.

41. Singletary SE, Robb GL. Oncologic safety of skin-sparing mastectomy. Ann Surg Oncol 2003;10(2):95–7.

42. Chagpar AB. Skin-sparing and nipple-sparing mastectomy: preoperative, intraoperative, and postoperative considerations. Am Surg 2004;70(5):425–32.

43. Fisher ER, Gregorio RM, Fisher B, et al. The pathology of invasive breast cancer: a syllabus derived from findings of the National Surgical Adjuvant Breast Project (protocol no. 4). Cancer 1975;36(1):1–85.

44. Wertheim U, Ozzello L. Neoplastic involvement of nipple and skin flap in carcinoma of the breast. Am J Surg Pathol 1980;4(6):543–9.

45. Ho CM, Mak CK, Lau Y, et al. Skin involvement in invasive breast carcinoma: safety of skin-sparing mastectomy. Ann Surg Oncol 2003;10(2):102–7.

46. Carlson GW, Bostwick J III, Styblo TM, et al. Skin-sparing mastectomy: oncologic and reconstructive considerations. Ann Surg 1997;225(5):570–5 [discussion: 5–8].

47. Kroll SS, Khoo A, Singletary SE, et al. Local recurrence risk after skin-sparing and conventional mastectomy: a 6-year follow-up. Plast Reconstr Surg 1999; 104(2):421–5.

48. Newman LA, Kuerer HM, Hunt KK, et al. Presentation, treatment, and outcome of local recurrence after skin-sparing mastectomy and immediate breast reconstruction. Ann Surg Oncol 1998;5(7):620–6.

49. Kroll SS, Schusterman MA, Tadjalli HE, et al. Risk of recurrence after treatment of early breast cancer with skin-sparing mastectomy. Ann Surg Oncol 1997;4(3):193–7.

50. Rivadeneira DE, Simmons RM, Fish SK, et al. Skin-sparing mastectomy with immediate breast reconstruction: a critical analysis of local recurrence. Cancer J 2000;6(5):331–5.

51. Simmons RM, Fish SK, Gayle L, et al. Local and distant recurrence rates in skin-sparing mastectomies compared with non-skin-sparing mastectomies. Ann Surg Oncol 1999;6(7):676–81.

52. Carlson GW, Styblo TM, Lyles RH, et al. Local recurrence after skin-sparing mastectomy: tumor biology or surgical conservatism? Ann Surg Oncol 2003;10(2):108–12.

53. Cunnick GH, Mokbel K. Skin-sparing mastectomy. Am J Surg 2004;188(1):78–84.

54. Garcia-Etienne CA, Borgen PI. Update on the indications for nipple-sparing mastectomy. J Support Oncol 2006;4(5):225–30.

55. Laronga C, Kemp B, Johnston D, et al. The incidence of occult nipple-areola complex involvement in breast cancer patients receiving a skin-sparing mastectomy. Ann Surg Oncol 1999;6(6):609–13.

56. Opatt D, Morrow M. The dual role of nipple preservation. J Support Oncol 2006; 4(5):233–4.

57. Petit JY, Veronesi U, Orecchia R, et al. Nipple-sparing mastectomy in association with intraoperative radiotherapy (ELIOT): a new type of mastectomy for breast cancer treatment. Breast Cancer Res Treat 2006;96(1):47–51.

58. Crowe JP Jr, Kim JA, Yetman R, et al. Nipple-sparing mastectomy: technique and results of 54 procedures. Arch Surg 2004;139(2):148–50.

59. Gerber B, Krause A, Reimer T, et al. Skin-sparing mastectomy with conservation of the nipple-areola complex and autologous reconstruction is an oncologically safe procedure. Ann Surg 2003;238(1):120–7.

60. Simmons RM, Brennan M, Christos P, et al. Analysis of nipple/areolar involvement with mastectomy: can the areola be preserved? Ann Surg Oncol 2002;9(2):165–8.

61. Stolier AJ, Grube BJ. Areola-sparing mastectomy: defining the risks. J Am Coll Surg 2005;201(1):118–24.

62. Simmons RM, Hollenbeck ST, Latrenta GS. Two-year follow-up of areola-sparing mastectomy with immediate reconstruction. Am J Surg 2004; 188(4):403–6.

63. Zakaria S, Degnim AC. Prophylactic mastectomy. Surg Clin North Am 2007; 87(2):317–31.

64. National Cancer Institute statistics. Available at: http://www.cancer.gov/cancertopics/type/breast. Accessed July 1, 2008.

65. Harris RE, Lynch HT, Guirgis HA. Familial breast cancer: risk to the contralateral breast. J Natl Cancer Inst 1978;60(5):955–60.

66. Rosen PP, Groshen S, Kinne DW. Prognosis in T2N0M0 stage I breast carcinoma: a 20-year follow-up study. J Clin Oncol 1991;9(9):1650–61.

67. Rosen PP, Groshen S, Kinne DW, et al. Contralateral breast carcinoma: an assessment of risk and prognosis in stage I (T1N0M0) and stage II (T1N1M0) patients with 20-year follow-up. Surgery 1989;106(5):904–10.

68. Rebbeck TR, Friebel T, Lynch HT, et al. Bilateral prophylactic mastectomy reduces breast cancer risk in BRCA1 and BRCA2 mutation carriers: the PROSE Study Group. J Clin Oncol 2004;22(6):1055–62.

69. Grann VR, Jacobson JS, Thomason D, et al. Effect of prevention strategies on survival and quality-adjusted survival of women with BRCA1/2 mutations: an updated decision analysis. J Clin Oncol 2002;20(10):2520–9.

70. Metcalfe K, Lynch HT, Ghadirian P, et al. Contralateral breast cancer in BRCA1 and BRCA2 mutation carriers. J Clin Oncol 2004;22(12):2328–35.

71. van Sprundel TC, Schmidt MK, Rookus MA, et al. Risk reduction of contralateral breast cancer and survival after contralateral prophylactic mastectomy in BRCA1 or BRCA2 mutation carriers. Br J Cancer 2005;93(3):287–92.

72. Guillem JG, Wood WC, Moley JF, et al. ASCO/SSO review of current role of risk-reducing surgery in common hereditary cancer syndromes. J Clin Oncol 2006; 24(28):4642–60.

73. Narod SA, Brunet JS, Ghadirian P, et al. Tamoxifen and risk of contralateral breast cancer in BRCA1 and BRCA2 mutation carriers: a case-control study. Hereditary Breast Cancer Clinical Study Group. Lancet 2000;356(9245):1876–81.

74. Consensus statement on guidelines for performing sentinel lymph node dissection in breast cancer. 2005. Available at: http://www.breastsurgeons.org/slnd.shtml. Accessed July 1, 2008.

75. Schijven MP, Vingerhoets AJ, Rutten HJ, et al. Comparison of morbidity between axillary lymph node dissection and sentinel node biopsy. Eur J Surg Oncol 2003; 29(4):341–50.

76. Lyman GH, Giuliano AE, Somerfield MR, et al. American Society of Clinical Oncology guideline recommendations for sentinel lymph node biopsy in early-stage breast cancer. J Clin Oncol 2005;23(30):7703–20.

77. Krag DN, Anderson SJ, Julian TB, et al. Technical outcomes of sentinel-lymph-node resection and conventional axillary-lymph-node dissection in patients with clinically node-negative breast cancer: results from the NSABP B-32 randomised phase III trial. Lancet Oncol 2007;8(10):881–8.

78. Singletary SE, Allred C, Ashley P, et al. Revision of the American Joint Committee on cancer staging system for breast cancer. J Clin Oncol 2002;20(17): 3628–36.

79. Singletary SE, Greene FL. Revision of breast cancer staging: the 6th edition of the TNM classification. Semin Surg Oncol 2003;21(1):53–9.

80. Brogi E, Torres-Matundan E, Tan LK, et al. The results of frozen section, touch preparation, and cytological smear are comparable for intraoperative examination of sentinel lymph nodes: a study in 133 breast cancer patients. Ann Surg Oncol 2005;12(2):173–80.

81. Cserni G, Gregori D, Merletti F, et al. Meta-analysis of non-sentinel node metastases associated with micrometastatic sentinel nodes in breast cancer. Br J Surg 2004;91(10):1245–52.

82. van Rijk MC, Peterse JL, Nieweg OE, et al. Additional axillary metastases and stage migration in breast cancer patients with micrometastases or submicrometastases in sentinel lymph nodes. Cancer 2006;107(3):467–71.

83. Rutgers EJ. Sentinel node biopsy: interpretation and management of patients with immunohistochemistry-positive sentinel nodes and those with micrometastases. J Clin Oncol 2008;26(5):698–702.

84. Schwartz GF, Giuliano AE, Veronesi U. Proceedings of the consensus conference on the role of sentinel lymph node biopsy in carcinoma of the breast, April 19–22, 2001, Philadelphia, Pennsylvania. Cancer 2002; 94(10):2542–51.

85. Hansen NM, Grube BJ, Ye C, et al. The impact of micrometastases in the sentinel nodes of patients with invasive breast cancer. Breast Cancer Res Treat 2007; 106(Suppl 1):S15.

86. Chen SL, Hoehne FM, Giuliano AE. The prognostic significance of micrometastases in breast cancer: a SEER population-based analysis. Ann Surg Oncol 2007;14(12):3378–84.

87. Grube BJ, Giuliano AE. Observation of the breast cancer patient with a tumor-positive sentinel node: implications of the ACOSOG Z0011 trial. Semin Surg Oncol 2001;20(3):230–7.

88. Fant JS, Grant MD, Knox SM, et al. Preliminary outcome analysis in patients with breast cancer and a positive sentinel lymph node who declined axillary dissection. Ann Surg Oncol 2003;10(2):126–30.

89. Hwang RF, Gonzalez-Angulo AM, Yi M, et al. Low locoregional failure rates in selected breast cancer patients with tumor-positive sentinel lymph nodes who do not undergo completion axillary dissection. Cancer 2007;110(4):723–30.

90. Jeruss JS, Winchester DJ, Sener SF, et al. Axillary recurrence after sentinel node biopsy. Ann Surg Oncol 2005;12(1):34–40.

91. Naik AM, Fey J, Gemignani M, et al. The risk of axillary relapse after sentinel lymph node biopsy for breast cancer is comparable with that of axillary lymph

node dissection: a follow-up study of 4008 procedures. Ann Surg 2004;240(3): 462–8 [discussion: 8–71].

92. Van Zee/Memorial Sloan-Kettering Breast Cancer Nomogram. 2008. Available at: http://www.mskcc.org/mskcc/html/15938.cfm. Accessed July 1, 2008.

93. Van Zee KJ, Manasseh DM, Bevilacqua JL, et al. A nomogram for predicting the likelihood of additional nodal metastases in breast cancer patients with a positive sentinel node biopsy. Ann Surg Oncol 2003;10(10):1140–51.

94. Soran A, Evrensel T, Ahrendt G, et al. Use of the breast cancer nomogram to predict non-sentinel nodal positivity in patients having received pre-operative chemotherapy. Ann Surg Oncol 2007;14(1):165.

95. Xing Y, Foy M, Cox DD, et al. Meta-analysis of sentinel lymph node biopsy after pre-operative chemotherapy in patients with breast cancer. Br J Surg 2006;93(5):539–46.

96. Jeruss JS, Newman LA, Ayers GD, et al. Factors predicting additional disease in the axilla in patients with positive sentinel lymph nodes after neoadjuvant chemotherapy. Cancer 2008;112(12):2646–54.

97. Greene FL, Page DL, Fleming ID, et al, editors. AJCC cancer staging manual. 6th edition. New York: Springer; 2002. p. 221.

98. Benson JR, Querci della Rovere G. Management of the axilla in women with breast cancer. Breast 2007;16(2):130–6.

99. Sosa JA, Diener-West M, Gusev Y, et al. Association between extent of axillary lymph node dissection and survival in patients with stage I breast cancer. Ann Surg Oncol 1998;5(2):140–9.

100. Orr RK. The impact of prophylactic axillary node dissection on breast cancer survival: a Bayesian meta-analysis. Ann Surg Oncol 1999;6(1):109–16.

101. Cady B. Case against axillary lymphadenectomy for most patients with infiltrating breast cancer. J Surg Oncol 1997;66(1):7–10.

102. Khan SA. Does resection of an intact breast primary improve survival in metastatic breast cancer? Oncology (Williston Park) 2007;21(8):924–31 [discussion: 31–2, 34, 42, passim].

103. Babiera GV, Rao R, Feng L, et al. Effect of primary tumor extirpation in breast cancer patients who present with stage IV disease and an intact primary tumor. Ann Surg Oncol 2006;13(6):776–82.

104. Blanchard DK, Shetty PB, Hilsenbeck SG, et al. Association of surgery with improved survival in stage IV breast cancer patients. Ann Surg 2008;247(5):732–8.

105. Gnerlich J, Jeffe DB, Deshpande AD, et al. Surgical removal of the primary tumor increases overall survival in patients with metastatic breast cancer: analysis of the 1988-2003 SEER data. Ann Surg Oncol 2007;14(8):2187–94.

106. Newman LA, Mamounas EP. Review of breast cancer clinical trials conducted by the National Surgical Adjuvant Breast Project. Surg Clin North Am 2007; 87(2):279–305.

107. Fisher B, Bryant J, Dignam JJ, et al. Tamoxifen, radiation therapy, or both for prevention of ipsilateral breast tumor recurrence after lumpectomy in women with invasive breast cancers of one centimeter or less. J Clin Oncol 2002;20(20):4141–9.

108. Goyal S, Kearney T, Haffty BG. Current application and research directions for partial-breast irradiation. Oncology (Williston Park) 2007;21(4):449–61 [discussion: 61–2, 64, 70].

109. Hughes KS, Schnaper LA, Berry D, et al. Lumpectomy plus tamoxifen with or without irradiation in women 70 years of age or older with early breast cancer. N Engl J Med 2004;351(10):971–7.

110. Smith BD, Gross CP, Smith GL, et al. Effectiveness of radiation therapy for older women with early breast cancer. J Natl Cancer Inst 2006;98(10):681–90.

111. Arthur DW, Koo D, Zwicker RD, et al. Partial breast brachytherapy after lumpectomy: low-dose-rate and high-dose-rate experience. Int J Radiat Oncol Biol Phys 2003;56(3):681–9.

112. Morrow M, Strom EA, Bassett LW, et al. Standard for the management of ductal carcinoma in situ of the breast (DCIS). CA Cancer J Clin 2002;52(5):256–76.

113. Pawlik TM, Buchholz TA, Kuerer HM. The biologic rationale for and emerging role of accelerated partial breast irradiation for breast cancer. J Am Coll Surg 2004;199(3):479–92.

114. Polgar C, Major T, Fodor J, et al. High-dose-rate brachytherapy alone versus whole breast radiotherapy with or without tumor bed boost after breast-conserving surgery: seven-year results of a comparative study. Int J Radiat Oncol Biol Phys 2004;60(4):1173–81.

115. Jeruss JS, Vicini FA, Beitsch PD, et al. Initial outcomes for patients treated on the American Society of Breast Surgeons MammoSite clinical trial for ductal carcinoma-in-situ of the breast. Ann Surg Oncol 2006;13(7):967–76.

116. Sanders ME, Scroggins T, Ampil FL, et al. Accelerated partial breast irradiation in early-stage breast cancer. J Clin Oncol 2007;25(8):996–1002.

117. Taghian AG, Recht A. Update on accelerated partial-breast irradiation. Curr Oncol Rep 2006;8(1):35–41.

118. Patel RR, Arthur DW. The emergence of advanced brachytherapy techniques for common malignancies. Hematol Oncol Clin North Am 2006;20(1):97–118.

119. Keisch M, Vicini F, Kuske RR, et al. Initial clinical experience with the MammoSite breast brachytherapy applicator in women with early-stage breast cancer treated with breast-conserving therapy. Int J Radiat Oncol Biol Phys 2003;55(2):289–93.

120. Pawlik TM, Perry A, Strom EA, et al. Potential applicability of balloon catheter-based accelerated partial breast irradiation after conservative surgery for breast carcinoma. Cancer 2004;100(3):490–8.

121. Keisch M, Vicini F, Scroggins T, et al. Thirty-nine month results with MammoSite brachytherapy applicator: details regarding cosmesis, toxicity and local control in partial breast irradiation. Int J Radiat Oncol Biol Phys 2005;63(2):S6.

122. Veronesi U, Arnone P, Veronesi P, et al. The value of radiotherapy on metastatic internal mammary nodes in breast cancer: results on a large series. Ann Oncol 2008;19(9):1553–60.

123. Arthur D. Accelerated partial breast irradiation: a change in treatment paradigm for early stage breast cancer. J Surg Oncol 2003;84(4):185–91.

124. Consensus Statement for Accelerated Partial Breast Irradiation. 2005. Available at: http://www.breastsurgeons.org/apbi.shtml. Accessed July 1, 2008.

125. Vicini F, Arthur D, Polgar C, et al. Defining the efficacy of accelerated partial breast irradiation: the importance of proper patient selection, optimal quality assurance, and common sense. Int J Radiat Oncol Biol Phys 2003;57(5):1210–3.

126. Lee MC, Jagsi R. Postmastectomy radiation therapy: indications and controversies. Surg Clin North Am 2007;87(2):511–26.

127. Early Breast Cancer Trialists' Collaborative Group.Effects of radiotherapy and surgery in early breast cancer: an overview of the randomized trials. Early Breast Cancer Trialists' Collaborative Group. N Engl J Med 1995;333(22):1444–55.

128. Recht A, Edge SB, Solin LJ, et al. Postmastectomy radiotherapy: clinical practice guidelines of the American Society of Clinical Oncology. J Clin Oncol 2001;19(5):1539–69.

129. Pierce LJ. The use of radiotherapy after mastectomy: a review of the literature. J Clin Oncol 2005;23(8):1706–17.

130. Buchholz TA, Tucker SL, Masullo L, et al. Predictors of local-regional recurrence after neoadjuvant chemotherapy and mastectomy without radiation. J Clin Oncol 2002;20(1):17–23.
131. Bear HD, Anderson S, Smith RE, et al. Sequential preoperative or postoperative docetaxel added to preoperative doxorubicin plus cyclophosphamide for operable breast cancer: National Surgical Adjuvant Breast and Bowel project protocol B-27. J Clin Oncol 2006;24(13):2019–27.
132. Fisher B, Brown A, Mamounas E, et al. Effect of preoperative chemotherapy on local-regional disease in women with operable breast cancer: findings from National Surgical Adjuvant Breast and Bowel project B-18. J Clin Oncol 1997; 15(7):2483–93.
133. Fisher ER, Wang J, Bryant J, et al. Pathobiology of preoperative chemotherapy: findings from the National Surgical Adjuvant Breast and Bowel (NSABP) protocol B-18. Cancer 2002;95(4):681–95.
134. Buchholz TA, Lehman CD, Harris JR, et al. Statement of the science concerning locoregional treatments after preoperative chemotherapy for breast cancer: a National Cancer Institute conference. J Clin Oncol 2008;26(5): 791–7.
135. Carlson RW, Allred C, Andersen BO, et al. Members NBCP. NCCN clinical practice guidelines in oncology: breast cancer. Proceedings of the American Society of Clinical Oncology; 2008.
136. Oncotype DX. Genomic Health, Inc. 2008. Available at: http://www.genomi chealth.com/oncotype/. Accessed July 1, 2008.
137. Ravdin PM, Siminoff LA, Davis GJ, et al. Computer program to assist in making decisions about adjuvant therapy for women with early breast cancer. J Clin Oncol 2001;19(4):980–91.
138. Olivotto IA, Bajdik CD, Ravdin PM, et al. Population-based validation of the prognostic model ADJUVANT! for early breast cancer. J Clin Oncol 2005; 23(12):2716–25.
139. Early Breast Cancer Trialists' Collaborative Group. Polychemotherapy for early breast cancer: an overview of the randomised trials. Lancet 1998;352(9132): 930–42.
140. Early Breast Cancer Trialists' Collaborative Group. Effects of chemotherapy and hormonal therapy for early breast cancer on recurrence and 15-year survival: an overview of the randomised trials. Lancet 2005;365(9472):1687–717.
141. Berry DA, Cirrincione C, Henderson IC, et al. Estrogen-receptor status and outcomes of modern chemotherapy for patients with node-positive breast cancer. JAMA 2006;295(14):1658–67.
142. Dressler LG, Berry DA, Broadwater G, et al. Comparison of HER2 status by fluorescence in situ hybridization and immunohistochemistry to predict benefit from dose escalation of adjuvant doxorubicin-based therapy in node-positive breast cancer patients. J Clin Oncol 2005;23(19):4287–97.
143. Yamashiro H, Toi M. Update of evidence in chemotherapy for breast cancer. Int J Clin Oncol 2008;13(1):3–7.
144. Henderson IC, Berry DA, Demetri GD, et al. Improved outcomes from adding sequential paclitaxel but not from escalating doxorubicin dose in an adjuvant chemotherapy regimen for patients with node-positive primary breast cancer. J Clin Oncol 2003;21(6):976–83.
145. Mamounas EP, Bryant J, Lembersky B, et al. Paclitaxel after doxorubicin plus cyclophosphamide as adjuvant chemotherapy for node-positive breast cancer: results from NSABP B-28. J Clin Oncol 2005;23(16):3686–96.

146. Nabholtz J, Pienkowski T, mackey J, et al. Phase III trial comparing TAC (docetaxel, doxorubicin, cyclophosphamide) with FAC (5-fluorouracil, doxorubicin, cyclophosphamide) in adjuvant treatment of node positive breast cancer (BC) patients: interim analysis of the BCIRG 001 study. Proc Am Soc Clin Oncol 2002;21:141 [abstract].

147. Sparano JA, Wang M, Martino S, et al. Weekly paclitaxel in the adjuvant treatment of breast cancer. N Engl J Med 2008;358(16):1663–71.

148. Bhattacharyya A, Ear US, Koller BH, et al. The breast cancer susceptibility gene BRCA1 is required for subnuclear assembly of Rad51 and survival following treatment with the DNA cross-linking agent cisplatin. J Biolumin Chemilumin 2000;275(31):23899–903.

149. Fisher B, Bryant J, Wolmark N, et al. Effect of preoperative chemotherapy on the outcome of women with operable breast cancer. J Clin Oncol 1998;16(8):2672–85.

150. Smith IC, Heys SD, Hutcheon AW, et al. Neoadjuvant chemotherapy in breast cancer: significantly enhanced response with docetaxel. J Clin Oncol 2002; 20(6):1456–66.

151. Guarneri V, Frassoldati A, Giovannelli S, et al. Primary systemic therapy for operable breast cancer: a review of clinical trials and perspectives. Cancer Lett 2007;248(2):175–85.

152. Mauri D, Pavlidis N, Ioannidis JP. Neoadjuvant versus adjuvant systemic treatment in breast cancer: a meta-analysis. J Natl Cancer Inst 2005;97(3):188–94.

153. Mieog JS, van der Hage JA, van de Velde CJ. Neoadjuvant chemotherapy for operable breast cancer. Br J Surg 2007;94(10):1189–200.

154. Jeruss JS, Mittendorf EA, Tucker SL, et al. Staging of breast cancer in the neoadjuvant setting. Cancer Res 2008;68(16):6477–81.

155. Jeruss JS, Mittendorf EA, Tucker SL, et al. Combined use of clinical and pathologic staging variables to define outcomes for breast cancer patients treated with neoadjuvant therapy. J Clin Oncol 2008;26(2):246–52.

156. Engel RH, Kaklamani VG. HER2-positive breast cancer: current and future treatment strategies. Drugs 2007;67(9):1329–41.

157. Bange J, Zwick E, Ullrich A. Molecular targets for breast cancer therapy and prevention. Nat Med 2001;7(5):548–52.

158. Carter P, Presta L, Gorman CM, et al. Humanization of an anti-p185HER2 antibody for human cancer therapy. Proc Natl Acad Sci U S A 1992;89(10):4285–9.

159. Henson ES, Hu X, Gibson SB. Herceptin sensitizes ErbB2-overexpressing cells to apoptosis by reducing antiapoptotic Mcl-1 expression. Clin Cancer Res 2006; 12(3 Pt 1):845–53.

160. Slamon DJ, Leyland-Jones B, Shak S, et al. Use of chemotherapy plus a monoclonal antibody against HER2 for metastatic breast cancer that overexpresses HER2. N Engl J Med 2001;344(11):783–92.

161. Romond EH, Perez EA, Bryant J, et al. Trastuzumab plus adjuvant chemotherapy for operable HER2-positive breast cancer. N Engl J Med 2005;353(16): 1673–84.

162. Piccart-Gebhart MJ, Procter M, Leyland-Jones B, et al. Trastuzumab after adjuvant chemotherapy in HER2-positive breast cancer. N Engl J Med 2005;353(16): 1659–72.

163. Slamon DJ, Eiermann W, Robert NJ, et al. Phase III randomized trial comparing doxorubicin and cyclophosphamide followed by docetaxel (AC®T) with doxorubicin and cyclophosphamide followed by docetaxel and trastuzumab (AC®TH) with docetaxel, carboplatin and trastuzumab (TCH) in HER2 positive early breast cancer patients: BCIRG 006 study. Breast Cancer Res Treat 2005;94:S5.

164. Joensuu H, Kellokumpu-Lehtinen PL, Bono P, et al. Adjuvant docetaxel or vinorelbine with or without trastuzumab for breast cancer. N Engl J Med 2006;354(8):809–20.
165. Tan-Chiu E, Yothers G, Romond E, et al. Assessment of cardiac dysfunction in a randomized trial comparing doxorubicin and cyclophosphamide followed by paclitaxel, with or without trastuzumab as adjuvant therapy in node-positive, human epidermal growth factor receptor 2-overexpressing breast cancer: NSABP B-31. J Clin Oncol 2005;23(31):7811–9.
166. Nahta R, Esteva FJ. HER2 therapy: molecular mechanisms of trastuzumab resistance. Breast Cancer Res 2006;8(6):215.
167. Longo R, Torino F, Gasparini G. Targeted therapy of breast cancer. Curr Pharm Des 2007;13(5):497–517.
168. Konecny GE, Pegram MD, Venkatesan N, et al. Activity of the dual kinase inhibitor lapatinib (GW572016) against HER-2-overexpressing and trastuzumab-treated breast cancer cells. Cancer Res 2006;66(3):1630–9.
169. Lin NU, Carey LA, Liu MC, et al. Phase II trial of lapatinib for brain metastases in patients with HER2+ breast cancer. J Clin Oncol 2006;24(18S):503.
170. Geyer CE, Forster J, Lindquist D, et al. Lapatinib plus capecitabine for HER2-positive advanced breast cancer. N Engl J Med 2006;355(26):2733–43.
171. Mayer EL, Lin NU, Burstein HJ. Novel approaches to advanced breast cancer: bevacizumab and lapatinib. J Natl Compr Canc Netw 2007;5(3):314–23.
172. Roy V, Pockaj BA, Northfelt DW, et al. N0338 phase II trial of docetaxel and carboplatin administered every two weeks as induction therapy for stage II or III breast cancer. J Clin Oncol 2008;26(15S):563.
173. Early Breast Cancer Trialists' Collaborative Group. Tamoxifen for early breast cancer: an overview of the randomised trials. Lancet 1998;351(9114):1451–67.
174. Mincey BA, Palmieri FM, Perez EA. Adjuvant therapy for breast cancer: recommendations for management based on consensus review and recent clinical trials. Oncologist 2002;7(3):246–50.
175. Howell A, Cuzick J, Baum M, et al. Results of the ATAC (Arimidex, Tamoxifen, Alone or in Combination) trial after completion of 5 years' adjuvant treatment for breast cancer. Lancet 2005;365(9453):60–2.
176. Coombes RC, Hall E, Gibson LJ, et al. A randomized trial of exemestane after two to three years of tamoxifen therapy in postmenopausal women with primary breast cancer. N Engl J Med 2004;350(11):1081–92.
177. Goss PE, Ingle JN, Martino S, et al. A randomized trial of letrozole in postmenopausal women after five years of tamoxifen therapy for early-stage breast cancer. N Engl J Med 2003;349(19):1793–802.
178. Vogel VG, Costantino JP, Wickerham DL, et al. Effects of tamoxifen versus raloxifene on the risk of developing invasive breast cancer and other disease outcomes: the NSABP Study of Tamoxifen and Raloxifene (STAR) P-2 trial. JAMA 2006;295(23):2727–41.
179. Folkman J. Tumor angiogenesis: therapeutic implications. N Engl J Med 1971;285(21):1182–6.
180. Salter JT, Miller KD. Antiangiogenic agents in breast cancer. Cancer Invest 2007;25(7):518–26.
181. Ferrara N, Davis-Smyth T. The biology of vascular endothelial growth factor. Endocr Rev 1997;18(1):4–25.
182. Heer K, Kumar H, Read JR, et al. Serum vascular endothelial growth factor in breast cancer: its relation with cancer type and estrogen receptor status. Clin Cancer Res 2001;7(11):3491–4.

183. Ragaz J, Miller K, Badve S, et al. Adverse association of expressed vascular endothelial growth factor (VEGF) with long-term outcome of stage I-III breast cancer (BrCa), with co-expression data of VEGF and Her2, Cox2, uPA and ER: results from the British Columbia Tissue Microarray Project. J Clin Oncol 2004;22(14S):524.

184. Willett CG, Boucher Y, di Tomaso E, et al. Direct evidence that the VEGF-specific antibody bevacizumab has antivascular effects in human rectal cancer. Nat Med 2004;10(2):145–7.

185. Shih T, Lindley C. Bevacizumab: an angiogenesis inhibitor for the treatment of solid malignancies. Clin Ther 2006;28(11):1779–802.

186. Miller KD, Wang M, gralow J, et al. A randomized phase III trial of paclitaxel versus paclitaxel plus bevacizumab as first-line therapy for locally recurrent or metastatic breast cancer: a trial coordinated by the Eastern Cooperation Oncology Group (E2100). Br Can Res Treat 2005;94:S6.

187. Spalding BJ. Thumbs up for Avastin. Nat Biotechnol 2008;26(4):365.

188. Hayes DF, Miller K, Sledge G. Angiogenesis as targeted breast cancer therapy. Breast 2007;16(Suppl 2):S17–9.

189. Curigliano G, Rescigno M, Goldhirsch A. Immunology and breast cancer: therapeutic cancer vaccines. Breast 2007;16(Suppl 2):S20–6.

190. Rosenberg SA, Yang JC, Restifo NP. Cancer immunotherapy: moving beyond current vaccines. Nat Med 2004;10(9):909–15.

191. Mittendorf EA, Peoples GE, Singletary SE. Breast cancer vaccines: promise for the future or pipe dream? Cancer 2007;110(8):1677–86.

192. Engelhorn ME, Guevara-Patino JA, Merghoub T, et al. Mechanisms of immunization against cancer using chimeric antigens. Mol Ther 2008;16(4):773–81.

193. Chopra A, Kim TS, OS I, et al. Combined therapy of an established, highly aggressive breast cancer in mice with paclitaxel and a unique DNA-based cell vaccine. Int J Cancer 2006;118(11):2888–98.

194. Avigan D, Vasir B, Gong J, et al. Fusion cell vaccination of patients with metastatic breast and renal cancer induces immunological and clinical responses. Clin Cancer Res 2004;10(14):4699–708.

195. Bruhn KW, Craft N, Miller JF. Listeria as a vaccine vector. Microbes Infect 2007; 9(10):1226–35.

196. Collins SA, Guinn BA, Harrison PT, et al. Viral vectors in cancer immunotherapy: which vector for which strategy? Curr Gene Ther 2008;8(2):66–78.

197. Freire T, Lo-Man R, Piller F, et al. Enzymatic large-scale synthesis of MUC6-Tn glycoconjugates for antitumor vaccination. Glycobiology 2006;16(5):390–401.

198. Mittendorf EA, Holmes JP, Ponniah S, et al. The E75 HER2/neu peptide vaccine. Cancer Immunol Immunother 2008;57(10):1511–21.

199. Elder EE, Brandberg Y, Bjorklund T, et al. Quality of life and patient satisfaction in breast cancer patients after immediate breast reconstruction: a prospective study. Breast 2005;14(3):201–8.

200. Alderman AK, Hawley ST, Waljee J, et al. Understanding the impact of breast reconstruction on the surgical decision-making process for breast cancer. Cancer 2008;112(3):489–94.

201. Djohan R, Gage E, Bernard S. Breast reconstruction options following mastectomy. Cleve Clin J Med 2008;75(Suppl 1):S17–23.

202. Reavey P, McCarthy CM. Update on breast reconstruction in breast cancer. Curr Opin Obstet Gynecol 2008;20(1):61–7.

203. Zienowicz RJ, Karacaoglu E. Implant-based breast reconstruction with allograft. Plast Reconstr Surg 2007;120(2):373–81.

204. Breuing KH, Warren SM. Immediate bilateral breast reconstruction with implants and inferolateral AlloDerm slings. Ann Plast Surg 2005;55(3):232–9.
205. Warren AG, Morris DJ, Houlihan MJ, et al. Breast reconstruction in a changing breast cancer treatment paradigm. Plast Reconstr Surg 2008;121(4):1116–26.
206. FDA breast implants home page. 2006. Available at: http://www.fda.gov/cdrh/breastimplants. Accessed July 1, 2008.
207. Hansen NM, Fen JW, Fine NA, et al. Plastic surgery: a component in the comprehensive care of cancer patients. Oncology 2002;16:1685–98.
208. Ascherman JA, Hanasono MM, Newman MI, et al. Implant reconstruction in breast cancer patients treated with radiation therapy. Plast Reconstr Surg 2006;117(2):359–65.
209. Keller A. The deep inferior epigastric perforator free flap for breast reconstruction. Ann Plast Surg 2001;46(5):474–9 [discussion: 9–80].
210. Granzow JW, Levine JL, Chiu ES, et al. Breast reconstruction with gluteal artery perforator flaps. J Plast Reconstr Aesthet Surg 2006;59(6):614–21.
211. Disa JJ, McCarthy CM, Mehrara BJ, et al. Immediate latissimus dorsi/prosthetic breast reconstruction following salvage mastectomy after failed lumpectomy/ir radiation. Plast Reconstr Surg 2008;121(4):159e–64e.
212. Clough KB, Cuminet J, Fitoussi A, et al. Cosmetic sequelae after conservative treatment for breast cancer: classification and results of surgical correction. Ann Plast Surg 1998;41(5):471–81.
213. Waljee JF, Hu ES, Newman LA, et al. Predictors of breast asymmetry after breast-conserving operation for breast cancer. J Am Coll Surg 2008;206(2):274–80.
214. Bulstrode NW, Shrotria S. Prediction of cosmetic outcome following conservative breast surgery using breast volume measurements. Breast 2001;10(2):124–6.
215. Audretsch W, Rezai M, Kolotas C, et al. Tumor-specific immediate reconstruction in breast cancer patients. Perspectives in plastic surgery 1998;11:71–100.
216. Asgeirsson KS, Rasheed T, McCulley SJ, et al. Oncological and cosmetic outcomes of oncoplastic breast conserving surgery. Eur J Surg Oncol 2005;31(8):817–23.
217. Baildam AD. Oncoplastic surgery for breast cancer. Br J Surg 2008;95(1):4–5.
218. Rietjens M, Urban CA, Rey PC, et al. Long-term oncological results of breast conservative treatment with oncoplastic surgery. Breast 2007;16(4):387–95.
219. Gradishar WJ, Hellmund R. A rationale for the reinitiation of adjuvant tamoxifen therapy in women receiving fewer than 5 years of therapy. Clin Breast Cancer 2002;2(4):282–6.
220. Arnon J, Meirow D, Lewis-Roness H, et al. Genetic and teratogenic effects of cancer treatments on gametes and embryos. Hum Reprod Update 2001;7(4):394–403.
221. Falcone T, Attaran M, Bedaiwy MA, et al. Ovarian function preservation in the cancer patient. Fertil Steril 2004;81(2):243–57.
222. Lutchman Singh K, Muttukrishna S, Stein RC, et al. Predictors of ovarian reserve in young women with breast cancer. Br J Cancer 2007;96(12):1808–16.
223. Gupta PB, Kuperwasser C. Contributions of estrogen to ER-negative breast tumor growth. J Steroid Biochem Mol Biol 2006;102(1–5):71–8.
224. Lee SJ, Schover LR, Partridge AH, et al. American Society of Clinical Oncology recommendations on fertility preservation in cancer patients. J Clin Oncol 2006;24(18):2917–31.
225. Telfer EE, McLaughlin M, Ding C, et al. A two-step serum-free culture system supports development of human oocytes from primordial follicles in the presence of activin. Humanit Rep 2008;23(5):1151–8.

226. Xu M, Kreeger PK, Shea LD, et al. Tissue-engineered follicles produce live, fertile offspring. Tissue Eng 2006;12(10):2739–46.

227. Badgwell BD, Povoski SP, Abdessalam SF, et al. Patterns of recurrence after sentinel lymph node biopsy for breast cancer. Ann Surg Oncol 2003;10(4): 376–80.

228. Blanchard DK, Donohue JH, Reynolds C, et al. Relapse and morbidity in patients undergoing sentinel lymph node biopsy alone or with axillary dissection for breast cancer. Arch Surg 2003;138(5):482–7.

229. Chung MA, Steinhoff MM, Cady B, et al. Clinical axillary recurrence in breast cancer patients after a negative sentinel node biopsy. Am J Surg 2002;184(4): 310–4.

230. Giuliano AE, Haigh PI, Brennan MB, et al. Prospective observational study of sentinel lymphadenectomy without further axillary dissection in patients with sentinel node-negative breast cancer. J Clin Oncol 2000;18(13):2553–9.

231. Heuts EM, van der Ent FW, Hulsewe KW, et al. Incidence of axillary recurrence in 344 sentinel node negative breast cancer patients after intermediate follow-up. A prospective study into the accuracy of sentinel node biopsy in breast cancer patients. Acta Chir Belg 2007;107(3):279–83.

232. Palesty JA, Foster JM, Hurd TC, et al. Axillary recurrence in women with a negative sentinel lymph node and no axillary dissection in breast cancer. J Surg Oncol 2006;93(2):129–32.

233. Reitsamer R, Peintinger F, Prokop E, et al. Sentinel lymph node biopsy alone without axillary lymph node dissection–follow up of sentinel lymph node negative breast cancer patients. Eur J Surg Oncol 2003;29(3):221–3.

234. Roumen RM, Kuijt GP, Liem IH, et al. Treatment of 100 patients with sentinel node-negative breast cancer without further axillary dissection. Br J Surg 2001;88(12):1639–43.

235. Schrenk P, Hatzl-Griesenhofer M, Shamiyeh A, et al. Follow-up of sentinel node negative breast cancer patients without axillary lymph node dissection. J Surg Oncol 2001;77(3):165–70.

236. Smidt ML, Janssen CM, Kuster DM, et al. Axillary recurrence after a negative sentinel node biopsy for breast cancer: incidence and clinical significance. Ann Surg Oncol 2005;12(1):29–33.

The Multidisciplinary Management of Rectal Cancer

Kenneth L. Meredith, MD[a], Sarah E. Hoffe, MD[b],
David Shibata, MD, FACS[a],*

KEYWORDS

- Multidisciplinary • Rectal cancer • Surgery
- Radiation therapy • Adjuvant chemotherapy

Colorectal cancer is the fourth most common noncutaneous malignancy in the United States and the second most frequent cause of cancer-related deaths. In 2008, an estimated 148,810 cases of colorectal cancer will be diagnosed and will account for 49,960 deaths.[1] Of these cancers, 70% will arise in the colon, whereas 30% (40,740) will occur in the rectum.[2] At diagnosis, approximately 25% of colon cancers are noted to have local extension through the muscularis of the bowel wall. In contrast, 50% of cancers in the rectum exhibit this progression, with lymph node metastases seen in approximately two thirds of these cases.[3,4]

Significant variability exists in defining the junction between the colon and rectum for the purposes of assigning patients to treatment regimens. A National Cancer Institute consensus panel recommended that the colon be defined as greater than 12 cm and the rectum as 12 cm or less from the anal verge using rigid proctoscopy.[5] Colorectal cancers located above 12 cm behave like colon cancers with respect to recurrence patterns and prognosis.[6,7] Several anatomic considerations also distinguish rectal cancers from those that occur in the colon. The extraperitoneal rectum resides within the narrow and bony confines of the pelvis, making surgical resection more difficult. Additionally, the absence of serosa below the peritoneal reflection facilitates deeper tumor growth in the perirectal fat and may contribute to higher rates of locoregional failure.[8]

The mainstay of treatment for patients who have rectal cancer has been curative surgical resection, with emphasis on minimizing morbidity and mortality. Significant improvements in local control and overall survival have been seen in patients who have resectable rectal cancer.[9–14] However, a greater understanding of the natural

[a] Department of Gastrointestinal Oncology, Moffitt Cancer Center and Research Institute, Tampa, FL 33612, USA
[b] Department of Radiation Oncology, Moffitt Cancer Center and Research Institute, Tampa, FL 33612, USA
* Corresponding author. H. Lee Moffitt Cancer Center and Research Institute, MCC 12505, 12902 Magnolia Drive, Tampa, FL 33612.
E-mail address: David.Shibata@moffitt.org (D. Shibata).

Surg Clin N Am 89 (2009) 177–215
doi:10.1016/j.suc.2008.09.021
0039-6109/08/$ – see front matter © 2009 Elsevier Inc. All rights reserved.

history of the disease, patterns of recurrence, and more precise histopathologic reporting have helped define patients who have a high risk for local recurrence and disease progression after curative resection. This knowledge has prompted a progression in the multidisciplinary approach to treatment, with the integration of expertise from additional disciplines such as pathology, medical and radiation oncology, gastroenterology, and radiology. The combination of anatomic and biologic factors contributes to the complex and often challenging nature of treating rectal cancers. Optimal management and outcomes of patients depends greatly on the successful communication and collaboration of a multidisciplinary treatment team.

STAGING

Pathologic stage represents the most important prognostic factor for patients who have rectal cancer. The tumor-node-metastasis (TNM) system, as defined by the American Joint Committee on Cancer (AJCC), is the most commonly used staging system and is based on depth of local invasion, extent of regional lymph node involvement, and presence of distant sites of disease (**Box 1**).[15,16] As the AJCC stage increases from stage I to stage IV, 5-year overall survival declines from greater than 90% to less than 10% (**Table 1**).[17,18] Synchronous polyps or cancers may be present in 4% to 15% of patients.[19] Fukatsua and colleagues[20] retrospectively reviewed 3061 patients and found an 8% incidence of synchronous colorectal cancers. Therefore, complete endoscopic evaluation of the entire colon is essential not only for visualization, localization, and biopsy of the primary rectal tumor but also to exclude additional lesions.

LOCAL

Establishing the extent of local and locoregional involvement is imperative for patients who have rectal cancer, particularly those who have locally advanced disease and are

---

Box 1
Tumor-node-metastasis (TNM) staging system for rectal cancer

Primary tumor (T)

Tx-Primary tumor cannot be assessed

Tis-Tumor invades submucosa

T1-Tumor invades muscularis propria

T3-Tumor invades through the muscularis propria into the subserosa

T4-Tumor invades other organs or structures, or perforates visceral peritoneum

Regional lymph nodes

Nx-Regional lymph nodes cannot be assessed

N0-No regional lymph node metastasis

N1-Metastasis in one to three regional lymph nodes

N2-Metastasis in four or more regional lymph nodes

Distant metastasis

Mx-Presence or absence of distant disease cannot be determined

M0-No distant metastasis detected

M1-Distant metastasis detected

Data from Greene FL, Page DL, Fleming, ID, et al. AJCC Cancer Staging Manual, Sixth Edition. New York: Springer; 2002.

Table 1
Stage-specific survival

Stage	Grouping	Five-Year Survival
I	T1-2, N0, M0	>90%
IIA	T3, N0, M0	60%–85%
IIB	T4, N0, M0	60%–85%
IIIA	T1-2, N1, M0	55%–60%
IIIB	T3-4, N1, M0	35%–42%
IIIC	T-1-4, N1, M0	25%–27%
IV	T1-4, N0-2, M1	5%–7%

at higher risk for recurrence and disease progression. Identifying these patients allows for the selection of treatment options, such as neoadjuvant chemoradiation which can improve recurrence-free survival, overall survival, and increase the likelihood of sphincter preservation.[21–29]

Simple history and physical examination may yield some clues as to the extent of local progression. Although many patients who have early rectal cancer are asymptomatic and detected by screening, more advanced tumors in the rectum are often associated with a group of common symptoms, such as rectal bleeding, change in the caliber of stools, and tenesmus. Rectal pain may indicate more distal involvement of the anal canal or possibly of the sacral bone or nerves. Digital rectal examination (DRE) is particularly important in determining the likelihood of sphincter preservation and can identify fixation and involvement of the sphincter complex, the distance from the anorectal ring, and the size of the tumor.[30] However, when establishing depth of invasion, other modalities are required, because the overall accuracy of DRE in staging of rectal cancer is only approximately 65%.[30]

ULTRASOUND

The most common technique for assessing the depth of rectal wall invasion is transrectal ultrasound (TRUS); 360° viewing transducers are available for use with either a flexible or rigid assembly. An integrated water-filled balloon enables close transducer contact and distension of the rectal wall.[31]

Meta-analysis of 90 articles describing TRUS in staging of rectal cancer yielded a sensitivity and specificity of 94% and 86%, respectively, for muscularis invasion, and 94% and 69%, respectively, for perirectal tissue invasion.[32] Therefore, TRUS is ideal for staging T1/T2 tumors being considered for local, nonradical surgery. However, caution must be exercised in interpreting imaging for large, locally invasive, or desmoplastic tumors, which make true tumor infiltration from tissue reaction difficult to discern and may result in overstaging.[33] Other limitations of TRUS include the staging of stenotic circumferential rectal tumors that are unable to be traversed by endoscope, or lesions treated with preoperative radiotherapy, which decreases the accuracy for T-staging secondary to increased echogenicity of the rectal wall.[34] The overall accuracy of TRUS for T staging is reported to range from 80% to 95%.[8,35–40]

Nodal staging using TRUS is more challenging because metastasis is difficult to detect within a lymph node, and consequently sensitivity and specificity are approximately 55% and 78%, respectively.[32,41] Sonographic lymph node changes associated with malignant involvement include a hypoechoic appearance, round nodal shape, and nodal diameter of 1 cm or greater.[42] Lymph nodes greater than

0.5 cm in diameter have a 50% to 70% possibility of being metastatic, whereas those smaller than 4 mm have a less than 20% likelihood of harboring metastasis.[43] The overall accuracy of TRUS in determining metastatic perirectal nodal involvement is approximately 70% to 75%.[34]

MRI

The use of MRI for the local staging of rectal cancer, particularly with an endorectal coil technique, has been well described.[44,45] MRI offers several theoretic advantages compared with TRUS: it permits a larger field of view, tends to be less operator- and technique-dependent, and allows for the study of stenotic tumors.[33,46,47] Reports on MRI in the T-staging of patients who have rectal cancer yielded scattered accuracies ranging from 50% to 95%.[44,45] However, a meta-analysis of 90 articles between 1995 and 2002 comparing the use of MRI, TRUS, and CT for staging with histopathologic findings as the reference standard came to the following conclusions: for T1/T2 lesions, TRUS and MRI had similar sensitivity but specificity was higher in TRUS (86 versus 69%), and for T3 tumors, the sensitivity of TRUS was significantly higher than that of MRI or CT.[32]

MRI can also be used toevaluate mesorectal nodal involvement. Rather than size criteria alone, lymph nodes can be characterized by imaging features. In their study of MRI with histologic correlation, Brown and colleagues[48] identified an irregular contour and in-homogeneous signal to be the most reliable MRI criteria for lymph node metastasis. MRI may also be useful for identifying nodal metastasis outside the mesorectum that may not be included in the resected specimen.[49] However, as with TRUS, MRI has shown less accuracy in predicting perirectal nodal involvement. Sensitivity and specificity are approximately 64% and 58%, respectively, with an overall accuracy in nodal staging ranging from 60% to 70%.[34,50]

In addition to traditional T- and N-staging of rectal cancer, MRI has been shown to have additional capabilities of characterizing the degree of mesorectal invasion by the primary tumor. Newer techniques such as high-resolution, thin-section MRI are better able to differentiate malignant tissue from the muscularis propria and define tumor infiltration of the mesorectal fascia (circumferential margin).[44,49] The Magnetic Resonance Imaging and Rectal Cancer European Equivalence study (MERCURY) prospectively evaluated the depth of extramural tumor invasion in patients who had rectal cancer while comparing it with the histopathologic results as the gold standard. MRI assessment of tumor invasion was considered equivalent to conventional histopathologic evaluation to within 0.5 mm.[51] Therefore, either high-resolution MRI or TRUS is an acceptable method to determine preoperative tumor stage. In Europe, both MRI and TRUS are performed preoperatively to evaluate not only T-stage but also likelihood of achieving a negative circumferential margin.[52] This decision is based on data illustrating that distance from the primary tumor to the mesorectal fascia on MRI before neoadjuvant therapy accurately predicted surgical margin and mesorectal status and subsequently correlated with survival and local recurrence patterns.[53]

CT SCANNING

Local staging with CT remains inferior to both TRUS and MRI because of its inability to distinguish the layers of the rectal wall and the inherent soft tissue planes, although it remains useful for the local relationships of high rectal tumors to pelvic structures.[8] The sensitivity of CT in local tumor staging of rectal cancer is 79%, only slightly better than that reported for DRE, and is significantly inferior to that of MRI or TRUS.[30] Therefore, either high-resolution MRI or TRUS is an acceptable method to determine preoperative tumor stage. For both techniques, T-staging is very accurate; however, the assessment of nodal status remains somewhat more difficult.

EVALUATION OF DISTANT METASTASIS

Establishing the presence or absence of distant metastases has significant implications for decision making in patients with newly diagnosed rectal cancer. The choice of optimal treatment (eg, neoadjuvant chemoradiation versus systemic chemotherapy alone) depends on the accurate assessment of distant disease. Approximately 50% to 60% of patients who have undergone treatment for rectal cancer will develop metastasis.[54] Hepatic (20%–25%), pulmonary (10%–20%), bone (6%–10%), and brain (3%) represent the most common sites of distant disease.[53,55] Although CT scanning may not be as useful as other modalities for local staging, CT of the chest, abdomen, and pelvis using oral and intravenous contrast is routinely performed to assess the presence of distant metastasis and represents the gold standard.[56]

Interest is increasing in the use of positron emission tomography (PET) as an additional imaging modality in patients who have rectal cancer. Nahas and colleagues[57] prospectively evaluated the ability PET to detect distant disease in patients who have locally advanced rectal cancer who were otherwise eligible for combined modality therapy. The overall accuracy, sensitivity, and specificity of PET in detecting distant disease were 93.7%, 77.8%, and 98.7%, respectively. Greatest accuracy occurred in detecting liver (accuracy, 99.9%; sensitivity, 100%; specificity, 98.8%) and lung (accuracy, 99.9%; sensitivity, 80%; specificity, 100%) disease. PET detected 11/12 confirmed malignant sites in liver and lung, whereas abdominopelvic CT scans accurately detected only 9 patients who had M1 disease. The authors concluded that PET may play a significant role in defining extent of distant disease in selected cases, thus impacting the choice of neoadjuvant therapy. Gearhart and colleagues[58] evaluated the use of PET/CT for primary rectal cancer and identified discordant findings in 14 patients (38%), which resulted in upstaging of 7 patients (50%) and downstaging of 3 (21%). Discordant PET/CT findings were significantly more common in patients who had a low rectal cancer than in those who had mid or high rectal cancer (13 versus 1; $P = .0027$). Currently, PET scanning in patients who have rectal cancer is not routinely recommended in the absence of synchronous metastasis.[56]

SURGICAL CONSIDERATIONS
Historical Perspective

The surgical approach to patients who have rectal cancer has evolved dramatically over the past hundred years. Surgeons such as Kocher, Kraske, Babcock, and Lisfranc[60] were the first to use sphincter-preserving techniques more than a century ago. Resections were generally achieved using local excision with transperineal, transcoccygeal, or transsacral approaches and were associated with significant morbidity and high recurrence rates.[59] In 1908, Miles[59] revolutionized the oncologic principles of rectal cancer by contending that existing local perineal approaches for rectal resection, which often spared the sphincters, did not address the "zone of upward spread" of cancer cells through the lymphatic channels. Furthermore, he noted the high rate of local recurrence, and cited postmortem examinations that frequently showed recurrences in the pelvic peritoneum, and lymph nodes along the left common iliac artery.[60] Miles suggested that the principles applied to en bloc resection for breast cancer, and that associated axillary lymph nodes should similarly be applied to the therapy of rectal cancer through a combined abdominal and perineal approach. These principles included the construction of an "abdominal anus" (colostomy), resection of the entire pelvic colon with the pelvic mesocolon and associated lymph nodes up to the level of the iliac bifurcation, and wide perineal excision.[59] The abdominoperineal resection (APR) quickly gained acceptance, becoming the gold standard for rectal cancers at any level proximal to the anus and supplanting existing surgical techniques.

Thirty years later, Dixon[61] described his low anterior resection (LAR) technique for patients who have rectal cancer, emphasizing adequate lateral and proximal mesenteric resections with the preservation of gastrointestinal continence. The use of LAR as an alternative to APR allowed surgeons to offer sphincter preservation without compromising survival or local recurrence.[14,62] The advent of the circular end to end anastomosis (EEA) has subsequently made LAR with even lower pelvic anastomosis technically more feasible, and its use has become routine.[63]

RADICAL SURGERY

The type and extent of surgery performed on patients who have rectal cancer largely depends on the preoperative tumor stage, the distance from the anorectal sphincter complex, the use of neoadjuvant therapy, histopathologic features, and the patient's projected ability to tolerate radical surgery. For tumors of the mid to upper rectum, low anterior resection is generally the preferred approach. For lesions of the lower rectum, either APR or LAR may be performed, depending on involvement of the sphincter mechanism. The goal with all surgical approaches is an R0 resection with negative distal and radial margins, which are important determinants of surgical outcome, overall survival, and recurrence-free survival.[7,9,10,64–70]

TOTAL MESORECTAL EXCISION

The technique of total mesorectal excision (TME) performed in concert with APR or LAR allows for precise dissection and removal of the entire rectal mesentery, including that distal to the tumor as an intact unit. Conventional blunt dissection techniques resulted in unacceptable inadequate surgical clearance and likely explained high local failure rates. Because TME is performed sharply under direct visualization with a focus on autonomic nerve preservation and avoidance of mesorectal envelope violation, all tumor satellites should be contained, improving likelihood of local control. In most series, local recurrence rates are less then 7% in patients undergoing TME even when no adjuvant therapy is given.[71–73]

One concern regarding early reports of TME was the high rate of anastomotic leak associated with this technique.[74] This adverse effect was believed to have occurred because of the application of TME for proximal rectal cancers with subsequent ischemia of a long rectal stump. Subsequently, experts have advocated that TME be used for mid and distal rectal cancers and that a partial mesorectal excision is acceptable for proximal lesions. The length of mesorectum beyond the primary tumor that must be removed is approximately 3 to 5 cm.[56] In several studies, tumor implants were seen no farther than 4 cm from the distal edge of the tumor within the mesorectum and no implants were seen beyond 1 cm in T1 or T2 lesions.[75,76] For proximal rectal cancers, a mesorectal excision to 5 cm below the lower border of the tumor is believed to be an adequate oncologic resection, whereas for distal rectal cancers less than 5 cm from the anorectal complex, TME with a negative bowel wall margin of 1 to 2 cm confirmed with frozen section may be acceptable.[77]

DISTAL MARGIN

The adequate length of the distal margin for a radical rectal cancer resection remains somewhat controversial. Although the primary area of extension for rectal cancer is upward along the lymphatics, tumors below the peritoneal reflection can spread distally through intramural or extramural lymphovascular routes. The use of APR for low rectal cancers has traditionally been based on the need for a 5-cm distal margin of normal tissue. However, subsequent retrospective studies have shown that margins as short as 1 cm are not associated with an increased risk for local recurrence.[14,78] Distal intramural spread is usually limited to within 2 cm of the tumor unless the lesion is poorly differentiated or metastatic.[11,69,79,80]

Williams and colleagues[80] showed that only 12 of 50 APR specimens with distal margins greater than 5 cm had distal intramural extension beyond the confines of the tumor edge (7 spread within 1 cm and 5 beyond 1 cm), 10 of which were from patients who had stage III disease. Furthermore, all five patients who had intramural extension beyond 1 cm had tumors that were poorly differentiated, who had node-positive disease, and whose mortality was related to distant rather then local recurrence. Additionally, no difference was seen in survival or recurrence rates between patients whose distal resection margin was greater than 5 cm and those whose margin was less than 5 cm. Similarly, others have found that tumor lymphatic extension beyond 1 cm represents a poor prognostic sign and that more radical operations are not beneficial.[81]

National Surgical Adjuvant Breast and Bowel Project (NSABP) R-01 was a prospective randomized trial designed to evaluate the efficacy of adjuvant therapy in rectal carcinoma in which 232 and 181 patients underwent APR and LAR, respectively.[14] A subgroup analysis evaluating the length of the distal resection margin in patients undergoing sphincter-preserving operations indicated that treatment failure and survival were not significantly different in patients whose margins were less than 2 cm, 2 to 2.9 cm, or greater than or equal to 3 cm.[14] As a result, a 1- to 2-cm margin has become acceptable; however, this should be confirmed as negative through frozen section and accompanied by adequate mesorectal excision.[56]

With confirmation of the oncologic safety of shorter distal margins, surgeons have been able adopt a more aggressive approach to sphincter preservation. Techniques such as hand-sewn or stapled coloanal anastomosis after ultra-low anterior resection and even intersphincteric (ISR) resection have been described.[66,82–85] Long-term results show no compromise of disease-free or overall survival, although poor functional outcomes can occur.[64,86] Functional status may be improved with an increased neo-rectal reservoir achieved through construction of a colonic pouch at resection.[82,84,87] At least 50% of the patients have acceptable functional continence after ISR, with medical and biofeedback treatments improving continence in another 25% of patients.[88] These methods should be considered carefully and on an individual basis.

RADIAL OR CIRCUMFERENTIAL MARGIN

Although the traditional concerns of achieving acceptable distal margins are warranted, the importance of obtaining adequate circumferential or radial margins has been shown to play a more critical role in determining local control. Positive radial margins may occur from extension of the primary tumor, extension of involved lymph nodes, or mesorectal tumor deposits.[12,89] A positive radial margin from inadequate TME is an independent predictor of local recurrence and survival.[9,10,12,75,90,91] Hall and colleagues[67] reported not only a 24% recurrence rate in patients who had a negative radial resection margin, compared with 50% in those having a positive margin, but also a worse disease-free and overall survival in the positive margin cohort.

LATERAL NODE DISSECTION

The use of more aggressive or extended lymphadenectomy for rectal cancer has been proposed as a means to improve local control and outcome. Advocates of the lateral lymph node dissection (LLND), which includes removal of all nodal tissue along the common and internal iliac artery, have cited improved local control and overall survival.[92] A survival benefit was reported in patients who had positive lateral lymph nodes who underwent LLND.[93] However, other reports have shown that LLND is not associated with improved outcome.[94–96] Further examination of this issue was reported by Nagawa and colleagues[96] in a prospective randomized controlled fashion in which patients underwent preoperative radiation followed by surgery with or without LLND. LLND provided no additional benefit in local recurrence or survival. This radical approach to lymphadenectomy has been associated with increased postoperative morbidity, such as urinary dysfunction in 18% of patients and sexual dysfunction in as many as 50%.[97–99] Until further data are available, the routine use of LLND is not warranted in patients who have no clinical evidence of suspicious lateral lymph nodes.

LAPAROSCOPIC RECTAL CANCER SURGERY

The use of laparoscopic-assisted colectomy for colon cancer is well established, with supporting evidence from several prospective clinical trials. Preliminary results are now available from four large prospective randomized clinical trials: Colon Cancer Laparoscopic or Open (COLOR), Conventional versus Laparoscopic Assisted Surgery in Colorectal Cancer (CLASICC), Clinical Outcomes of Surgical Therapy Study Group (COSTSG), and Barcelona.[100–103] These trials have uniformly and consistently shown this technique to be associated with a significant reduction in the use of narcotics, oral analgesics, and length of hospital stay, and a faster return of diet and bowel function. The Barcelona and COSTSG trials have sufficient maturation and follow-up to report recurrence and survival data, with neither showing a survival disadvantage in patients treated with laparoscopic colectomy. Results of the Barcelona trial suggest a cancer-related survival advantage in patients treated with laparoscopic colectomy, based solely on differences in patients who have stage III disease, but this is not confirmed by the COSTSG trial.[102,103] Results of the CLASICC and COLOR trials, and 5-year data from the COSTSG trial, should definitively address survival differences.

The equivalent applicability of laparoscopic techniques for the treatment of rectal cancer remains unclear. Early reports of laparoscopic-assisted LAR and APR in patients who have rectal cancer show that the approaches are technically feasible and are not associated with worse survival or recurrence patterns.[104–106] The investigational experience with laparoscopic rectal cancer is not as mature; the subset of patients in the CLASICC trial who had rectal cancer (n = 253) provides the only available randomized controlled trial data. The initial short-term reporting of the CLASICC trial was an intent-to-treat report that documented an equal number of patients who had stages IIIB and IIIC on final pathologic diagnoses. The hospital mortality was 5%, and patients requiring conversion from laparoscopic-assisted to open surgery had more complications, and those who underwent laparoscopic low anterior resections for rectal cancer had an increased number of involved resection margins (twice that of the open) and increased port site recurrence (nine times that of open).[100,107]

Additionally, long-term bladder dysfunction has been reported in 3.1% of patients after laparoscopic rectal resection and sexual dysfunction among 44% of male patients.[108] Laparoscopic colectomy in patients who have curable cancer is accepted as an alternative to open colectomy, whereas the applicability of laparoscopic rectal cancer resection requires further investigation. Until the aforementioned prospective randomized trials are completed, laparoscopic approaches for rectal cancer should be limited to participation in clinical trials.[56,107,109]

LOCAL EXCISION

Local excision is generally accepted as an option for the treatment of T1 adenocarcinomas of the rectum with favorable clinical and histologic features and is associated with low rates of recurrence and surgical morbidity.[110–114] Additional criteria for eligibility for treatment of rectal cancer by transanal excision include (1) well- to moderately differentiated cancer, (2) absence of lymphovascular or perineural invasion, (3) lesion is within 8 to 10 cm from the anal verge, and (4) tumor smaller than 3 to 4 cm and occupying less than one third of the circumference of the rectal lumen.[115,116] Traditionally, excision is achieved through a transanal technique, although transcoccygeal and transsphincteric approaches can be used.[115,117,118]

The use of local excision for more advanced lesions (T2 and T3) has been reported to have unacceptably high rates of recurrence (17%–62%), even with the use of adjuvant chemoradiation strategies.[119–124] However, in select circumstances, local excision can be offered as a surgical option for patients who refuse APR with permanent colostomy, have significant comorbidities, or have distant metastasis with a short life expectancy.[70,125]

Transanal excision can be performed with minimal morbidity and mortality. Recovery is rapid; a temporary or permanent ostomy is not necessary and long-term bowel function is generally excellent.[126,127] In contrast, radical surgery, even in experienced hands, confers a significant risk of perioperative morbidity, may require a stoma, usually necessitates several weeks of recovery, and frequently leaves patients with compromised bowel or sexual function.[128–131]

The technique of transanal excision involves complete full-thickness excision of the rectal cancer down to the perirectal fat, with a minimum lateral margin of 1 cm. Intraoperative frozen section evaluation of the peripheral and deep margins is performed. Single layer, primary closure of the defect is usually performed. As noted, the conventional transanal approach is limited to low to mid-rectal lesions within 8 to 10 cm from the anal verge. Minimally invasive endoscopic techniques, such as transanal endoscopic microsurgery (TEM), have expanded the range of transanal excision to otherwise inaccessible lesions that are within reach of the endoscope.[132–134] Using TEM, full-thickness excisions can be performed up to 15 cm posteriorly, 12 cm laterally, and 10 cm anteriorly.[132–138] Oncologic results seem to be similar to those of the traditional transanal approach, or anterior resection, particularly for early-stage rectal cancers, but patient selection is critical.[111,114,135,136]

Several retrospective reviews have raised some concern regarding the oncologic safety of local excision for rectal cancer, citing local recurrence rates of 17% to 21% and 26% to 47% for T1 and T2 lesions, respectively.[123,139] Additionally, retrospective review of long-term results of transanal excision showed local recurrence and 10-year survival rates for T1 rectal cancers to be 17% and 74%, respectively, with corresponding rates of 26% and 72% for T2 tumors, raising concern that cancer mortality may be higher than generally appreciated for local excison.[139] However, in a multiinstitutional prospective trial (CALGB 8984) Steele and colleagues[127] showed that local excision for T1 lesions was associated with an acceptable 5% local recurrence rate, although the corresponding recurrence rate for T2 lesions was 14%.

Recently, long-term follow-up data for CALGB 8984 were reported, with a median follow-up of 7.1 years (2.1–11.4 years). Patients who had T1 and T2 tumors had 10-year overall survival rates of 84% and 66%, respectively, and disease-free survival of 75% and 64%, respectively. The local recurrence rates for patients who had T1 tumors were reported to be 8% compared with 18% for those who had T2 tumors. The authors concluded that local excision for T1 rectal adenocarcinomas is associated with durable local control and acceptable overall survival. However, T2 tumors even with adjuvant chemoradiation exhibited higher recurrence rates. Given that salvage rates for recurrent disease can be less than 50%,[121,123,125,139,140] patients who have T2 disease should be offered radical resection with total mesorectal excision unless enrolled in a clinical trial. One such trial is the current American College of Surgeons Oncology Group (ACOSOG) Z6041 trial that is designed to assess outcomes of patients who have T2 rectal cancers treated with neoadjuvant chemoradiation followed by local excision.

PATHOLOGIC CONSIDERATIONS
Histopathologic Features and Node Sampling

Poorly differentiated histology, lymphovascular invasion, perineural invasion, T4 tumor stage, clinical obstruction or perforation, and an elevated preoperative carcinoembryonic antigen (CEA) are associated with increased recurrence rates and worse survival in patients who have rectal cancer.[141–145] In addition to unfavorable histopathologic features, the examination of an inadequate number of lymph nodes has also been linked to increased mortality in patients who have both node-negative and -positive rectal cancer.[21,146,147] Inadequate sampling of lymph nodes may reflect a less-complete surgical resection or inadequate inspection of the pathologic specimen, which may lead to understaging with higher-than-expected relapse rates because of potential omission of adjuvant therapy. Current guidelines recommend the identification of 12 or more lymph nodes in the specimen for accurate staging.[16,148]

TECHNIQUE FOR ASSESSING RADIAL MARGINS

A description of the gross appearance of the mesorectum and radial or circumferential margin assessment are critical features of the pathologic evaluation of a surgically resected rectal specimen. The techniques of radial margin assessment and mesorectal evaluation[90] have been used in recent trials, including the MRC CLASSIC trial[100] and MRC CRO7,[149] and in historic trials, such as the Dutch Rectal Cancer trial.[150] Subsequently, a qualitative scale was instituted that graded that completeness of the mesorectal excision, with grade 1 designating incomplete excision, grade 2 nearly complete excision, and grade 3 complete excision.

The specimens should be received intact and unopened as soon as possible after resection to allow for further inspection and location of the primary tumor and to note any obvious macroscopic perforations. The nonperitonealized surgical resection margin in the vicinity of the tumor is then inked or painted with a suitable marker to enable the subsequent identification of margin involvement. This margin represents the "bare" area in the connective tissue at the surgical plane of excision that is not covered by a serosal surface. This closest radial margin between the deepest penetration of the tumor and the edge of the resected soft tissue around the rectum is termed the *circumferential resection margin* (CRM). Low rectal tumors will be completely surrounded by a nonperitonealized margin CRM, whereas upper rectal tumors will have a nonperitonealized margin posterolaterally, which is inked, and a peritonealized (serosal) surface anteriorly, which is not inked.

After the margin is inked, the specimen is opened along the anterior surface 1 to 2 cm above and below the tumor, pinned to a cork board, and fixed in formalin for 48 hours. The specimen is then sectioned at 3- to 4-mm intervals (bread-loaf slicing technique) to include the tumor, adjacent lymph nodes, serosa, and nonperitonealized CRM. At least four blocks are submitted to show the deepest tumor penetration into the bowel wall, involvement of the serosal surface, invasion of extramural veins, and involvement of adjacent organs. An additional block illustrating the closest approximation of the tumor to the CRM, either in continuity with the main tumor mass or a separate extramural deposit or tumor in a lymph node, whichever is closest, is examined for CRM determination and measured in millimeters.[90,150]

Quirke[151] found that despite extensive surgical training, only 57% of operations were judged to be complete excision, with nearly one quarter (24%) being classified as incomplete excisions. Additionally, tumors deemed incompletely removed through suboptimal surgery had a significantly higher rate of margin involvement (44% versus 27% for complete resections). Abdominoperineal excisions were particularly poor, in that complete resection was achieved in only 34% of cases, compared with 73% for anterior resections. When combining resections classed as grade 3 (complete) and 2 (nearly complete) and comparing them with grade 1 (incomplete), incomplete resections had a significantly higher overall recurrence rate (36% versus 22%; $P = .01$).[151] The frequency of local recurrence alone was almost halved (from 15% to 9%) with better resections.

Accurate reporting of CRM status is critical because of its significant prognostic implications. The frequency of histologic involvement of the CRM is strongly associated with local recurrence and poor survival.[90,152–154] A debate in ongoing about when to call the CRM positive. Tumor within 1 mm of the CRM has been shown to substantially increase the risk for recurrence,[9,12,155] whereas other studies have shown that at 2 mm the risk for recurrence is less, but still high.[156] The TNM definition of a positive margin (R1) is a microscopically incomplete resection with 0 mm clearance; in most cases, CRM is considered positive when tumor is noted 1 mm or less from the margin of resection. Based on the prognostic value for local recurrence, 2 mm has also been considered as a cutoff point.[89]

With non-TME surgery, 36% of all patients and 25% of those undergoing a curative operation showed CRM involvement; however, when TME was implemented and performed by surgeons who have adequate training, these rates fell.[90] In patients who have a positive CRM, assessing the quality of surgery adds nothing to the prediction of local recurrence above CRM involvement alone. However, in patients who have a negative CRM and incomplete resection, the overall recurrence rate doubles from 15% to 29% and survival decreases from 91% to 77% ($P<.05$).[151]

DEGREE OF PATHOLOGIC RESPONSE

Currently, preoperative combined modality therapy regimens are associated with a pathologic complete response (pCR) rate of approximately 4% to 33%.[157–161] When using hematoxylin and eosin staining and light-microscopic analysis, areas of tumor treatment response can be characterized by the replacement of neoplastic glands with loosely collagenized fibrous tissue and scattered chronic inflammatory cells: a pathologic observation previously reported.[162,163] A pathologic complete response is defined by no evidence of viable tumor cells on pathologic analysis, whereas tumors that display any evidence of residual cancer cells in the resection specimen are defined as having a partial pathologic response (pPR).[157,160,164] Stipa and colleagues[157] showed a 5-year relapse-free survival of 96% for patients experiencing a pCR compared with only 54% in the group showing no degree of pathologic down-staging (P<.0001). Moreover, 5-year overall survival improved in patients who had a pCR (90% versus 68%; P = .009), with an associated enhancement of sphincter preservation rates (91% versus 76%; P = .01), compared with those who exhibited no pathologic downstaging.

Chan and colleagues[153] reported similar data from Canada for 128 patients undergoing preoperative combined modality therapy for locally advanced rectal cancer. On multivariate analysis, tumor stage after the preoperative therapy was the most statistically significant independent predictor of survival (P = .003) and relapse-free survival (P<.001). In summary, communication between surgeons and pathologists is essential to optimize both the surgical treatment and pathologic evaluation of rectal cancer specimens. Mutual feedback can enhance quality of care provided by both disciplines, with the goal of improving patient outcomes.

NEOADJUVANT AND ADJUVANT THERAPY
Radiation

Before 1980, surgery alone was the standard treatment for all stages of colorectal cancer. The observation that high rates of locoregional recurrence were associated with locally advanced rectal cancer[165] led to the development of randomized trials exploring the possible benefit of postoperative chemotherapy and radiotherapy in this subset of high-risk patients.

The first United States trials were conducted by the Gastrointestinal Tumor Study Group (GITSG), the National Surgical Adjuvant Breast and Bowel Project (NSABP), and the North Central Cancer Treatment Group (NCCTG). In 1975, the GITSG's GI-7175 trial began randomizing patients to a four-arm trial after a "curative" resection for rectal adenocarcinoma.[166] Patients (n = 227) underwent no further therapy, radiation (40–48 Gy over 5 weeks), chemotherapy alone (fluorouracil and semustine or methyl-CCNU), or a combination of chemotherapy and radiotherapy. Patients undergoing the combined radiation therapy and chemotherapy regimen showed a statistically significant advantage in disease-free and overall survival compared with the surgery-alone group.

The NSABP R-01 adjuvant therapy trial randomized patients (n = 500) with pathologic T3, T4, or node-positive disease to surgery alone versus adjuvant 5-fluoruracil (FU), semustine, and vincristine (MOF) versus adjuvant pelvic radiation to 46 to 47 Gy with a possible tumor bed boost to a maximum of 53 Gy.[167] The trial showed improved disease-free and overall survival in the chemotherapy group compared with surgery-alone group. The adjuvant radiation group experienced a reduction in locoregional recurrence from 25% to 16% compared with the surgery-alone group without a survival benefit.

Subsequently, the NCCTG initiated an adjuvant trial randomizing 200 postoperative patients to radiation therapy alone or radiation combined with semustine and 5-FU. After a median follow-up of 7 years, the combined-therapy arm showed a 34% reduction in tumor relapse and 36% reduction in cancer-related deaths.[168] These two positive randomized trials from the GITSG and the NCCTG set a new standard of care for the postoperative management of high-risk rectal cancer.

Subsequent studies were then designed to determine the optimal adjuvant regimen for surgically resected rectal cancer. The NCCTG group performed a subsequent trial exploring the question as to whether semustine was necessary by comparing it with continuous infusion versus bolus 5-FU.[169] Data from more than 600 patients were analyzed in this four-arm randomized trial. Semustine did not improve local control or survival and was subsequently abandoned. This trial also showed that continuous infusional 5-FU was superior to bolus infusion when administered concurrently with pelvic radiation. Infusional 5-FU, when compared with bolus infusion, showed a significant reduction in the overall rate of tumor relapse from 47% to 37% and distant metastasis from 40% to 31%.[169]

The NSABP questioned the benefit of radiation to chemotherapy compared with chemotherapy alone in the R-02 randomized trial.[170] Patients who had stage II and III rectal cancer had been randomized to either postoperative chemotherapy alone or chemotherapy with postoperative radiation. The treatment arms trial consisted of 5-FU plus leucovorin for all female patients and either MOF or 5-FU plus leucovorin for male patients. During radiation, all patients received bolus 5-FU during the first 3 and last 3 days of treatment. This trial showed that postoperative chemoradiation compared with chemotherapy alone reduced the cumulative incidence of locoregional relapse from 13% to 8% at 5-year follow-up.

PREOPERATIVE VERSUS POSTOPERATIVE APPROACH

Although postoperative regimens were being optimized in the United States, investigators in Europe were exploring the potential benefits of treatment given in the preoperative setting. The Stockholm Colorectal Cancer Study Group randomized patients (n = 849) to surgery alone versus a short-course neoadjuvant regimen of 25 Gy in five fractions of 5 Gy per treatment followed by surgery (Stockholm I).[171] The radiation was delivered to a large treatment field encompassing L1–2 superiorly to 1 cm below the anal verge inferiorly, with two beams directed anterior to posterior and posterior to anterior (APPA). This trial showed no difference in survival; however, a significant reduction in pelvic recurrences was seen among irradiated patients in all stages. The irradiated group also showed a significantly prolonged interval to local recurrence or distant metastasis. However, radiation was associated with increased mortality (8% versus 2%; $P = .01$) and an increase in long-term complications, such as venous thromboembolism, postoperative fistulas, intestinal obstruction, and femoral neck and pelvic fractures.[172]

Data from the Stockholm Colorectal Cancer Study group led to the evolution of the Swedish Rectal Cancer trial (SRCT). In this era before TME, the SRCT accrued from greater than 70 hospitals in Sweden more than 1000 patients younger than 80 years who had resectable rectal cancer.[26] The SRCT also addressed the benefit of short-course neoadjuvant radiation; however, the technique and volume of tissue irradiated were altered to decrease the risk for complications. Instead of an APPA technique, treatments were designed using three to four fields. Through incorporating lateral fields into the beam arrangement, larger portions of small bowel were able to be blocked from the field. Additionally, the superior border was lowered from L1–2 to the L4–5 level.

Patients randomized to the preoperative radiation arm received a dose of 25 Gy in five fractions 1 week before resection. Patients undergoing preoperative radiation experienced a decreased risk for local failure (11% versus 27%; $P<.001$) and an increase in both 5-year overall survival (58% versus 48%; $P = .004$) and 9-year cancer-specific survival (74% versus 65%; $P = .002$). Patients experienced no increase in mortality from the preoperative radiotherapy in this trial. Additional follow-up to a median of 13 years, has shown that the local control (9% versus 26%; $P<.001$) and survival (38% versus 30%; $P = .008$) benefits have remained durable.[24,26]

One of the criticisms of the SRCT was the very high rate of recurrence in the surgery-alone arm. Concurrent to these studies was the development of the TME technique, which in itself resulted in a dramatic reduction in local recurrence compared with historical rates.[73] Subsequently, the TME technique was incorporated into the Dutch CKVO 95-04 trial in which 1805 patients who had resectable rectal cancer were randomized to preoperative radiation consisting of 25 Gy in five fractions plus TME surgery versus TME surgery alone.[29] This trial confirmed the local control benefit of preoperative radiation even in the setting of optimal surgery. The overall 5-year rate of local recurrence was 12% for TME alone compared with 6% for radiation plus TME ($P<.001$).

In the 1990s, data from the European studies began to be incorporated into preoperative treatment regimens in the United States. Encouraged by the European data, interest increased in the United States to study the benefits of neoadjuvant chemoradiation in the preoperative setting. This approach was attractive because of several theoretic benefits, such as enhanced radiosensitivity, increased sphincter preservation rates, improved likelihood of resection, and less acute and late toxicity.[173–175]

Some of these potential benefits were confirmed in early trials by Willet and colleagues,[176] who showed down-staging in 31% of patients, and Minsky and colleagues[177] who illustrated a 90% sphincter preservation rate in patients initially believed to require APR. Unfortunately two national multiinstitutional trials, NSABP R03 and RTOG 94-01, comparing neoadjuvant with adjuvant chemoradiation were closed because of lack of accrual.

This specific issue was addressed by the German Rectal Cancer Trial in which 823 patients who had stage II and III rectal cancer were randomized to preoperative versus postoperative chemoradiotherapy.[178] This study incorporated conventional radiation dosing of 1.8 Gy per fraction along with concurrent infusional 5-FU chemotherapy. The treatment arms compared preoperative 5-FU, 50.4 Gy of pelvic radiation, and TME surgery to TME surgery followed by the same postoperative therapy, except that a boost to the tumor bed of 5.4 Gy was delivered after the 50.4 Gy to the whole pelvis. Although no difference was seen in survival between groups, a significant reduction in local failure (6% versus 13%, $P = .006$), less acute toxicity (27% versus 40% $P = .001$), and less chronic toxicity (14% versus 24% $P = .01$) occurred in the preoperative group. In addition, among the 194 patients who had tumors that were determined by the surgeon before randomization to require an APR, a statistically significant increase in sphincter preservation was seen among patients who underwent preoperative chemoradiotherapy (39% versus 19%; $P = .004$).

Based on these randomized results, the preferred standard of care for preoperatively staged greater than T3 or node-positive disease is neoadjuvant combined modality therapy. In the United States, standard doses of 45 Gy are delivered to the whole pelvis in 25 fractions of 1.8 Gy per fraction, with consideration of a 5.4 to 9.0 Gy boost to the site of local disease. This regimen is typically performed in conjunction with continuous-infusion 5-FU, although selective substitution with oral 5-FU agents has been described.[179]

INTRAOPERATIVE RADIATION THERAPY

Patients who have borderline resectable and unresectable rectal cancer are generally treated with pelvic radiation and chemotherapy and may be considered for intraoperative radiation therapy (IORT) when available.[180] With IORT, the tumor bed at highest risk can be focally irradiated with a single-boost dose. Advantages of this technique include the ability to displace the normal tissue away from the region at risk during surgery, which allows a radiobiologically higher dose to be delivered to the tumor. IORT has been associated with improved local control and survival in this patient population, especially those in whom a gross total resection can be achieved.[181]

For patients who have experienced recurrence in the setting of prior pelvic radiation, data support reirradiation. Valentini and colleagues[182] reported one third of patients who experienced local recurrence in the setting of prior pelvic radiation were able to undergo R0 resection after additional preoperative radiation therapy, with an overall 5-year survival of 39%.

ADVANCES IN RADIATION THERAPY

Technologic advances in radiation oncology are now being investigated for application in the treatment of rectal cancer. PET/CT fusion in the treatment position has enhanced targeting of the tumor.[183] Emerging developments, such as intensity-modulated radiation therapy (IMRT), image-guided radiation therapy (IGRT), and stereotactic body radiation therapy (SBRT), are being evaluated for clinical efficacy.[184,185] These techniques offer the ability to deliver more reliable conformal radiation treatment with concomitant improved sparing of normal tissues. A critical objective of newer technologies is to combine with established and novel radiation sensitizers to enhance the complete pathologic response rate with an attenuation of short- and long-term toxicities.

ADJUVANT CHEMOTHERAPY

The benefit of adjuvant chemotherapy for stage III colon cancer is well established.[17,186–189] A pooled analysis of seven clinical trials involving patients who had stage III colon cancer showed that adjuvant chemotherapy increased the probability of remaining disease-free from 42% to 58% and improved 5-year overall survival from 51% to 64%.[187,190]

The use of adjuvant chemotherapy for stage II colon cancer remains somewhat more controversial. Overall survival after surgery alone is 70% and 80%, with a disease-free survival of 65% and 73% for stage IIA and 51% and 60% for stage IIB colon cancer.[191] The Intergroup (Int 0035)[192] trial randomized patients who had stage II and III colon cancer to undergo surgery alone or surgery with adjuvant chemotherapy. At 7-year follow-up, no differences in survival were seen between treatment groups in patients who had stage II disease; however, the study was underpowered to detect a reduction in recurrences less than 50%.[192,193]

This finding led to the Intergroup (Int 0089)[146] trial in which 3759 patients who had high-risk stage II colon cancer, defined by bowel obstruction, perforation, or invasion of adjacent organs, were randomized to undergo adjuvant therapy after surgery. The investigators found no evidence of benefit from additional treatment. Much of the controversy that exists for stage II disease stems from the pooled results from four NSABP trials (C01–C04) of adjuvant therapy in stage II and III colon cancer, which showed an overall 30% reduction in mortality in patients who had stage II disease. This response was greater than that seen in patients who had stage III disease treated with adjuvant therapy (18%).[189] The reduction in mortality was seen in all patients who had stage II disease regardless of the presence or absence of high-risk features. However, only the C01 and C02 had true surgery-alone control groups. Despite these limitations, the NSABP subsequently recommended the routine use of adjuvant treatment for patients who had stage II colon cancer. However, this approach generally has not been uniformly accepted. Currently, it is recommended that adjuvant chemotherapy be considered for patients who have stage II disease with unfavorable histologic or clinical features.[56]

The evidence for the role of adjuvant chemotherapy in patients who have rectal cancer is not as well developed as that for colon cancer. The NSABP R-01 trial randomized 528 patients to either postoperative MOF chemotherapy, radiation therapy, or surgery alone. This trial showed a significant increase in 5-year disease-free survival (42% versus 30%; $P = .006$) and overall survival (53% versus 43%; $P = .05$) in patients undergoing adjuvant chemotherapy compared with those undergoing surgery alone.[170]

Decision making regarding the application of adjuvant therapy is more complicated for patients who have rectal cancer who have been treated with neoadjuvant chemoradiation. The equivocal accuracy of preoperative staging and frequent downstaging of both the primary tumor and regional lymph nodes leads to uncertainty regarding the true original stage.[194–197] The European Organisation for Research and Treatment of Cancer Radiotherapy Group Trial (EORTC) 22921 randomized 1011 patients to preoperative radiation (PrXRT), preoperative chemoradiation (PrCXRT), preoperative radiation and postoperative chemotherapy (PrXrt/PoC), or preoperative chemoradiation and postoperative chemotherapy (PrCXRT/PoC). The 5-year survival did not differ among patients undergoing adjuvant chemotherapy and those who did not (63.2% versus 67.2%; $P = .12$).[198] Chemotherapy, regardless of whether administered pre- or postoperatively did show a benefit with respect to local recurrence; 17.1% for those not treated with chemotherapy, 8.7% for PrCXRT, 9.6% for PrXRT/PoC, and 7.6% in the PrCXRT/PoC group ($P = .002$). However, criticism of this trial, which did not show a survival benefit in the adjuvant chemotherapy cohorts, relates to the poor adherence of patients in the adjuvant chemotherapy arms (42.9%) compared with those undergoing preoperative therapy (82%).

Given the lack of strong evidence in the setting of rectal cancer, support for the use of adjuvant chemotherapy in patients who had rectal cancer is generally an extrapolation from the data available for colon cancer.[199,200] In the setting of rectal cancer not treated with neoadjuvant chemoradiation, pathologic stage is considered accurate and adjuvant chemotherapy generally reserved for patients who have stage III disease. However, for patients who have preoperative stage II and III rectal cancer treated with neoadjuvant chemoradiation, the current recommendations include the use of adjuvant chemotherapy for approximately 6 months, regardless of final pathologic stage.[56]

SPECIFIC AGENTS
5-Fluorouracil

The mainstay of adjuvant chemotherapy in colorectal cancer is 5-FU, a fluorinated pyrimidine that acts by inhibiting thymidylate synthase, the rate-limiting enzyme in pyrimidine nucleotide synthesis.[192] Multiple randomized trials have shown that intravenous 5-FU or 5-FU plus leucovorin improves outcomes in patients who have stage III colon cancer.[201–203] Historically, 5-FU was combined with levamisole, an antihelminthic agent; however, because of increased efficacy, 5-FU is currently administered with leucovorin, a reduced folate that stabilizes the binding of fluorouracil to thymidylate synthase, thereby enhancing the inhibition of DNA synthesis.[193,201,203–205]

In patients who have advanced colorectal cancer, treatment with 5-FU and leucovorin reduces tumor size by 50% or more in approximately 20% of patients, and prolongs median survival from 6 months without treatment to 11 months with treatment.[206–208]

The major side effects associated with 5-FU depend on the method of administration. When the drug is given in bolus form for five consecutive days every 4 to 5 weeks, neutropenia and stomatitis are the most common side effects, whereas when it is given in weekly boluses, diarrhea is more frequent. In contrast, continuous infusions are associated with less hematologic and gastrointestinal toxicity but hand–foot syndrome is more common.[188,209,210]

Oral 5-FU

Early attempts to administer fluorouracil orally proved unsuccessful in randomized trials secondary to its erratic intestinal absorption and differing amounts of mucosal dihydropyrimidine dehydrogenase (DPD).[211] Strategies to circumvent this issue included development of a prodrug that is not catabolized by DPD (capecitabine) and coadministration with an inhibitor of DPD (tegafur uracil). Capecitabine is a prodrug of fluorouracil that is absorbed intact in the gastrointestinal mucosa and undergoes a three-step enzymatic conversion to 5-FU.[212] Capecitabine has been found to be therapeutically equivalent to bolus fluorouracil and leucovorin in the adjuvant treatment of patients who have stage III colorectal cancer.[200] Similar results were reported in the setting of metastatic disease, although these studies showed a higher incidence of hand–foot syndrome and hyperbilirubinemia but less stomatitis and neutropenia.[200] Tegafur uracil, an inhibitor of DPD that allows for more uniform absorption, has shown similar results in disease-free and overall survival compared with 5-FU/leucovorin. Although it was withdrawn by its manufacturer in the United States because of reports of severe side effects, it remains commercially available in Europe and Asia.[213]

Irinotecan

Irinotecan, a semisynthetic derivative of the natural alkaloid camptothecin, inhibits topoisomerase I, an enzyme that catalyzes the breakage and rejoining of DNA strands during replication.[214] The efficacy of single-agent irinotecan was established in the second-line treatment of patients who have metastatic disease and showed a 2- to 3-month increase in median survival versus supportive care or infusional 5-FU.[215,216] Diarrhea, myelosuppression, and alopecia were the side effects most commonly observed.

Subsequent trials have shown the additional benefits of combining irinotecan with either bolus or infusional 5-FU and leucovorin.[217,218] Based on these encouraging results, irinotecan was anticipated to be useful in the adjuvant treatment of colorectal cancer. Three randomized trials of adjuvant irinotecan with either bolus or infusional 5-FU have been reported. The CALGB randomized 1264 patients who had resectable stage III disease to receive 5-FU/leucovorin or irinotecan with weekly bolus 5-FU and leucovorin (IFL). Although IFL was proven superior in patients who have metastatic disease, it did not improve disease-free or overall survival when administered as adjuvant therapy.[219]

The Pan European Trials in Adjuvant Colon Cancer 3 (PETACC 3) trial randomized 3278 patients who had resectable stage II or III disease to receive infusional 5-FU/leucovorin with or without irinotecan.[220] After a median follow-up of 32 months, the addition of irinotecan did not significantly improve 3-year disease-free survival (63.3% versus 60.3%). A smaller European trial, Accord 02, randomized 400 patients who had resected high-risk stage III disease (>3 involved lymph nodes or any number lymph nodes and obstruction or perforation) to undergo adjuvant therapy with 5-FU/leucovorin alone or with irinotecan.[221] After a median follow-up 36 months, the rate of 3-year disease-free survival was poorer in patients who received irinotecan (53% versus 59%). The addition of irinotecan to 5-FU in each of these clinical trials resulted in increased toxicity without a meaningful improvement in outcome.

Oxaliplatin

Oxaliplatin is a diaminocyclohexane platinum compound that forms DNA adducts leading to impaired DNA replication and cellular apoptosis.[222] In patients who have metastatic colorectal cancer, single-agent oxaliplatin has limited efficacy, but clinical benefit has been observed when administered with 5-FU/leucovorin.[223–225] Oxaliplatin was evaluated in patients who had metastatic colorectal cancer in two phase III clinical trials that showed that adding oxaliplatin to infusional 5-FU/leucovorin increased response rate and disease-free survival, with a trend toward improving overall survival.[226–228]

Three clinical trials were initiated to evaluate oxaliplatin in the adjuvant setting. In the Multicenter International Study of Oxaliplatin/Fluorouracil/Leucovorin in the Adjuvant treatment of Colon Cancer (MOSAIC) study, 2246 patients who had stage II or III disease were randomized to receive 6 months of infusional 5-FU/leucovorin with or without oxaliplatin.[199,229] After a median follow-up of 49 months, the 4-year disease-free survival in patients who had stage III disease was statistically superior in those who received oxaliplatin (69.7% versus 61%).[186,190] Although a statistically significant benefit was not observed in patients who had stage II disease, a 5.4% absolute improvement in disease-free survival was noted in those who had high-risk stage II disease, defined as presence of T4 tumor, bowel obstruction, tumor perforation, poorly differentiated histology, venous invasion, or less than 10 nodes sampled.[190]

In a second study, the NSABP randomized 2407 patients who had resected stage II or III disease to undergo adjuvant therapy with bolus 5-FU/leucovorin with or without oxaliplatin.[230] After a median follow-up of 34 months, the 3-year disease-free survival was significantly improved in patients who received oxaliplatin (76.5% versus 71.6%) by an identical amount as seen in the MOSAIC trial. This outcome is noteworthy as the NSABP administered 5-FU in a bolus fashion rather then the infusional regimen used in the MOSAIC study. However, The addition of oxaliplatin in each trial resulted in additional treatment-related toxicity, including grade 3 or 4 neutropenia, grade 3 paresthesias, and grade 3 neurotoxicity.

Because disease recurrence is fatal in the vast majority of patients, disease-free survival has been proposed as a surrogate for overall survival. In an analysis of individualized patient data from 18 randomized controlled trials of adjuvant fluorouracil-based chemotherapy, 3-year disease-free survival was highly correlated with 5-year overall survival.[231] The MOSAIC and NSABP trials have shown improved disease-free survival when oxaliplatin is added to 5-FU/leucovorin; however, an overall survival benefit has yet to be observed in either study (**Table 2**).[231]

EPIDERMAL GROWTH FACTOR RECEPTOR INHIBITORS

The epidermal growth factor receptor (EGFR) is a transmembrane glycoprotein that interacts with signaling pathways affecting cellular growth, proliferation, and programmed cell death.[232] It is expressed in malignancies of the colon, lung, breast, and head and neck.[233] In colorectal cancer, EGFR expression has been shown in up to 80% of tumors and is associated with a poorer prognosis.[234,235] Cetuximab, a chimeric monoclonal antibody that inhibits EGFR, has shown promise in patients who have colorectal cancer. In an initial phase II study of 121 patients who had metastatic colorectal carcinoma whose tumors expressed EGFR and were refractory to irinotecan, the addition of cetuximab to irinotecan resulted in a response rate of 17%.[236] To determine whether this antineoplastic effect was caused by synergy or independent activity of cetuximab, a randomized phase III trial was performed of 329 patients refractory to irinotecan, showing a 22.9% response rate with combination

Table 2 Efficacy of adjuvant fluorouracil, leucovorin, and oxaliplatin in patients with resected stage ii or iii disease						
		Three-Year Disease-Free Survival			Overall Survival	
Trial	Treatment Arms	Patients	%	P Value	%	P Value
MOSAIC	FOLFOX	1123	78.2	.002	87.7	NS
	5FU/LV	1123	72.9		86.6	
NSABP C-07[a]	FLOX	1200	76.5	.004	NR	
	5FU/LV	1207	71.6		NR	

Multi-center International Study of Oxaliplatin/5-fluorouracil/Leucovor in the Adjuvant Treatment of Colon Cancer (MOSAIC). (NSABP) National Surgical Adjuvant Breast and Bowel Project C-07.
[a] Given as Roswell Park Regimen of bolus fluorouracil 500 mg/m^2 + Leucovorin 500 mg/m^2 given 6 of 8 weeks.

therapy compared with 10.8% with cetuximab alone.[237] The role of cetuximab in the adjuvant setting has yet to be defined. The NCCTG and EORTC are each randomizing more than 2000 patients who have stage III disease to receive FOLFOX alone or in combination with cetuximab; these trials will provide data on its efficacy in the adjuvant setting. The most common side effects of cetuximab are dermatologic, including acne-like rash, xerosis (dry-skin), and fissures of the skin.[237]

Panitumumab is a humanized monoclonal antibody to EGFR that has shown similar single-agent activity as cetuximab in metastatic colorectal cancer. In a phase II trial, 9% of 148 patients who had progressive disease after 5-FU and either irinotecan or oxaliplatin experienced a partial response to panitumumab.[238] This response rate is comparable to those observed in clinical trials of cetuximab in a similar patient population.[236,237] In a randomized phase III trial of 463 patients who had previously treated metastatic colorectal cancer, preliminary results suggest a progression-free survival benefit for panitumumab compared with best supportive care.[239]

Recently, there has been insight into predicting which patients will respond to EGFR inhibitors by identifying the status of K-RAS mutations.[240–242] A phase III randomized controlled trial[240] showed that median progression-free survival for patients treated with panitumumab who had wild-type K-RAS was 12.3 weeks, with a corresponding survival of 7.4 weeks for those who had mutated K-RAS. The median progression-free survival for patients in both K-RAS groups who underwent best supportive care only was 7.3 weeks. Among patients who had wild-type K-RAS who were treated with panitumumab, 17% responded and 34% had stable disease. Among patients who had the mutated K-RAS gene, 0% responded and 12% had stable disease. When the two treatment groups were combined, the overall survival was longer in patients who had wild-type K-RAS than in those who had mutated K-RAS.

Bevacizumab

The inhibition of new blood vessel formation has been explored as a strategy to control malignant proliferation and spread.[243] Currently the most successful antiangiogenic therapy has focused on inhibiting vascular endothelial growth factor (VEGF), a soluble protein that stimulates blood vessel proliferation.[244] Bevacizumab is a humanized monoclonal antibody directed against VEGF that has been examined in patients who had metastatic colorectal cancer. In a randomized phase III trial of 815 untreated patients who had metastatic disease, the addition of bevacizumab to IFL led to a statistically significant improvement in response rate (44.8% versus 34.8%) and a 4.7- month prolongation in median overall survival (20.3 versus 15.6 months).[245] Similarly, the addition of bevacizumab to FOLFOX regimens in patients who had metastatic colorectal carcinoma also demonstrated statistically significant improvements in disease-free and overall survival when compared with FOLFOX alone.[246] Bevacizumab was well tolerated in both trials, with reversible hypertension and proteinuria representing the two most common adverse events. The role of bevacizumab in the adjuvant setting is under examination in the United States and Europe (**Table 3**). Until the results of these trials are available, recommending its use as a part of adjuvant therapy for colorectal cancer is not advisable.

SPECIFIC CLINICAL CONTROVERSIES
Obstructing Lesions

Obstructing rectal cancer presents a unique clinical dilemma with respect to appropriate treatment options. Historically, management has consisted of an initial operation, such as a Hartmann's procedure with resection and temporary colostomy, followed by adjuvant treatment as indicated and reanastomosis. However, with the evolution of neoadjuvant chemoradiation as the preferred approach for rectal cancer, other temporizing solutions have become more prevalent. The use of gastrointestinal diversion without resection is one option and can be performed using either conventional or laparoscopic-assisted techniques.[64,72,84,105]

Endoscopic stenting represents a nonsurgical alternative for managing obstructing rectal lesions. This approach requires the ability to thread a guidewire across the lumen of the tumor and is limited to tumors lying 5 cm from the anal verge.[247] Morbidity and mortality in patients requiring emergency surgery for obstructing colorectal cancer were 39% and 12%, respectively, compared with 23% and 3.5% for patients who were treated with stenting and converted to elective surgery.[248] A pooled analysis of 54 studies of colorectal stenting showed technical and clinical success rates of 94% and 91%, respectively, with minimal morbidity (3.5%) and mortality (0.58%).[249,250] In addition to its ability to convert emergency surgery to a safer elective scenario, studies have shown that neoadjuvant chemoradiation may be safely administered in the presence of a rectal stent.[251,252]

Table 3		
Ongoing adjuvant clinical trials		
Clinical Trial	**American Joint Committee on Cancer Stage**	**Randomization**
NCCTG N0147	III	FOLFOX versus FOLFOX + cetuximab
PETACC 8	III	FOLFOX versus FOLFOX + cetuximab
NSABP C-08	II, III	FOLFOX versus FOLFOX + bevacizumab
AVANT	II, III	FOLFOX versus FOLFOX + bevacizumab versus capecitabine + oxaliplatin + bevacizumab
ECOG E5202	II	Molecular high-risk (MSS or MSI and 18q LOH) FOLFOX versus FOLFOX + bevacizumab standard risk observation

Abbreviations: NCCTG NO 147, North Central Cancer Treatment Group; PETACC 8, Pan European Trials in Alimentary Tract Cancer; NSABP c-08, National Surgical Adjuvant Breast and Bowel Project; AVANT, Avastin as Adjuvant Therapy; ECOG E5202, Eastern Cooperative Oncology Group.

RECTAL CANCER WITH SYNCHRONOUS RESECTABLE LIVER METASTASIS

The presence of liver metastases at initial diagnosis of a rectal cancer primary represents a particularly difficult dilemma for clinical decision making. Despite the presence of generalized guidelines, patients are extremely heterogeneous with respect to characteristics of the primary and metastatic sites, and each situation must be highly individualized. Therefore, a comprehensive multidisciplinary approach to determine the incorporation and timing of surgery, chemotherapy, and radiation therapy is essential in treating these patients.

Approximately 50% to 60% of patients diagnosed with colorectal cancer will develop liver metastases,[54] and of these, 15% to 20% will present in the synchronous setting. Unfortunately, only 10% to 20% of patients who have colorectal liver metastasis are candidates for curative-intent hepatic surgery.[253] However, in these patients, 5-year overall survival rates may exceed 50% after liver resection.[254]

As long as the primary tumor is amenable to resection, the initial critical step is to determine the resectability of the liver metastases. This determination will help determine whether to pursue an aggressive curative versus a more palliative objective. In patients who have unresectable metastases and an asymptomatic primary rectal cancer, standard chemotherapy for advanced disease should be initiated. In the setting of significant symptoms, maneuvers such as surgical diversion, stenting, chemoradiation, or even resection may be required before systemic treatment.

The approach to patients who have resectable rectal cancer and synchronous hepatic metastases is framed by the extent of disease at the primary and metastatic sites. Acceptable options for initial treatment include staged or synchronous surgical resection of the primary and metastatic disease; neoadjuvant chemoradiation; and combination bevacizumab-containing chemotherapy regimens.

Staged or Synchronous Surgical Resection of the Primary and Metastatic Disease

Simultaneous resection may be most appropriate in the setting of minimal disease at both sites. An important consideration for this approach is that the synchronous presentation of metastases may indicate a more disseminated disease state and harbor a worse prognosis than disease that develops metachronously.[255] Therefore, experts have argued that initial chemotherapy may be more prudent.[256–258] Furthermore, Reddy and colleagues[259] showed that morbidity and mortality of synchronous resections of the liver and colon/rectum increased significantly when major hepatic resections (greater than a lobe) were performed in a simultaneous versus staged approach, and thus recommended caution in performing simultaneous approaches in patients requiring extensive hepatic resections. In a staged approach, after resection of the primary, hepatic surgery may be performed 4 to 6 weeks after resection of the primary or, alternatively, chemotherapy can be administered first followed by reevaluation.

Neoadjuvant Chemoradiation

The administration of neoadjuvant chemoradiation to the primary site as an initial step may be considered, particularly in the setting of symptomatic (eg, near-obstructing, bleeding) locally advanced disease and, ideally, with concomitant low-volume liver disease. This approach can reduce patient symptoms and improve local control. Chemoradiation may be followed by staged or synchronous resection as described previously. Alternatively, a course of systemic chemotherapy may be administered first, followed by reevaluation. However, chemoradiation can result in reduced tolerance to bevacizumab, thereby altering potential treatment of metastatic disease.[260]

Combination Bevacizumab-Containing Chemotherapy Regimens

The initial administration of systemic chemotherapy is also an acceptable option for patients who have synchronous liver metastases. Chemotherapy may be followed by staged or synchronous resection or, alternatively, by chemoradiation, depending on the extent of disease at the primary and distant sites. Neoadjuvant chemotherapy serves to address systemic disease but may also impact the primary tumor.[261] Moreover, response to neoadjuvant chemotherapy before hepatic resection has been correlated with overall survival. Allen and colleagues[262] showed that 5-year survival was statistically similar between patients undergoing neoadjuvant chemotherapy before hepatic surgery and those who did not (43% versus 35%; $P = .49$); however, those receiving neoadjuvant chemotherapy whose disease did not progress experienced significantly improved survival (85% versus 35%; $P = .03$).[261]

In this setting, several issues require communication between surgeons and medical oncologists. Bevacizumab may be associated with an increased risk for surgical bleeding and therefore experts recommend that it be stopped at least 6 to 8 weeks before major surgery and only initiated at least 4 weeks postoperatively.[56] An additional issue pertains to the increased risk for hepatotoxicity with prolonged administration of systemic chemotherapy.[263–266] Fernandez and colleagues[265] examined liver biopsies for nonalcoholic steatohepatitis (NASH) from 37 patients undergoing irinotecan/oxaliplatin (IRI-OXALI) regimens, 5-FU, or no chemotherapy. Biopsy scores were significantly worse for IRI-OXALI compared with no chemotherapy or 5-FU-only for NASH score ($P = .003$). Moreover, in patients undergoing hepatic surgery, Vauthey and colleagues[266] showed an increased 90-day mortality in those who had evidence of steatohepatitis compared with those who did not (14.7% versus 1.6%, respectively; $P = .001$). Therefore, hepatic resection, if feasible, should be considered after four to six cycles of systemic chemotherapy.

For patients undergoing successful resections of the primary tumor and liver metastases in the absence of pelvic radiation, the use of adjuvant chemoradiation may be considered. In the infrequent circumstance of pT1/T2 N0 M1 disease, the risk for additional metastases is higher than locoregional failure and, therefore systemic chemotherapy should be given and radiation may be omitted.

T3N0M0

Historically, local recurrence rates after surgery for rectal cancer were approximately 20%.[8,9,66,68,69,77,90,168] However, with the advent of the TME technique, local recurrence rates have been reduced dramatically and are now routinely less than 10%.[9,12,24,65,67,75,128,156,267,268] Consequently, the issue has been raised as to whether optimal surgery alone (without adjuvant treatment) is adequate for the local control of T3N0 rectal cancer. In an analysis of 95 pT3N0 patients treated with TME surgery alone, the 5-year actuarial recurrence rate was 12%, with 5-year disease-specific and overall survival rates reported as 86.6% and 75%, respectively.[71] Experts suggested that adjuvant chemoradiation may be omitted in select patients who have T3N0 rectal cancer.

Currently, neoadjuvant combined modality therapy remains the preferred treatment for cT3N0 rectal cancer. A major concern in this setting has been the overtreatment of individuals who may be overstaged by pretreatment staging modalities. The German Rectal Cancer study showed that 18% of patients deemed suitable for preoperative treatment by endorectal ultrasound may be overstaged.[178] In a recent evaluation of 188 patients who had cT3N0 rectal cancer treated with preoperative chemoradiation, Guillem and colleagues[269] showed that on final pathologic analysis, 22% of patients harbored residual, undetected mesorectal lymph node involvement, suggesting the inaccurate nature of pretreatment staging techniques. Although a subset of patients will be overstaged and thus overtreated, experts suggest that even a larger number of patients will have nodal understaging. In the absence of neoadjuvant treatment, the group with nodal understaging would subsequently require postoperative chemoradiation, which is associated with significantly worse local control, higher toxicities, and inferior bowel function.[178] Currently, the recommended approach is to administer neoadjuvant combined modality treatment to patients who have cT3N0 rectal cancer.[56]

CONSERVATIVE MANAGEMENT OF T2/T3 TUMORS AFTER NEOADJUVANT THERAPY

Local excision is generally accepted as an option for the treatment of T1 adenocarcinomas of the rectum with favorable features and is associated with low rates of recurrence and surgical morbidity.[111,112] Local excision for more advanced lesions (T2 and T3) has been reported to have unacceptably high rates of recurrence (17%–62%), even with the use of adjuvant chemoradiation strategies.[121–123,160] Therefore, enthusiasm for local excision for T2 and T3 lesions has waned significantly. However, with the increasing use of neoadjuvant chemoradiation for locally advanced rectal cancers, renewed interest has been shown in the application of local excision for select situations.

Associated with the use of neoadjuvant treatment is the observation that a complete pathologic response may be achieved in up to 30% of patients.[160,270] Radical surgery is still considered standard care for these patients but may result in significant morbidity, including infection, anastomotic leak, need for ostomy, and genitourinary complications.[68,99,104,128,271] Consequently, the question has been raised as to whether radical surgery can be avoided in patients who have a significant response to preoperative combined modality therapy.[164] Habr-Gama and colleagues[272] reported a controversial treatment strategy, based on the clinical response to neoadjuvant therapy. In patients (n = 256) who had distal rectal cancer deemed resectable and underwent neoadjuvant chemoradiation, those who had an incomplete clinical response were referred for radical surgery, whereas those who experienced a complete clinical response were observed. Rates of 5-year overall and disease-free survival were 88% and 83%, respectively, in the resection group and 100% and 92%, respectively, in the observation group.

An important concern is that a complete clinical response is highly inaccurate in predicting a complete pathologic response. Guillem and colleagues[163,269] reported that DRE underestimated response in 78% of patients undergoing neoadjuvant therapy and, similarly, other investigators have shown that radiologic imaging such as transrectal ultrasound, MRI, and PET scanning have not been reliable in predicting response.[273,274]

Others have explored the application of local excision for patients who have T2/T3 tumors exhibiting substantial response to neoadjuvant therapy, although few studies are found in the literature and these were limited by relatively low numbers of patients and short follow-up. These studies, which contain heterogeneous groups of T2, T3, and T4 tumors, have reported local and distant recurrence rates ranging from 0% to 12.5% and 0% to 20%, respectively.[275–277]

Recently, Nair and colleagues[164] reported outcomes for patients who had T2/T3 tumors undergoing local excision after neoadjuvant therapy. They showed a 9% local recurrence after neoadjuvant therapy and 5-year survival rates of 84% for T2/3 N0 and 81% for T2/3 N1 lesions. Despite these promising results, in the absence of prospective randomized data, local excision for T2/T3 tumors after neoadjuvant chemoradiation should remain reserved for patients who are unable to tolerate or refuse radical surgery, or in the setting of clinical trials. The ongoing ACOSOG Z6041 trial will shed additional light on the role of local excision of T2 rectal cancer after preoperative combined modality therapy.

SUMMARY

Accurate preoperative staging with transrectal ultrasound or MRI is important in properly selecting patients who have rectal cancer for immediate surgery or neoadjuvant therapy. Radical surgical approaches, such as APR or LAR, should incorporate TME and focus on achieving adequate distal and radial margins. Local excision through conventional transanal or TEM approaches may be performed selectively on T1 tumors with fully favorable clinical and histopathologic features. Laparoscopic-assisted rectal cancer surgery seems promising, with preliminary data suggesting surgical and oncologic safety. However, until further results are reported of prospective trials specific to rectal cancer, these techniques should remain limited to enrollment in clinical trials. Multiple agents are available in the adjuvant setting for patients who have stage II and III rectal cancer. However, the current adjuvant standard is the combination of 5-FU/LV and oxaliplatin (FOLFOX), a regimen that was initially shown to improve disease-free and overall survival in metastatic colorectal carcinoma. In patients who have stage III disease, adjuvant FOLFOX has also yielded improved disease-free survival but has yet to translate into an overall survival benefit. Newer agents, such as VEGF and EGFR inhibitors, are routinely used in the setting of metastatic disease, but currently no data support their use in the adjuvant setting. Management of rectal cancer can be complex and is optimized when approached in a coordinated manner by an experienced multidisciplinary cancer treatment team.

REFERENCES

1. Jemal A, Siegel R, Ward E, et al. Cancer statistics, 2008. CA Cancer J Clin 2008; 58(1):71–96.
2. Wolpin BM, Meyerhardt JA, Mamon HJ, et al. Adjuvant treatment of colorectal cancer. CA Cancer J Clin 2007;57(3):168–85.
3. Ellenhorn D, Coia L, Alberts S, et al, editors. Colorectal and anal cancers. Coia L, Hoskins W, editors. Cancer management: a multidisciplinary approach. Melville (NY): PRR Inc; 2002.
4. Cohen SM, Neugut AI, Cohen SM, et al. Adjuvant therapy for rectal cancer in the elderly. Drugs Aging 2004;21(7):437–51.
5. Nelson H, Petrelli N, Carlin A. Guidelines 2000 for colon and rectal cancer surgery. J Natl Cancer Inst 2001;93(8):583–96.
6. Tjandra JJ, Kilkenny JW, Buie WD, et al. Practice parameters for the management of rectal cancer. Dis Colon Rectum 2005;48(3):411–23.
7. Pilipshen SJ, Heilweil M, Quan SH, et al. Patterns of pelvic recurrence following definitive resections of rectal cancer. Cancer 1984;53:1354–62.
8. Glynne-Jones R, Mathur P, Elton C, et al. The multidisciplinary management of gastrointestinal cancer. Multimodal treatment of rectal cancer. Best Pract Res Clin Gastroenterol 2007;21(6):1049–70.
9. Adam IJ, Mohamdee MO, Martin IG, et al. Role of circumferential margin involvement in the local recurrence of rectal cancer. Lancet 1994;344(8924):707–11.
10. Arbman G, Nilsson E, Hallbook O, et al. Local recurrence following total mesorectal excision for rectal cancer. Br J Surg 1996;83(3):375–9.
11. Goligher JC, Dukes CE, Bussey HJ. Local recurrences after sphincter saving excisions for carcinoma of the rectum and rectosigmoid. Br J Surg 1951;39(155):199–211.

12. de Haas-Kock DF, Baeten CG, Jager JJ, et al. Prognostic significance of radial margins of clearance in rectal cancer. Br J Surg 1996;83(6):781–5.
13. Rich T, Gunderson LL, Lew R, et al. Patterns of recurrence of rectal cancer after potentially curative surgery. Cancer 1983;52(7):1317–29.
14. Wolmark N, Fisher B. An analysis of survival and treatment failure following abdominoperineal and sphincter-saving resection in Dukes' B and C rectal carcinoma. A report of the NSABP clinical trials. National Surgical Adjuvant Breast and Bowel Project. Ann Surg 1986;204(4):480–9.
15. Greene F, Page D, Fleming I, editors. AJCC cancer staging handbook. 6th edition. New York: Springer; 2002.
16. Greene FL, Stewart AK, Norton HJ. New tumor-node-metastasis staging strategy for node-positive (stage III) rectal cancer: an analysis. J Clin Oncol 2004;22(10):1778–84.
17. Meyerhardt JA, Mayer RJ. Systemic therapy for colorectal cancer. N Engl J Med 2005;352(5):476–87.
18. O'Connell JB, Maggard MA, Ko CY. Colon cancer survival rates with the new American Joint Committee on Cancer sixth edition staging. J Natl Cancer Inst 2004;96(19):1420–5.
19. Hideya T, Tomohiro T, Nagasaki S, et al. Synchronous multiple colorectal adenocarcinomas. Journal of Surgical Oncology 1997;64:304–7.
20. Fukatsua H, Katoa J, Nasub J, et al. Clinical characteristics of synchronous colorectal cancer are different according to tumour location. Dig Liver Dis 2007;39(1):40–6.
21. Stocchi L, Nelson H, Sargent DJ, et al. Impact of surgical and pathologic variables in rectal cancer: a United States community and cooperative group report. J Clin Oncol 2001;19(18):3895–902.
22. Higgins GA, Humphrey EW, Dwight RW, et al. Preoperative radiation and surgery for cancer of the rectum. Veterans Administration Surgical Oncology Group Trial II. Cancer 1986;58(2):352–9.
23. Roswit B, Higgins GA, Keehn RJ. Preoperative irradiation for carcinoma of the rectum and rectosigmoid colon: report of a National Veterans Administration randomized study. Cancer 1975;35(6):1597–602.
24. Folkesson J, Birgisson H, Pahlman L, et al. Swedish rectal cancer trial: long lasting benefits from radiotherapy on survival and local recurrence rate. J Clin Oncol 2005;23(24):5644–50.
25. Wong RKS, Tandan V, De Silva S, et al. Pre-operative radiotherapy and curative surgery for the management of localized rectal carcinoma. Cochrane Database Syst Rev 2007;(2):CD002102.
26. Swedish Rectal Cancer Trial. Improved survival with preoperative radiotherapy in resectable rectal cancer. N Engl J Med 1997;336(14):980–7.
27. Kim NK, Baik SH, Seong JS, et al. Oncologic outcomes after neoadjuvant chemoradiation followed by curative resection with tumor-specific mesorectal excision for fixed locally advanced rectal cancer: impact of postirradiated pathologic downstaging on local recurrence and survival. Ann Surg 2006;244(6):1024–30.
28. Boller A-M, Cima RR. Impact of pre- and postoperative multimodality therapy on rectal cancer. J Surg Oncol 2007;96(8):665–70.
29. Kapiteijn E, Marijnen CA, Nagtegaal ID, et al. Preoperative radiotherapy combined with total mesorectal excision for resectable rectal cancer. N Engl J Med 2001;345(9):638–46.
30. Brown G, Davies S, Williams GT, et al. Effectiveness of preoperative staging in rectal cancer: digital rectal examination, endoluminal ultrasound or magnetic resonance imaging? Br J Cancer 2004;91(1):23–9.

31. Zoumpoulis P, Tragea H, Pahos K, et al. How to efficiently perform transrectal ultrasound (TRUS) and TRUS guided biopsy of the prostate. Ultrasound Med Biol 2006;32(Suppl 5):248.
32. Bipat S, Glas AS, Slors FJ, et al. Rectal cancer: local staging and assessment of lymph node involvement with endoluminal US, CT, and MR imaging—a meta-analysis. Radiology 2004;232(3):773–83.
33. Hulsmans FJ, Tio TL, Fockens P, et al. Assessment of tumor infiltration depth in rectal cancer with transrectal sonography: caution is necessary [see comment]. Radiology 1994;190(3):715–20.
34. Siddiqui A, Fayiga Y, Huerta S. The role of endoscopic ultrasound in the evaluation of rectal cancer. Int Semin Surg Oncol 2006;3(36):1–7.
35. Beynon J, Foy DM, Roe AM, et al. Endoluminal ultrasound in the assessment of local invasion in rectal cancer. Br J Surg 1986;73(6):474–7.
36. Hunerbein M, Pegios W, Rau B, et al. Prospective comparison of endorectal ultrasound, three-dimensional endorectal ultrasound, and endorectal MRI in the preoperative evaluation of rectal tumors. Preliminary results. Surg Endosc 2000;14(11):1005–9.
37. Karantanas AH, Yarmenitis S, Papanikolaou N, et al. Preoperative imaging staging of rectal cancer. Dig Dis 2007;25(1):20–32.
38. Meyenberger C, Huch Boni RA, Bertschinger P, et al. Endoscopic ultrasound and endorectal magnetic resonance imaging: a prospective, comparative study for preoperative staging and follow-up of rectal cancer. Endoscopy 1995;27(7):469–79.
39. Starck M, Bohe M, Fork FT, et al. Endoluminal ultrasound and low-field magnetic resonance imaging are superior to clinical examination in the preoperative staging of rectal cancer. Eur J Surg 1995;161(11):841–5.
40. Tankova L, Kadnian K, Draganov V, et al. [Endoluminal echography in rectal cancer—preoperative staging and postoperative control]. Khirurgiia 2003;59(5):26–30 [Russian].
41. Kulinna C, Scheidler J, Strauss T, et al. Local staging of rectal cancer: assessment with double-contrast multislice computed tomography and transrectal ultrasound. J Comput Assist Tomogr 2004;28(1):123–30.
42. Hulsmans F, Bosma A, Mulder P, et al. Perirectal lymph nodes in rectal cancer: in vitro correlation of sonographic parameters and histopathologic findings. Radiology 1992;184:553–60.
43. Beynon J, Mortensen NJ, Foy DM, et al. Pre-operative assessment of local invasion in rectal cancer: digital examination, endoluminal sonography or computed tomography? Br J Surg 1986;73(12):1015–7.
44. Brown G, Radcliffe AG, Newcombe RG, et al. Preoperative assessment of prognostic factors in rectal cancer using high-resolution magnetic resonance imaging. Br J Surg 2003;90(3):355–64.
45. Gualdi GF, Casciani E, Guadalaxara A, et al. Local staging of rectal cancer with transrectal ultrasound and endorectal magnetic resonance imaging: comparison with histologic findings. Dis Colon Rectum 2000;43(3):338–45.
46. Hildebrandt U, Feifel G. Preoperative staging of rectal cancer by intrarectal ultrasound. Dis Colon Rectum 1985;28(1):42–6.
47. Orrom WJ, Wong WD, Rothenberger DA, et al. Endorectal ultrasound in the preoperative staging of rectal tumors. A learning experience. Dis Colon Rectum 1990;33(8):654–9.
48. Brown G, Richards CJ, Bourne MW. Morphologic predictors of lymph node status in rectal cancer with use of high-spatial-resolution MR imaging with histopathologic comparison. Radiology 2003;227(2):371–7.

49. Brown G, Kirkham A, Williams GT, et al. High-resolution MRI of the anatomy important in total mesorectal excision of the rectum. AJR Am J Roentgenol 2004; 182(2):431–9.

50. Chun HK, Choi D, Kim MJ, et al. Preoperative staging of rectal cancer: comparison of 3-T high-field MRI and endorectal sonography. AJR Am J Roentgenol 2006;187(6):1557–62.

51. Mercury Study Group. Extramural depth of tumor invasion at thin-section MR in patients with rectal cancer: results of the MERCURY study. Radiology 2007; 243(1):132–9.

52. Wieder HA, Rosenberg R, Lordick F, et al. Rectal cancer: MR imaging before neoadjuvant chemotherapy and radiation therapy for prediction of tumor-free circumferential resection margins and long-term survival. Radiology 2007;243(3): 744–51.

53. Satoshi A, Masaru M, Hiroshi I, et al. Resection of hepatic and pulmonary metastases in patients with colorectal carcinoma. Cancer 2000;82(2):274–8.

54. Yoo PS, Lopez RI, Longo WE, et al. Liver resection for metastatic colorectal cancer in the age of neoadjuvant therapy and bevacizumab. Clin Colorectal Cancer 2006;6:202–7.

55. Sundermeyeer M, Meropol NJ, Rogatko A, et al. Changing patterns of colorectal metastases: a 10-year retrospective review (abstract). Proc Am Soc Clin Oncol 2004;23:257a.

56. NCCN Clinical Practice Guidelines in Oncology. Rectal Cancer 2008;3:1–69.

57. Nahas CS, Ankhurst T, Yeung H, et al. Positron emission tomography detection of distant metastatic or synchronous disease in patients with locally advanced rectal cancer receiving preoperative chemoradiation. Ann Surg Oncol 2008; 15(4):704–11.

58. Gearhart SL, Frassica D, Rosen R, et al. Improved staging with pretreatment positron emission tomography/computed tomography in low rectal cancer. Ann Surg Oncol 2006;13(3):397–404.

59. Miles EW. A method of performing abdominoperineal excision for carcinoma of the rectum and the terminal portion of the pelvic colon. Lancet 1908;2: 1812–3.

60. Yeatman TJ, Bland KI. Sphincter-saving procedures for distal carcinoma of the rectum. Ann Surg 1989;209(1):1–18.

61. Dixon CF. Surgical removal of lesions occurring in the sigmoid and rectosigmoid. Am J Surg 1939;46:12–7.

62. Mayo CW, Laberge MY, Hardy WM. Five-year survival after anterior resection for carcinoma of the rectum and rectosigmoid. Surg Gynecol Obstet 1958;105: 695–8.

63. Fain SN, Patin S, Morganstern L. Use of mechanical apparatus in low colorectal anastomosis. Arch Surg 1975;110:1079–82.

64. Baik SH, Kim NK, Lee KY, et al. Hand-sewn coloanal anastomosis for distal rectal cancer: long-term clinical outcomes. J Gastrointest Surg 2005;9(6):775–80.

65. Bolognese A, Cardi M, Muttillo IA, et al. Total mesorectal excision for surgical treatment of rectal cancer. J Surg Oncol 2000;74(1):21–3.

66. Gamagami RA, Liagre A, Chiotasso P, et al. Coloanal anastomosis for distal third rectal cancer: prospective study of oncologic results. Dis Colon Rectum 1999; 42(10):1272–5.

67. Hall NR, Finan PJ, al-Jaberi T, et al. Circumferential margin involvement after mesorectal excision of rectal cancer with curative intent. Predictor of survival but not local recurrence? Dis Colon Rectum 1998;41(8):979–83.

68. Lavery IC, Lopez-Kostner F, Fazio VW, et al. Chances of cure are not compromised with sphincter-saving procedures for cancer of the lower third of the rectum. Surgery 1997;122(4):779–84.

69. Pollett WG, Nicholls RJ. The relationship between the extent of distal clearance and survival and local recurrence rates after curative anterior resection for carcinoma of the rectum. Ann Surg 1983;198(2):159–63.

70. Tytherleigh MG, Warren BF, Mortensen NJ. Management of early rectal cancer. Br J Surg 2008;95(4):409–23.

71. Merchant NB, Guillem JG, Paty PB, et al. T3N0 rectal cancer: results following sharp mesorectal excision and no adjuvant therapy. J Gastrointest Surg 1999; 3(6):642–7.

72. Leo E, Belli F, Andreola S, et al. Total rectal resection, mesorectum excision, and coloendoanal anastomosis: a therapeutic option for the treatment of low rectal cancer. Ann Surg Oncol 1996;3(4):336–43.

73. Heald RJ, Husband EM, Ryal RD. The mesorectum in rectal cancer surgery—clue to pelvic recurrence? Br J Surg 1982;69:613–8.

74. Heald RJ. Rectal cancer: the surgical options. Eur J Cancer 1995;31:1189–92.

75. Scott N, Jackson P, al-Jaberi T, et al. Total mesorectal excision and local recurrence: a study of tumour spread in the mesorectum distal to rectal cancer. Br J Surg 1995;82(8):1031–3.

76. Hida J, Yasutomi M, Maruyama T, et al. Lymph node metastases detected in the mesorectum distal to carcinoma of the rectum by the clearing method: justification of total mesorectal excision. J Am Coll Surg 1997;184(6):584–8.

77. Bokey EL, Ojerskog B, Chapuis PH, et al. Local recurrence after curative excision of the rectum for cancer without adjuvant therapy: role of total anatomical dissection. Br J Surg 1999;86(9):1164–70.

78. Vernava AM, Moran M, Rothenberger DA, et al. A prospective evaluation of distal margins in carcinoma of the rectum. Surg Gynecol Obstet 1992;175: 333–6.

79. Black WA, Waugh JM. The intramural extension of carcinoma of the descending colon, sigmoid, and rectosigmoid: a pathologic study. Surg Gynecol Obstet 1948;87:457–64.

80. Williams NS, Dixon MF, Johnson D. Reappraisal of the 5 cm rule of distal excision for carcinoma of the rectum; a study of distal intramural spread and of patients' survival. Br J Surg 1983;70:150–4.

81. Grinnell RS. Lymphatic block with atypical and retrograde lymphatic metastasis and spread in carcinoma of the colon and rectum. Ann Surg 1966;163:272–80.

82. Guillem JG. Ultra-low anterior resection and coloanal pouch reconstruction for carcinoma of the distal rectum. World J Surg 1997;21(7):721–7.

83. Hassan I, Larson DW, Cima RR, et al. Long-term functional and quality of life outcomes after coloanal anastomosis for distal rectal cancer. Dis Colon Rectum 2006;49(9):1266–74.

84. Tytherleigh MG, Mc CMNJ, Tytherleigh MG, et al. Options for sphincter preservation in surgery for low rectal cancer. Br J Surg 2003;90(8):922–33.

85. Rullier E, Zerbib F, Laurent C, et al. Intersphincteric resection with excision of internal anal sphincter for conservative treatment of very low rectal cancer. Dis Colon Rectum 1999;42:1168–75.

86. Bretagnol F, Rullier E, Laurent C, et al. Comparison of functional results and quality of life between intersphincteric resection and conventional coloanal anastomosis for low rectal cancer. Dis Colon Rectum 2004;47:832–8.

87. Ho YH, Seow-Choen F, Tan M, et al. Colonic J-pouch function at six months versus straight coloanal anastomosis at two years: randomized controlled trial. World J Surg 2001;25(7):876–81.

88. Rullier E, Laurent C, Bretagnol F, et al. Sphincter saving resection: end of the 2 cm rule? Ann Surg 2005;242(6):903–4.

89. Nagtegaal ID, Quirke P. What is the role for the circumferential margin in the modern treatment of rectal cancer? J Clin Oncol 2008;26(2):303–12.

90. Quirke P, Durdey P, Dixon MF, et al. Local recurrence of rectal adenocarcinoma due to inadequate surgical resection. Histopathological study of lateral tumour spread and surgical excision. Lancet 1986;2(8514):996–9.

91. Cawthorn SJ, Parums DV, Gibbs NM, et al. Extent of mesorectal spread and involvement of lateral resection margin as prognostic factors after surgery for rectal cancer [see comment]. Lancet 1990;335(8697):1055–9.

92. Fujita S, Yamamoto S, Akasu T, et al. Lateral pelvic lymph node dissection for advanced lower rectal cancer. Br J Surg 2003;90(12):1580–5.

93. Shiozawa M, Akaike M, Yamada R, et al. Lateral lymph node dissection for lower rectal cancer. Hepatogastroenterology 2007;54(76):1066–70.

94. Kim JC, Takahashi K, Yu CS, et al. Comparative outcome between chemoradiotherapy and lateral pelvic lymph node dissection following total mesorectal excision in rectal cancer. Ann Surg 2007;246(5):754–62.

95. Mann B. Lateral lymph node dissection in rectal cancer patients: is there any indication? Int J Colorectal Dis 2004;19(3):195–6.

96. Nagawa H, Muto T, Sunouchi K, et al. Randomized, controlled trial of lateral node dissection vs. nerve-preserving resection in patients with rectal cancer after preoperative radiotherapy. Dis Colon Rectum 2001;44(9):1274–80.

97. Kumar A. Observations on rectal cancer practice in Japan. Eur J Surg Oncol 2002;29(7):630–1.

98. Michelassi F, Block G. Morbidity and mortality of wide pelvic lymphadenectomy for rectal adenocarcinoma. Dis Colon Rectum 1992;35(12):1143–7.

99. Kyo K, Sameshima S, Takahashi M, et al. Impact of autonomic nerve preservation and lateral node dissection on male urogenital function after total mesorectal excision for lower rectal cancer. World J Surg 2006;30(6):1014–9.

100. Guillou PJ, Quirke P, Thorpe H, et al. JM, MRC CLASICC Trial Group. Short-term endpoints of conventional versus laparoscopic assisted surgery in patients with colorectal cancer (MRC CLASICC trial): multicentre, randomized controlled study. Lancet 2005;365:1718–29.

101. Clinical Outcomes of Surgical Therapy Study Group. A comparison of laparoscopically assisted and open colectomy for colon cancer. N Engl J Med 2004; 350(20):2050–9.

102. Veldkamp R, Kuhry E, Hop WC. Colon cancer Laparoscopic or Open Resection Study Group (COLOR). Laparoscopic surgery versus open surgery for colon cancer: short-term outcomes of a randomized trial. Lancet Oncol 2005;6(7): 477–84.

103. Lacy AM, Garcia-Valdecasas JC, Delgado S. Laparoscopy-assisted colectomy versus open colectomy for treatment of non-metastatic colon cancer: a randomised trial. Lancet Oncol 2002;359:2224–9.

104. Leung KL, Kwok SP, Lau WY, et al. Laparoscopic-assisted abdominoperineal resection for low rectal adenocarcinoma. Surg Endosc 2000;14(1):67–70.

105. Liang JT, Lai HS, Lee PH, et al. Laparoscopic pelvic autonomic nerve-preserving surgery for patients with lower rectal cancer after chemoradiation therapy. Ann Surg Oncol 2007;14(4):1285–7.

106. Reza MM, Blasco JA, Andradas E, et al. Systematic review of laparoscopic versus open surgery for colorectal cancer. Br J Surg 2006;93(8):921–8.
107. Wagman LD. Laparoscopic and open surgery for colorectal cancer: reaching equipoise? J Clin Oncol 2007;25(21):2996–8.
108. Rullier E, Sa Cunha A, Couderc P. Laparoscopic intersphincteric resection with coloplasty and coloanal anastomosis for mid and low rectal cancer. Br J Surg 2003;90(4):445–51.
109. Boller AM, Nelson H. Colon and rectal cancer: laparoscopic or open? Clin Cancer Res 2007;13(22):6894–6.
110. Sengupta S, Tjandra JJ. Local excision of rectal cancer: what is the evidence? Dis Colon Rectum 2001;44(9):1345–61.
111. Heintz A, Morschel M, Junginger T. Comparison of results after transanal endoscopic microsurgery and radical resection for T1 carcinoma of the rectum. Surg Endosc 1998;12(9):1145–8.
112. Palma P, Freudenberg S, Samel S, et al. Transanal endoscopic microsurgery: indications and results after 100 cases. Colorectal Dis 2004;6(5):350–5.
113. Varma MG, Rogers SJ, Schrock TR, et al. Local excision of rectal carcinoma. Arch Surg 1999;134(8):863–8.
114. Winde G, Nottberg H, Kellerr Schmid KW, et al. Surgical cure for early rectal carcinomas (T1). Transanal endoscopic microsurgery vs. anterior resection. Dis Colon Rectum 1996;39(9):969–76.
115. Bleday R. Local excision of rectal cancer. World J Surg 1997;21(7):706–14.
116. Morson BC, Bussey HJ, Samoorian S. Policy of local excision for early cancer of the colorectum. Gut 1977;18(12):1045–50.
117. Bleday R. Local excision of small distal rectal cancers. Clin Colon Rectal Surg 2002;15:163–8.
118. Greenberg J, Bleday R. Local excision of rectal cancer oncologic results. Semin Colon Rectal Surg 2005;16(1):40–6.
119. Garcia-Aguilar J, Mellgren A, Sirivongs P. Local excision of rectal cancer without adjuvant therapy: a word of caution. Ann Surg 2000;231(3):345–51.
120. Madbouly KM, Remzi FH, Erkek BA, et al. Recurrence after transanal excision of T1 rectal cancer: should we be concerned? Dis Colon Rectum 2005;48(4): 711–21.
121. Chakravarti A, Compton CC, Shellito PC, et al. Long-term follow-up of patients with rectal cancer managed by local excision with and without adjuvant irradiation. Ann Surg 1999;230(1):49–54.
122. Lezoche E, Guerrieri M, Paganini A, et al. Is transanal endoscopic microsurgery (TEM) a valid treatment for rectal tumors? Surg Endosc 1996;10(7):736–41.
123. Mellgren A, Sirivongs P, Rothenberger DA, et al. Is local excision adequate therapy for early rectal cancer? Dis Colon Rectum 2000;43(8):1064–74.
124. Minsky BD, Rich T, Recht A, et al. Selection criteria for local excision with or without adjuvant radiation therapy for rectal cancer. Cancer 1989;63(7):1421–9.
125. Koscinski T, Malinger S, Drews M, et al. Local excision of rectal carcinoma not-exceeding the muscularis layer. Colorectal Dis 2003;5(2):159–63.
126. Greenberg JA, Shibata D, Herndon JE, et al. Local excision of distal rectal cancer: an update of cancer and leukemia group b 8984. Dis Colon Rectum 2008;0:1–10.
127. Steele GD Jr, Herndon JE, Bleday R, et al. Sphincter-sparing treatment for distal rectal adenocarcinoma. Ann Surg Oncol 1999;6(5):433–41.
128. Enker WE, Thaler HT, Cranor ML, et al. Total mesorectal excision in the operative treatment of carcinoma of the rectum. J Am Coll Surg 1995;181(4):335–46.

129. Maas CP, Moriya Y, Steup WH, et al. A prospective study on radical and nerve-preserving surgery for rectal cancer in the Netherlands. Eur J Surg Oncol 2000; 26(8):751–7.
130. Masui H, Ike H, Yamaguchi S, et al. Male sexual function after autonomic nerve-preserving operation for rectal cancer. Dis Colon Rectum 1996; 39(10):1140–5.
131. Shirouzu K, Ogata Y, Araki Y, et al. Oncologic and functional results of total mesorectal excision and autonomic nerve-preserving operation for advanced lower rectal cancer. Dis Colon Rectum 2004;47(9):1442–7.
132. Neary P, Makin GB, White TJ, et al. Transanal endoscopic microsurgery: a viable operative alternative in selected patients with rectal lesions. Ann Surg Oncol 2003;10(9):1106–11.
133. Gavagan JA, Whiteford MH, Swanstrom LL, et al. Full-thickness intraperitoneal excision by transanal endoscopic microsurgery does not increase short-term complications. Am J Surg 2004;187(5):630–4.
134. Kennedy ML, Lubowski DZ, King DW, et al. Transanal endoscopic microsurgery excision: is anorectal function compromised? Dis Colon Rectum 2002;45(5): 601–4.
135. Lee W, Lee D, Choi S, et al. Transanal endoscopic microsurgery and radical surgery for T1 and T2 rectal cancer. Surg Endosc 2003;17(8):1283–7.
136. Stipa F, Lucandri G, Ferri M, et al. Local excision of rectal cancer with transanal endoscopic microsurgery (TEM). Anticancer Res 2004;24(2C):1167–72.
137. Wang HS, Lin JK, Yang SH, et al. Prospective study of the functional results of transanal endoscopic microsurgery. Hepatogastroenterology 2003;50(53): 1376–80.
138. Guillem JG, Chessin DB, Jeong SY, et al. Contemporary applications of transanal endoscopic microsurgery: technical innovations and limitations. Clin Colorectal Cancer 2005;5(4):268–73.
139. Paty PB, Nash GM, Baron P, et al. Long-term results of local excision for rectal cancer. Ann Surg 2002;236(4):522–30.
140. Friel CM, Cromwell JW, Marra C, et al. Salvage radical surgery after failed local excision for early rectal cancer. Dis Colon Rectum 2002;45(7):875–9.
141. Compton C, Fenoglio-Preiser CM, Pettigrew N, et al. American Joint Committee on Cancer Prognostic Factors Consensus Conference: Colorectal Working Group. Cancer 2000;88(7):1739–57.
142. Krasna MJ, Flancbaum L, Cody RP, et al. Vascular and neural invasion in colorectal carcinoma. Incidence and prognostic significance. Cancer 1988;61(5): 1018–23.
143. Wanebo HJ, Rao B, Pinsky CM, et al. Preoperative carcinoembryonic antigen level as a prognostic indicator in colorectal cancer. N Engl J Med 1978; 299(9):448–51.
144. Nakagoe T, Sawai T, Ayabe H, et al. Prognostic value of carcinoembryonic antigen (CEA) in tumor tissue of patients with colorectal cancer. Anticancer Res 2001;21(4B):3031–6.
145. Wolmark N, Fisher B, Wieand HS, et al. The prognostic significance of preoperative carcinoembryonic antigen levels in colorectal cancer. Results from NSABP (National Surgical Adjuvant Breast and Bowel Project) clinical trials. Ann Surg 1984;199(4):375–82.
146. Le Voyer TE, Sigurdson ER, Hanlon AL, et al. Colon cancer survival is associated with increasing number of lymph nodes analyzed: a secondary survey of intergroup trial INT-0089. J Clin Oncol 2003;21(15):2912–9.

147. Swanson RS, Compton CC, Stewart AK, et al. The prognosis of T3N0 colon cancer is dependent on the number of lymph nodes examined. Ann Surg Oncol 2003;10(1):65–71.
148. Tepper JE, O'Connell MJ, Niedzwiecki D, et al. Impact of number of nodes retrieved on outcome in patients with rectal cancer. J Clin Oncol 2001;19(1): 157–63.
149. Colorectal Cancer Working Party CR07. Pathology guided treatment in rectal cancer: a randomised trial comparing preoperative radiotherapy and selective postoperative chemoradiotherapy in rectal cancer. Clinical Protocol 2005.
150. Nagetaal ID, Van de Velde CH, Van der Worp E. Macroscopic evaluation of rectal cancer resection specimen: clinical significance of the pathologist in quality control. Pathology review committee for the cooperative clinical investigators of the Dutch colorectal group. J Clin Oncol 2002;20:1729–34.
151. Quirke P. Training and quality assurance for rectal cancer: 20 years of data is enough. Lancet Oncol 2003;4(11):695–701.
152. Birbeck KF, Macklin CP, Tiffin NJ. Rates of circumferential margin involvement vary between surgeons and predict outcomes in rectal cancer surgery. Ann Surg 2002;235:449–57.
153. Chan AK, Wong A, Jenken D, et al. Posttreatment TNM staging is a prognostic indicator or survival and recurrence in tethered or fixed rectal carcinoma after preoperative chemotherapy and radiotherapy. Int J Radiat Oncol Biol Phys 2005;61(3):665–77.
154. Chan KW, Boey J, Wong SKC. A method of reporting radial invasion and surgical clearance of rectal carcinoma. Histopathology 1985;9:1319–27.
155. Wibe A, Rendedal PR, Svensson E. Prognostic significance of the circumferential resection margin following total mesorectal excision for rectal cancer. Br J Surg 2002;89:327–34.
156. Nagetaal ID, Marijnen CAM, Kranenbarg EK. Circumferential margin involvement is still an important predictor of local recurrence in rectal carcinoma. Not one millimetre but two millimetres is the limit. Am J Surg Pathol 2002;26:350–7.
157. Stipa F, Chessin DB, Shia J. A pathologic complete response of rectal cancer to preoperative combined-modality therapy results in improved oncological outcome with those who achieve no downstaging on the basis of preoperative endorectal ultrasonography. Ann Oncol 2006;13(8):1047–53.
158. Ahmad NR, Nagle D. Long-term results of preoperative radiation therapy alone for stage T3 and T4 rectal cancer. Br J Surg 1997;84(10):1445–8.
159. Mehta VK, Poen J, Ford J, et al. Radiotherapy, concomitant protracted-venous-infusion 5-fluorouracil, and surgery for ultrasound-staged T3 or T4 rectal cancer. Dis Colon Rectum 2001;44(1):52–8.
160. García-Aguilar J, Hernandez de Anda E, Sirivongs P, et al. A pathologic complete response to preoperative chemoradiation is associated with lower local recurrence and improved survival in rectal cancer patients treated by mesorectal excision. Dis Colon Rectum 2003;46(3):298–304.
161. Guillem JG, Chessin DB, Cohen AM, et al. Long-term oncologic outcome following preoperative combined modality therapy and total mesorectal excision of locally advanced rectal cancer. Ann Surg 2005;241(5):829–36.
162. Ruo L, Tickoo S, Klimstra DS, et al. Long-term prognostic significance of extent of rectal cancer response to preoperative radiation and chemotherapy. Ann Surg 2002;236:75–81.
163. Guillem JG, Puig-La Calle J Jr, Akhurst T. Prospective assessment of primary rectal cancer response to preoperative radiation and chemotherapy using

18-fluorodeoxyglucose positron emission tomography. Dis Colon Rectum 2000; 43:18–24.

164. Nair R, Siegel E, Chen DT, et al. Long-term results of transanal excision after neoadjuvant chemoradiation for T2 and T3 adenocarcinomas of the rectum. J Gastrointest Surg 2008;12:1797–805.

165. Gunderson LL, Sosin H. Areas of failure found at reoperation (second or symptomatic look) following "curative surgery" for adenocarcinoma of the rectum. Cancer 1974;34(4):1278–92.

166. Thomas PR, Lindblad AS. Adjuvant postoperative radiotherapy and chemotherapy in rectal carcinoma: a review of the Gastrointestinal Tumor Study Group experience. Radiother Oncol 1988;13(4):245–52.

167. Fisher B, Wolmark N, Rockette H, et al. Postoperative adjuvant chemotherapy or radiation therapy for rectal cancer: results from NSABP protocol R-01. J Natl Cancer Inst 1988;80(1):21–9.

168. Krook JE, Moertel CG, Gunderson LL, et al. Effective surgical adjuvant therapy for high-risk rectal carcinoma. N Engl J Med 1991;324(11):709–15.

169. O'Connell M, Martenson JA, Wieand HS, et al. Improving adjuvant therapy for rectal cancer by combining protracted-infusion fluorouracil with radiation therapy after curative surgery. N Engl J Med 1994;333(8):502–7.

170. Wolmark N, Wieand HS, Hyams DM, et al. Randomized trial of postoperative adjuvant chemotherapy with or without radiotherapy for carcinoma of the rectum: National Surgical Adjuvant Breast and Bowel Project Protocol R-02 [see comment]. J Natl Cancer Inst 2000;92(5):388–96.

171. Cedermark B, Johansson H, Rutqvist LE, et al. The Stockholm I trial of preoperative short term radiotherapy in operable rectal carcinoma. A prospective randomized trial. Cancer 1995;75(9):2269–75.

172. Holm T, Singnomklao T, Rutqvist LE, et al. Adjuvant preoperative radiotherapy in patients with rectal carcinoma. Adverse effects during long term follow-up of two randomized trials. Cancer 1996;78(5):968–76.

173. Martenson JA, Gunderson LL. "Colon and rectum" principles and practice of radiation oncology. 2nd edition. Philadelphia: J.B. Lippincott Company; 1992.

174. Minsky BD. Adjuvant therapy for rectal cancer—the transatlantic view. Colorectal Dis 2003;5(5):416–22.

175. Minsky BD. Adjuvant therapy of resectable rectal cancer. Cancer Treat Rev 2002;28(4):181–8.

176. Willett CG, Warland G, Coen J, et al. Rectal cancer: the influence of tumor proliferation on response to preoperative irradiation. Int J Radiat Oncol Biol Phys 1995;32(1):57–61.

177. Minsky BD, Cohen AM, Enker WE, et al. Phase I/II trial of preoperative radiation therapy and coloanal anastomosis in distal invasive resectable rectal cancer. Int J Radiat Oncol Biol Phys 1992;23(2):387–92.

178. Sauer R, Becker H, Hohenberger W, et al. German Rectal Cancer Study Group. Preoperative versus postoperative chemoradiotherapy for rectal cancer. N Engl J Med 2004;351(17):1731–40.

179. Dunst J, Reese T, Sutter T, et al. Phase I trial evaluating the concurrent combination of radiotherapy and capecitabine in rectal cancer. J Clin Oncol 2002; 20(19):3983–91.

180. Willett CG, Czito BG, Tyler DS. Intraoperative radiation therapy. J Clin Oncol 2007;25(8):971–7.

181. Hahnloser D, Haddock MG, Nelson H. Intraoperative radiotherapy in the multimodality approach to colorectal cancer. Surg Oncol Clin N Am 2003;12(4):993–1013.

182. Valentini V, Morganti AG, Gambacorta MA, et al. Preoperative hyperfractionated chemoradiation for locally recurrent rectal cancer in patients previously irradiated to the pelvis: a multicentric phase II study. Int J Radiat Oncol Biol Phys 2006;64(4):1129–39.
183. Ciernik I, Dizendorf E, Baumert B, et al. Radiation treatment planning with an integrated positron emission and computer tomography (PET/CT): a feasibility study. Int J Radiat Oncol Biol Phys 2003;57(3):853–63.
184. Laub W, Yan D, Robertson J, et al. Intensity modulated radiation therapy (IMRT) in the radiotherapy treatment of colo-rectal cancer. J Radiother Pract 2002;2: 189–98.
185. Vijayakumar S, Narayan S, Yang CC, et al. Introducing new technologies into the clinic. Front Radiat Ther Oncol 2007;40:180–92.
186. De Gramont A, Boni C, Navarro M. Oxaliplatin/5FU/LV in the adjuvant treatment of stage II and III colon cancer: efficacy results with median follow-up of 4 years. JCO 2005;23(16S):3501.
187. Gill S, Loprinzi CL, Sargent DJ, et al. Pooled analysis of fluorouracil-based adjuvant therapy for stage II and III colon cancer: who benefits and by how much? J Clin Oncol 2004;22(10):1797–806.
188. Lokich JJ, Ahlgren JD, Gullo JJ, et al. A prospective randomized comparison of continuous infusion fluorouracil with a conventional bolus schedule in metastatic colorectal carcinoma: a Mid-Atlantic Oncology Program Study. J Clin Oncol 1989;7(4):425–32.
189. Mamounas E, Wieand S, Wolmark N, et al. Comparative efficacy of adjuvant chemotherapy in patients with Dukes' B versus Dukes' C colon cancer: results from four National Surgical Adjuvant Breast and Bowel Project adjuvant studies (C-01, C-02, C-03, and C-04). J Clin Oncol 1999;17(5):1349–55.
190. Hickish T, Boni C, Navarro M. FOLFOX4 as adjuvant treatment for stage II colon cancer: subpopulation data from the MOSAIC trial. J Clin Oncol 2004;22(Suppl): [abstract 3619].
191. Grothey A, Sargent DJ. FOLFOX for stage II colon cancer? A commentary on the recent FDA approval of oxaliplatin for adjuvant therapy of stage III colon cancer. J Clin Oncol 2005;23(15):3311–3.
192. Sobrero A, Guglielmi A, Grossi F, et al. Mechanism of action of fluoropyrimidines: relevance to the new developments in colorectal cancer chemotherapy. Semin Oncol 2000;27(5 Suppl 10):72–7.
193. Poplin EA, Benedetti JK, Estes NC, et al. Phase III Southwest Oncology Group 9415/Intergroup 0153 randomized trial of fluorouracil, leucovorin, and levamisole versus fluorouracil continuous infusion and levamisole for adjuvant treatment of stage III and high-risk stage II colon cancer. J Clin Oncol 2005;23(9): 1819–25.
194. Dulabh K, Monga D, O'Connell M. Surgical adjuvant therapy for colorectal cancer: current approaches and future directions. Ann Surg Oncol 2006;13: 1021–34.
195. Bernini A, Deen K, Madoff R, et al. Preoperative adjuvant radiation with chemotherapy for rectal cancer: its impact on stage of disease and the role of endorectal ultrasound. Ann Surg Oncol 1996;3(2):131–5.
196. Rainer F, Gunther K. Adjuvant chemotherapy following neoadjuvant therapy of rectal cancer: the type of neoadjuvant therapy (chemoradiotherapy or radiotherapy) may be important for selection of patients. J Clin Oncol 2008;26(3):507–8.
197. Enker W. The elusive goal of preoperative staging in rectal cancer. Ann Surg Oncol 2004;11:245–6.

198. Bosset JF, Collete L, Calais G. Chemotherapy with preoperative radiotherapy in rectal cancer. N Engl J Med 2006;355:1114–23.
199. Andre T, Boni C, Mounedji-Boudiaf L, et al. Oxaliplatin, fluorouracil, and leucovorin as adjuvant treatment for colon cancer. N Engl J Med 2004;350(23): 2343–51.
200. Twelves C, Wong A, Nowacki MP, et al. Capecitabine as adjuvant treatment for stage III colon cancer. N Engl J Med 2005;352(26):2696–704.
201. Moertel CG, Fleming TR, Macdonald JS, et al. Intergroup study of fluorouracil plus levamisole as adjuvant therapy for stage II/Dukes' B2 colon cancer. J Clin Oncol 1995;13(12):2936–43.
202. Haller DG, Lefkopoulou M, Macdonald JS, et al. Some considerations concerning the dose and schedule of 5FU and leucovorin: toxicities of two dose schedules from the intergroup colon adjuvant trial (INT-0089). Adv Exp Med Biol 1993; 339:51–6.
203. Wolmark N, Rockette H, Mamounas E, et al. Clinical trial to assess the relative efficacy of fluorouracil and leucovorin, fluorouracil and levamisole, and fluorouracil, leucovorin, and levamisole in patients with Dukes' B and C carcinoma of the colon: results from National Surgical Adjuvant Breast and Bowel Project C-04. J Clin Oncol 1999;17(11):3553–9.
204. Zhang ZG, Harstrick A, Rustum YM, et al. Modulation of fluoropyrimidines: role of dose and schedule of leucovorin administration. Semin Oncol 1992;19(2 Suppl 3):10–5.
205. Moertel CG, Fleming TR, Macdonald JS, et al. Levamisole and fluorouracil for adjuvant therapy of resected colon carcinoma. N Engl J Med 1990;322(6):352–8.
206. Scheithauer W, Rosen H, Kornek GV, et al. Randomised comparison of combination chemotherapy plus supportive care with supportive care alone in patients with metastatic colorectal cancer. BMJ 1993;306(6880):752–5.
207. Smyth JF, Hardcastle JD, Denton G, et al. Two phase III trials of tauromustine (TCNU) in advanced colorectal cancer. Ann Oncol 1995;6(9):948–9.
208. Thirion P, Michiels S, Pignon JP, et al. Modulation of fluorouracil by leucovorin in patients with advanced colorectal cancer: an updated meta-analysis. J Clin Oncol 2004;22(18):3766–75.
209. de Gramont A, Bosset JF, Milan C, et al. Randomized trial comparing monthly low-dose leucovorin and fluorouracil bolus with bimonthly high-dose leucovorin and fluorouracil bolus plus continuous infusion for advanced colorectal cancer: a French intergroup study. J Clin Oncol 1997;15(2):808–15.
210. Anonymous. Efficacy of intravenous continuous infusion of fluorouracil compared with bolus administration in advanced colorectal cancer. J Clin Oncol 1998;16(1):301–8.
211. Hahn RG, Moertel CG, Schutt AJ, et al. A double-blind comparison of intensive course 5-flourouracil by oral vs. intravenous route in the treatment of colorectal carcinoma. Cancer 1975;35(4):1031–5.
212. Pentheroudakis G, Twelves C, Pentheroudakis G, et al. The rational development of capecitabine from the laboratory to the clinic. Anticancer Res 2002; 22(6B):3589–96.
213. Lembersky BC, Wieand HS, Petrelli NJ, et al. Oral uracil and tegafur plus leucovorin compared with intravenous fluorouracil and leucovorin in stage II and III carcinoma of the colon: results from National Surgical Adjuvant Breast and Bowel Project Protocol C-06. J Clin Oncol 2006;24(13):2059–64.
214. Iyer L, Ratain MJ, Iyer L, et al. Clinical pharmacology of camptothecins. Cancer Chemother Pharmacol 1998;42(Suppl):S31–43.

215. Rougier P, Van Cutsem E, Bajetta E, et al. Randomised trial of irinotecan versus fluorouracil by continuous infusion after fluorouracil failure in patients with metastatic colorectal cancer. Lancet 1998;352(9138):1407–12.

216. Van Cutsem E, Blijham GH, Van Cutsem E, et al. Irinotecan versus infusional 5-fluorouracil: a phase III study in metastatic colorectal cancer following failure on first-line 5-fluorouracil. V302 Study Group. Semin Oncol 1999;26(1):13–20.

217. Douillard JY, Cunningham D, Roth AD, et al. Irinotecan combined with fluorouracil compared with fluorouracil alone as first-line treatment for metastatic colorectal cancer: a multicentre randomised trial. Lancet 2000;355(9209):1041–7.

218. Saltz LB, Cox JV, Blanke C, et al. Irinotecan plus fluorouracil and leucovorin for metastatic colorectal cancer. Irinotecan Study Group. N Engl J Med 2000; 343(13):905–14.

219. Saltz LB, Niedzwieki D, Hollis D. Irinotecan plus fluorouracil / leucovorin (IFL) versus fluorouracil / leucovorin (FL) in stage III colon cancer (intergroup trial CALGB C89803). Proc Am Soc Clin Oncol 2004;22(Suppl):240s [abstract 3500].

220. Van Cutsem E, Labianca R, Hossfeld G. Randomized phase III trial comparing infused irinotecan/5-fluorouracil (5-FU)/folinic acid (IF) versus 5-FU/FA (F) in stage III colon cancer patients (PETACC 3). J Clin Oncol 2005;23(Suppl): [abstract 8].

221. Ychou MR, Raoul JL, Douillard JY. A phase III randomized trial of LV/5FU + CPT-11 vs LV/5FU alone in adjuvant high risk colon cancer. J Clin Oncol 2005;23(Suppl): [abstract 3502].

222. Raymond E, Chaney SG, Taamma A, et al. Oxaliplatin: a review of preclinical and clinical studies. Ann Oncol 1998;9(10):1053–71.

223. Becouarn Y, Ychou M, Ducreux M, et al. Phase II trial of oxaliplatin as first-line chemotherapy in metastatic colorectal cancer patients. Digestive Group of French Federation of Cancer Centers. J Clin Oncol 1998;16(8):2739–44.

224. Tournigand C, Andre T, Achille E, et al. FOLFIRI followed by FOLFOX6 or the reverse sequence in advanced colorectal cancer: a randomized GERCOR study. J Clin Oncol 2004;22(2):229–37.

225. Rothenberg ML, Oza AM, Bigelow RH, et al. Superiority of oxaliplatin and fluorouracil-leucovorin compared with either therapy alone in patients with progressive colorectal cancer after irinotecan and fluorouracil-leucovorin: interim results of a phase III trial. J Clin Oncol 2003;21(11):2059–69.

226. Giacchetti S, Bjarnason G, Garufi C, et al. Phase III trial comparing 4-day chronomodulated therapy versus 2-day conventional delivery of fluorouracil, leucovorin, and oxaliplatin as first-line chemotherapy of metastatic colorectal cancer: the European Organisation for Research and Treatment of Cancer Chronotherapy Group. J Clin Oncol 2006;24(22):3562–9.

227. Giacchetti S, Perpoint B, Zidani R, et al. Phase III multicenter randomized trial of oxaliplatin added to chronomodulated fluorouracil-leucovorin as first-line treatment of metastatic colorectal cancer. J Clin Oncol 2000;18(1):136–47.

228. de Gramont A, Figer A, Seymour M, et al. Leucovorin and fluorouracil with or without oxaliplatin as first-line treatment in advanced colorectal cancer. J Clin Oncol 2000;18(16):2938–47.

229. Andre T, Tournigand C, Achille E, et al. Adjuvant treatment of colon cancer MOSAIC study's main results. Bull Cancer 2006;93(1):5–9.

230. Wolmark N, Wieand HS, Keubler JP. A phase III trial comparing FULV to FULV + oxaliplatin in stage II or III carcinoma of the colon: results of NSABP protocol C-07. J Clin Oncol 2005;23(Suppl):[abstract 3500].

231. Sargent DJ, Wieand HS, Haller DG, et al. Disease-free survival versus overall survival as a primary end point for adjuvant colon cancer studies: individual patient data from 20,898 patients on 18 randomized trials. J Clin Oncol 2005; 23(34):8664–70.
232. Baselga J. Why the epidermal growth factor receptor? The rationale for cancer therapy. Oncologist 2002;7:2–8.
233. Spaulding DC, Spaulding BO. Epidermal growth factor receptor expression and measurement in solid tumors. Semin Oncol 2002;29:45–54.
234. Messa C, Russo F, Caruso MG, et al. EGF, TGF-alpha, and EGF-R in human colorectal adenocarcinoma. Acta Oncol 1998;37(3):285–9.
235. Mayer A, Takimoto M, Fritz E, et al. The prognostic significance of proliferating cell nuclear antigen, epidermal growth factor receptor, and mdr gene expression in colorectal cancer. Cancer 1993;71(8):2454–60.
236. Saltz LB, Rubin J, Hochster N, et al. Cetuximab (IMC-C225) plus irinotecan (CPT-11) is active in cpt-11-refractory colorectal cancer (CRC) that expresses epidermal growth factor receptor (EGFR). Proc Am Soc Clin Oncol 2001;20: 3a, Abstract 7.
237. Cunningham D, Humblet Y, Siena S, et al. Cetuximab monotherapy and cetuximab plus irinotecan in irinotecan-refractory metastatic colorectal cancer. N Engl J Med 2004;351(4):337–45.
238. Malik I, Hecht JR, Patnaik A. Safety and efficacy of panitumumab monotherapy in patients with metastatic colorectal cancer. J Clin Oncol 2005;23(Suppl):251s [abstract 3520].
239. Peeters M, Van Cutsem E, Siena S. A phase 3, multicenter, randomized controlled trial of panitumamab plus best supportive care versus best supportive care alone in patients with metastatic colorectal cancer. Paper presented at: American Association for Cancer Research (AACR). Washington, DC; April 1, 2006. 2006:[abstract CP-1].
240. Amado RG, Wolf M, Peeters M, et al. Wild-type KRAS is required for panitumumab efficacy in patients with metastatic colorectal cancer. J Clin Oncol 2008; 26(10):1626–34.
241. Lièvre A, Bachet J, Le Corre D, et al. KRAS mutation status is predictive of response to cetuximab therapy in colorectal cancer. Cancer Res 2006;66(8): 3992–5.
242. Messersmith W, Hidalgo M. Panitumumab, a monoclonal anti-epidermal growth factor receptor antibody in colorectal cancer: another one or the one. Clin Cancer Res 2007;13:4664–6.
243. Folkman J. Tumor angiogenesis: therapeutic implications. N Engl J Med 1971; 285:1182–6.
244. Ferrara N, Gerber HP, LeCouter J. The biology of VEGF and its receptors. Nat Med 2003;9:669–76.
245. Hurwitz H, Fehrenbacher L, Novotny W, et al. Bevacizumab plus irinotecan, fluorouracil, and leucovorin for metastatic colorectal cancer. N Engl J Med 2004; 350(23):2335–42.
246. Giantonio BJ, Catalano PJ, Meropol NJ, et al. Bevacizumab in combination with oxaliplatin, fluorouracil, and leucovorin (FOLFOX4) for previously treated metastatic colorectal cancer: results from the Eastern Cooperative Oncology Group Study E3200. J Clin Oncol Apr 20 2007;25(12):1539–44.
247. Ptok H, Meyer F, Marusch F, et al. Palliative stent implantation in the treatment of malignant colorectal obstruction. Surg Endosc 2006;20(6):909–14.

248. Leitman IM, Sullivan JD, Brams D, et al. Multivariate analysis of morbidity and mortality from the initial surgical management of obstructing carcinoma of the colon. Surg Gynecol Obstet 1992;174:513–8.

249. Sebastian S, Johnston S, Geoghegan T, et al. Pooled analysis of the efficacy and safety of self-expanding metal stenting in malignant colorectal obstruction. Am J Gastroenterol 2004;99:2051–7.

250. Simmons DT, Baron TH. Technological insight: enteral stenting and new technology. Nat Clin Pract Gastroenterol Hepatol 2005;2:365–74.

251. Suzuki N, Saunders BP, Thomas-Gibson S, et al. Colorectal stenting for malignant and benign disease: outcomes in colorectal stenting. Dis Colon Rectum 2004;47(7):1201–7.

252. Hünerbein M, Krause M, Moesta KT, et al. Palliation of malignant rectal obstruction with self-expanding metal stents. Surgery 2005;137(1):42–7.

253. Van Cutsem E, Nordlinger B, Adam R. Towards a pan-European consensus on the treatment of patients with colorectal liver metastasis. Eur J Cancer 2006;42:2212–21.

254. Choti MA, Sitzmann JV, Tiburi MF. Trends in long-term survival following liver resection for hepatic colorectal metastasis. Ann Surg 2002;235:759–66.

255. Tsai M, Su Y, Ho M. Clinicopathologic features and prognosis in resectable synchronous and metachronous colorectal liver metastasis. Ann Surg Oncol 2007;14:786–94.

256. Nordlinger B, Van Cutsem E, Rougier P, et al. Does chemotherapy prior to liver resection increase the potential for cure in patients with metastatic colorectal cancer? A report from the European Colorectal Metastases Treatment Group. Eur J Cancer 2007;43(14):2037–45.

257. Hewes J, Dighe S, Morris R, et al. Preoperative chemotherapy and the outcome of liver resection for colorectal metastases. World J Surg 2007;31(2):353–64.

258. Welsh FK, Tilney HS, Tekkis PP, et al. Safe liver resection following chemotherapy for colorectal metastases is a matter of timing. Br J Cancer 2007;96:1037–42.

259. Reddy S, Pawlik T, Zorzi D, et al. Simultaneous resections of colorectal cancer and synchronous liver metastases: a multi-institutional analysis. Ann Surg Oncol 2007;14:3481–91.

260. Aschele C, Lonardi S, Aschele C, et al. Multidisciplinary treatment of rectal cancer: medical oncology. Ann Oncol 2007;18(9):114–21.

261. Glynne-Jones R, Grainger J, Harrison M. Neoadjuvant chemotherapy prior to preoperative chemoradiation or radiation in rectal cancer: should we be more cautious? Br J Cancer 2006;94:363–71.

262. Allen PJ, Kemeny N, Jarnagin W, et al. Importance of response to neoadjuvant chemotherapy in patients undergoing resection of synchronous colorectal liver metastases. J Gastrointest Surg 2007;7(1):109–17.

263. Kooby DA, Fong Y, Suriawinata A, et al. Impact of steatosis on perioperative outcome following hepatic resection. J Gastrointest Surg 2003;7(8):1034–44.

264. Reddy SK, Morse M, Hurwitz HI. Addition of bevacizumab to irinotecan and oxaliplatin-based preoperative chemotherapy regimens does not increase morbidity after resection of colorectal liver metastases. J Am Coll Surg 2008;206:96–106.

265. Fernandez FG, Ritter J, Goodwin JW, et al. Effect of steatohepatitis associated with irinotecan or oxaliplatin pretreatment on resectability of hepatic colorectal metastases. J Am Coll Surg 2005;200(6):845–53.

266. Vauthey JN, Pawlik TM, Ribero D, et al. Chemotherapy regimen predicts steato-hepatitis and an increase in 90-day mortality after surgery for hepatic colorectal metastases. J Clin Oncol 2006;24(13):2065–72.

267. Marr R, Birbeck K, Garvican J, et al. The modern abdominoperineal excision: the next challenge after total mesorectal excision. Ann Surg 2005;242(1):74–82.

268. Tzardi M, Tzardi M. Role of total mesorectal excision and of circumferential resection margin in local recurrence and survival of patients with rectal carcinoma. Dig Dis 2007;25(1):51–5.

269. Guillem JG, Díaz-González JA, Minsky BD, et al. cT3N0 rectal cancer: potential overtreatment with preoperative chemoradiotherapy is warranted. J Clin Oncol 2008;26(3):368–73.

270. Willett CG, Hagan M, Daley W, et al. Changes of tumor proliferation of rectal cancer induced by preoperative 5-fluorouracil and irradiation. Dis Colon Rectum 1998;41(1):62–7.

271. den Dulk M, Marijnen CA, Putter H, et al. Risk factors for adverse outcome in patients with rectal cancer treated with an abdominoperineal resection in the total mesorectal excision trial. Ann Surg 2007;246(1):83–90.

272. Habr-Gama A, Oliva Perez R, Nadalin W, et al. Operative versus nonoperative treatment for stage 0 distal rectal cancer following chemoradiation therapy: long-term results. Ann Surg 2004;240(4):711–8.

273. Hiotis SP, Weber SM, Cohen AM, et al. Assessing the predictive value of clinical complete response to neoadjuvant therapy for rectal cancer: an analysis of 488 patients. J Am Coll Surg 2002;194(2):131–5 [discussion: 135–6].

274. Kuo LJ, Chern MC, Tsou MH, et al. Interpretation of magnetic resonance imaging for locally advanced rectal carcinoma after preoperative chemoradiation therapy. Dis Colon Rectum 2005;48(1):23–8.

275. Lezoche E, Guerrieri M, Paganini AM. Long-term results in patients with T2-3 N0 distal rectal cancer undergoing radiotherapy before transanal endoscopic microsurgery. Br J Surg 2005;92(12):1546–52.

276. Bonnen M, Crane C, Vauthey JN, et al. Long-term results using local excision after preoperative chemoradiation among selected T3 rectal cancer patients. Int J Radiat Oncol Biol Phys 2004;60(4):1098–105.

277. Ruo L, Guillem JG, Minsky BD, et al. Preoperative radiation with or without chemothreapy and full-thickness transanal excision for selected T2 and T3 distal rectal cancers. Int J Colorectal Dis 2002;17(1):54–8.

Multidisciplinary Treatment of Gastrointestinal Stromal Tumors

T. Peter Kingham, MD[a],*, Ronald P. DeMatteo, MD[b]

KEYWORDS

• Gastrointestinal stromal tumors • Diagnosis • Treatment

Gastrointestinal stromal tumor (GIST) is the most common mesenchymal tumor of the gastrointestinal tract. Although rare as a clinical entity, there is much interest in their pathology and treatment, because the *KIT* proto-oncogene mutation common to most GISTs can be inhibited by imatinib mesylate (Gleevec; Novartis Pharmaceutical, Basel, Switzerland). The utility of imatinib has marked a new era in treating solid tumors, with specific therapeutic molecular targeting. Diagnosing and treating GIST requires a multidisciplinary approach, given the combination of pathologic and radiographic evaluation, surgical treatment, and oncologic care required to successfully treat patients with GIST.

GIST has been recognized as a unique tumor only in the last decade. Originally, GISTs were thought to be derived from smooth muscle cells and were considered variations of leiomyosarcomas or leiomyomas. Immunohistochemical staining assisted in defining GIST as a distinct disease based on *KIT* (CD117) expression (found in 95% of GIST). Platelet-derived growth factor receptor alpha (*PDGFRα*) mutations have since been found in about 5% of GISTs that lack *KIT* expression.

EPIDEMIOLOGY

GISTs affect men more than women. They constitute 80% of all gastrointestinal mesenchymal tumors and approximately 20% of all small bowel malignant neoplasms, excluding lymphomas. It is difficult to judge the historical incidence of GIST. A population-based study in Sweden reported an incidence of approximately 13 cases per million persons per year.[1] Extrapolating from this, it is believed the US incidence is

[a] Department of Surgery, Memorial Sloan-Kettering Cancer Center, 303 E. 60th Street, Apt 28E, NY 10022, USA
[b] Department of Surgery, Memorial Sloan-Kettering Cancer Center, 1275 York Avenue, Box 203, NY 10065, USA
* Corresponding author.
E-mail address: kinghamt@mskcc.org (T.P. Kingham).

Surg Clin N Am 89 (2009) 217–233
doi:10.1016/j.suc.2008.10.003
0039-6109/08/$ – see front matter © 2009 Elsevier Inc. All rights reserved.

surgical.theclinics.com

3,000 to 5,000 cases per year. GISTs generally occur in older adults, between 40 and 80 years of age.[2–6] The median age at diagnosis is approximately 60. GIST can occur in children, especially girls, and typically has lymph node metastasis, gastric location, and wild-type *KIT/PDGFRα* genotype.[7]

GIST is usually sporadic, although there are recognized kindreds with familial GIST throughout the world. Most familial GISTs have a germline *KIT* mutation in exon 11.[8] GIST can occur in young women in the context of "Carney's triad." This rare syndrome occurs in young women and includes functioning extra-adrenal paragangliomas, pulmonary chondromas, and gastric GIST. GIST can also occur in patients with the Neurofibromatosis type-1 (NF1) syndrome, and these GISTs usually are found in the small intestine. The origin of these GISTs may be different than sporadic GIST, because of the lack of identified *KIT* or *PDGFRα* mutations in patients with NF1.

MOLECULAR BASIS OF DISEASE

GISTs are related to the interstitial cells of Cajal. Their behavior ranges from benign to malignant, and there are several histologic subtypes, including spindle cell (70%), epithelioid (20%), and pleomorphic types.[9] Ninety-five percent of GISTs have gain-of-function *KIT* mutations or *PDGFRα* mutations. *KIT* encodes for a transmembrane receptor glycoprotein with tyrosine kinase function and normally participates in cell growth and survival. Most *KIT* mutations cause ligand-independent activation of the receptor tyrosine kinase function. Identifying *KIT* and *PDGFRα* mutations are useful for both the diagnosis and treatment of GIST. *KIT* mutations occur most frequently in exon 11 (70%), the juxtamembrane domain of the *KIT* protein. Mutations can also occur in exon 9 (10%), the extracellular domain of the *KIT* protein. It is helpful to identify the location of the *KIT* mutation, given that exon 9 mutant GISTs do not respond as well to imatinib as exon 11 mutant GISTs. Rarely, *KIT* exon 13 and 17 mutations can occur. These locations, in addition to exon 14, are also areas of mutation in GIST that can be associated with imatinib resistance.

Approximately 5% of GISTs do not express the *KIT* protein. In the 3% of GISTs with *PDGFRα* mutations, the mutation generally is present in exon 18 (80%) or exon 12. *PDGFRα* mutations are more common in gastric GISTs. The location of the *PDGFRα* mutation is important given that most exon 18 mutant GISTs are resistant to imatinib, whereas the exon 12 mutant GISTs are sensitive to imatinib. GISTs that do not have identifiable mutations are considered wild-type, and their pathogenesis is unclear.

MALIGNANCY AND GASTROINTESTINAL STROMAL TUMOR LOCATIONS

GIST behavior occupies a wide spectrum from benign to malignant. Malignancy is most common in intestinal GIST (40%) and lowest in gastric GIST (20%). GISTs occur from the esophagus to the anus. Gastric GISTs are the most common (60%), and have many different forms and mutations. Treatment ranges from wedge resection to total gastrectomy, depending on the location. Gastric tumors can adhere to surrounding structures in the lesser sac, such as the pancreas and transverse colon. Duodenal GISTs occur most commonly in the second portion. They resemble small intestine GISTs histologically. Thirty percent of GISTs are in the jejunum or ileum, and ileal tumors are slightly less common than jejunal tumors.[10] GIST can also occur in the rectum but rarely in the colon.

CLINICAL PRESENTATION

The clinical presentation of GIST often depends on its size and location. GIST may not induce symptoms and can be found incidentally during physical examination or during an invasive procedure. When symptoms do arise, they generally are caused by mass effect, given the extraluminal location of GIST. The mean duration of symptoms is 4 to 6 months. In Sweden, approximately 70% of GISTs were associated with symptoms.[1] The median size of GIST in those with symptoms was 8.9 cm compared with 2.7 cm in those who were asymptomatic. Most symptoms consisted of nausea, emesis, pain, early satiety, or abdominal distension. Patients can present with microcytic anemia and fatigue when GISTs erode into the intestinal tract lumen and cause subclinical gastrointestinal bleeding. Up to 25% of patients with GIST can present with significant bleeding, either caused by erosion into the gastrointestinal tract or intraperitoneal rupture.

DIAGNOSIS

GISTs often are diagnosed only after resection and pathologic examination. Imaging has become more common in the evaluation of patients with abdominal symptoms, so contrast-enhanced computed tomography (CT) scans and magnetic resonance imaging (MRI) are more frequently able to suggest the diagnosis of GIST. On MRI, GISTs have low signal intensity on T1-weighted images, high intensity on T2-weighted images, and are enhanced with gadolinium contrast.[11] GISTs usually involve the muscularis propria of the gastrointestinal wall, so the characteristic image is that of a well-circumscribed, smooth, intramural mass with exophytic growth. The organ of origin can be often identified by focal mural thickening. Smaller primary GISTs usually are well circumscribed with neovascularity and are associated with the stomach or small intestine. Larger GISTs (>10 cm) have borders of various thickness and can have heterogeneous central areas of necrosis or hemorrhage. As gastric GISTs enlarge, they extend into the gastrohepatic, gastrocolic, or gastrosplenic ligament. Small intestine GIST can extend into the small bowel mesentery as they grow, which can make preoperative diagnosis difficult because of similarities with lymphoma and other sarcomas. Axial imaging also allows for evaluation of the liver and peritoneum, the most common sites of metastasis. Given the rarity of metastatic spread to the thorax, a chest radiograph is adequate to assess the thorax for metastatic disease. Lymphatic spread is rare with metastatic GIST, so lymphadenopathy generally is not encountered on physical examination or imaging studies.[12] Staging of GIST relies primarily on CT imaging. CT supplies the necessary information to determine whether surgical resection is feasible. [18]Fluorodeoxyglucose (FDG) positron emission tomography (PET) uptake is sensitive, but not specific, when used to diagnose GIST. It is generally not necessary in most patients but can be used as an early test of treatment response **(Fig. 1)**.[13]

Once the diagnosis of GIST has been suggested on axial imaging, endoscopy can be useful in determining the presence of a gastric or colorectal submucosal mass. Endoscopic ultrasound scan can delineate the full depth of the tumor, although it is not able to predict tumor behavior. Preoperative biopsy generally is not indicated for several reasons. First, GISTs are fragile and can theoretically rupture and spread tumor cells when biopsied. Second, given their hypervascular nature, a biopsy can cause intratumoral hemorrhage. Perhaps most important, pathologists often cannot diagnose GIST from fine-needle aspirates, especially when the area sampled is necrotic. Endoscopic biopsy is less likely to cause hemorrhage and is useful only to confirm the diagnosis; exclude the diagnosis of lymphoma, which can have a similar radiologic

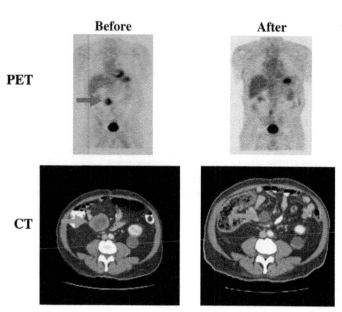

Fig.1. PET scan response of recurrent GIST to imatinib. The peritoneal recurrence (*lower left*) had increased uptake of PET scan (*upper left*). Imatinib was used for several weeks, and there was a partial response, with a reduction in tumor size (*lower right*) and absence of PET uptake (*upper right*). (*From* DeMatteo RP. The GIST of targeted cancer therapy: a tumor (gastrointestinal stromal tumor), a mutated gene (c-kit), and a molecular inhibitor (STI571). Ann Surg Oncol 2002;9:831; with permission.)

appearance; or allow for neoadjuvant imatinib therapy for a marginally resectable tumor.

PATHOLOGIC DIAGNOSIS AND PROGNOSIS

In the multidisciplinary approach to diagnosing and treating patients with GIST, pathologic review plays a central role in initiating treatment algorithms. Determining KIT receptor positivity on immunohistochemistry is vital. Other immunohistochemical characteristics used in the diagnosis of GIST are CD34, a hematopoietic progenitor cell antigen (present in 60% to 70% of GIST); smooth-muscle actin (30%–40%); and S-100 protein (5%).[14] On rare occasions, GIST can express desmin, similar to smooth muscle tumors, but it is generally isolated to small focal areas of the tumor.[9] In KIT-negative tumors, protein kinase C theta, a protein kinase activated downstream in the KIT pathway, may be useful to differentiate GIST from other tumor types, given its predilection for GIST.[15]

The prognosis of GIST is quite variable. The stage of disease is significant, demonstrated by a lower survival rate in patients with metastatic disease.[2] The most pertinent variables that affect the prognosis of primary, nonmetastatic GIST, are tumor site, size, and number of mitoses (per 50 high-power fields [HPF], **Table 1**). All GISTs are potentially malignant, except perhaps small (<1 cm) tumors. In one historical series from Memorial Sloan-Kettering Cancer Center (MSKCC), multivariate analysis found the significance of tumor size as an independent prognostic factor of survival. In patients with large GIST (>10 cm), the 5-year actuarial survival rate was only 20% (**Fig. 2**). Similar findings were reported by MD Anderson Cancer Center (MDACC).[16] The importance of tumor size is also shown by a high tumor-related mortality rate seen with

Table 1
Rates of metastases or tumor-related death in GISTs of stomach and small intestine by tumors grouped by mitotic rate and tumor size

	Tumor Parameters		Percentage of Patients with Progressive Disease During Long-Term Follow-up and Characterization of Risk for Metastasis			
Group	Size	Mitotic Rate	Gastric GISTS	Jejunal and Ileal GISTS	Duodenal GISTS	Rectal GISTS
1	≤2 cm	≤5 per 50 HPF	0, None	0, None	0, None	0, None
2	>2cm ≤5 cm	≤5 per 50 HPFs	1.9, Very low	4.3, Low	8.3, Low	8.5, Low
3a	>5cm ≤10 cm	≤5 per 50 HPF	3.6, Low	24, Moderate		
3b	>10 cm	≤5 per 50 HPF	12, Moderate	52, High	34, High[a]	57, High[a]
4	≤2 cm	>5 per 50 HPF	0	50		54, High
5	>2cm ≤5 cm	>5 per 50 HPF	16, Moderate	73, High	50, High	52, High
6a	>5cm ≤10 cm	>5 per 50 HPF	55, High	85, High		
6b	>10 cm	>5 per 50 HPF	86, High	90, High	86, High[a]	71, High[a]

[a] Groups 3a and 3b or 6a and 6b are combined in duodenal and rectal GISTs because of small number of cases.
From Miettinen M, Lasota J. Gastrointestinal stromal tumors: Pathology and prognosis at different sites. Semin Diagnostic Pathol 2006;23:70; with permission.

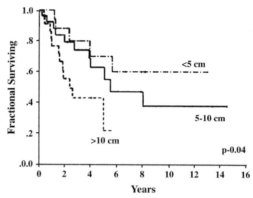

Fig. 2. Disease-specific survival and tumor size after complete resection of primary GIST (n = 80). (*From* DeMatteo RP, Lewis JJ, Leung D, et al. Two hundred gastrointestinal stromal tumors: recurrence patterns and prognostic factors for survival. Ann Surg 2000;231(1):51–8; with permission.)

GIST larger than 5 cm and with a mitotic rate greater than 5 per 50 HPF. Median survival can be 1 to 2 years in this subset of patients, in the absence of tyrosine kinase inhibitor therapy. Mitotic rate and tumor location are also predictors of outcome in patients with GIST.[7] GISTs of the stomach are less aggressive than GISTs in other locations. Gastric tumors less than 5 cm with less than 5 mitoses per 50 HPF have a lower than 2% rate of malignancy compared with GIST with similar mitotic rates in other anatomic sites, which have higher rates.[17] Long-term follow-up for GIST is necessary because there is an unpredictable metastatic pattern. Small tumors have been known to metastasize 10 years after diagnosis.

Whether a *KIT* mutation is present and what type of mutation it is are also prognostic. Recurrence after primary resection is more common in patients with a deletion/insertion mutation of exon 11.[18] GIST with regulatory-type mutations in the juxtamembrane and extracellular ligand binding domains that leave the enzymatic site that binds to imatinib intact respond to imatinib. GIST with an enzymatic site mutation can alter the sequence of the kinase catalytic moiety and thus prevent effective response to imatinib.[19] In addition to these variables, alternative prognostic factors have been studied. Tumor rupture before or during resection predicts a poor outcome and increased peritoneal recurrence.[16] The completeness of resection and tumor size also have been correlated with survival.[20,21] Aneuploidy has been identified as another marker of malignancy.[22,23] Telomerase expression has been identified in 29% of a cohort of 24 patients with primary GIST and all patients with metastatic disease.[16] Despite all of the prognostic variables that have been identified for GIST, it remains difficult for pathologists to confidently identify benign GIST. Instead, pathologists often characterize GIST as low or high risk for malignancy.[24] Commonly accepted guidelines for classifying a GIST as malignant are size greater than 5 to 10 cm, with more than 5 mitoses per 50 HPF.

Although there are many predictors for the malignant potential of primary GIST, there are few predictors of the site of first recurrence. Several studies have looked at historical data to describe recurrence patterns. At MSKCC, the first recurrence in patients with complete resection of a primary GIST was the peritoneum (52%), liver (63%), or both (15%).[2] Similar findings were described from MDACC, with approximately 40% of recurrences identified as peritoneal.[25] The only reliable predictor appears to be tumor rupture, which leads to a higher peritoneal metastasis rate. Overall survival at 5 years for patients with GIST at MSKCC was 35%.[2] The 5-year disease-specific survival rate in patients with a primary GIST who undergo complete resection ranges from 40% to 65%.[2,16,26,27] This decreases to 9 to 12 months in patients with incomplete resections.[2,26] Peritoneal disease occurred in 52% of patients, with a 2-year median time to recurrence after a complete resection.[2,16] Median survival in patients with a local recurrence was 12 months and in patients with metastases was 19 months. Although approximately half of all patients who undergo complete resection survive more than 5 years, given the high local and distant recurrence rate, adjuvant therapy is now a key factor in successful long-term treatment of GIST.

TREATMENT

Imatinib mesylate is the first targeted small molecule inhibitor used for solid tumors. It competitively inhibits the *KIT*, *PDGFRα*, and *BCR-ABL* kinases. By binding to the ATP-binding pocket of the kinases, it blocks the transfer of a phosphate group to the substrate and thus blocks the transduction of signals initiated by *KIT* or *PDGFRα* activation. For imatinib to bind effectively, the activation loop of the kinase (encoded on *KIT* exon 17) must be in an inactive conformation.[28] Imatinib is metabolized in the liver via the cytochrome P450 pathway. Fifty percent to 70% of patients with GIST have a partial response to imatinib, and 15% to 30% are maintained with stable disease.[29,30] Tumor volume reduction occurs at a median of 3 to 4 months. PET scan with [18]FDG can reveal diminished uptake within days of imatinib treatment.[31] The location of the *KIT* or *PDGFRα* mutation can predict response to imatinib. *KIT* exon 11 mutations are the most sensitive to imatinib treatment. Approximately 70% to 80% of these patients undergo partial remission compared with 40% to 50% with exon 9 mutation.[30,32] Wild-type GIST, without a recognized *KIT* or *PDGFRα* mutation have a lower response rate (23%–39%) to imatinib that patients with *KIT* exon 11 mutations.[30,33] Given these findings, regardless of the *KIT* or *PDGFRα* mutation status, imatinib is the first-line treatment of metastatic GIST. One of the few exceptions to this is in GIST with *PDGFRα* exon 18 D842 V mutations that are known to be resistant to imatinib.[34]

Imatinib should be administered without interruption. This was seen in a study of 58 patients with metastatic or unresectable GIST who had stable or responsive disease after 1 year of treatment with imatinib and were followed up in a prospective multicenter trial that randomly assigned them to discontinue use of imatinib.[35] Patients randomly assigned to the interrupted arm were able to cross over to the treatment arm if their disease progressed. Eighty-one percent of patients in the interrupted group had disease progression in a median evaluation period of 21 months compared with 31% of patients in the continuous treatment group. Ninety-two percent of patients who had disease progression in the interrupted group responded to imatinib when it was restarted. Reported side effects of imatinib are diarrhea, nausea, abdominal pain, fatigue, and rash. Approximately 95% of patients tolerate treatment.

PRIMARY RESECTABLE DISEASE

Surgery traditionally has been the cornerstone of treatment for resectable GIST. In the post-imatinib era, surgery shares a role in a multidisciplinary treatment plan (**Fig. 3**). In primary disease, complete surgical resection provides the chance of cure (**Table 2**). There are several important principles that guide surgical resection. Because GIST can be fragile with extensive necrosis or hemorrhage, meticulous dissection is vital to avoid tumor rupture during the procedure, which can increase the risk of intraperitoneal recurrence. GISTs normally are surrounded by a pseudocapsule that should be

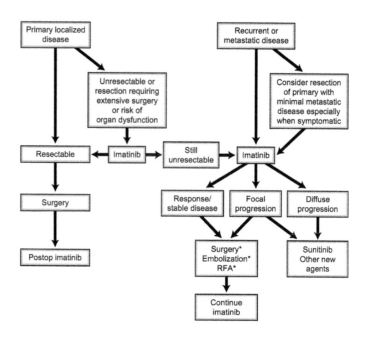

RFA = Radiofrequency ablation

* If all gross disease or all imatinib-resistant disease is treatable

Fig. 3. GIST treatment algorithm. (*From* Gold JS, DeMatteo RP. Combined surgical and molecular therapy: the gastrointestinal stromal tumor model. Ann Surg 2006;244:176; with permission.)

intact after resection. Given the normal exophytic growth pattern of GIST within the gastrointestinal tract, wedge or segmental resections often are possible. GISTs adhere to surrounding structures, so additional organ resections may be required for complete resection. Margins of resection should be microscopically negative. To achieve this, a 1-cm gross margin is generally sufficient. A positive microscopic margin forces the surgeon to consider whether the margin is truly positive and decide

Table 2						
Outcome in large series of complete surgical resection of primary localized GIST						
Author	Year	No. of Patients	No. with Completely Resected Primary Localized Disease	Median Follow-up (mo)	No. with Recurrence (%)	5-Year Survival
DeMatteo et al[2]	2000	200	80	24	32 (40%)	54% DSS
Wong et al[61]	2003	108	108	43		42% OS, 29% RFS
Kim et al[3]	2004	101	86	36	29 (34%)	78% OS
Martin et al[4]	2005	162	162	42	42 (26%)	68% RFS
Wu et al[5]	2006	100	85	33	44 (44%)	44% DFS
Bumming et al[6]	2006	259	221		38 (17%)	

Abbreviations: DSS, disease-specific survival; OS, overall survival; RFS, recurrence-free survival; disease-free survival.

From Gold JS, DeMatteo RP. Combined surgical and molecular therapy: the gastrointestinal stromal tumor model. Ann Surg 2006;244:176; with permission.

if it can be identified and resected a second time. Laparoscopy is a useful modality to resect small gastric GIST, especially because lymphadenectomy is rarely required.

Complete resection is possible in 85% of patients with primary GIST.[2,3,6] In completely resected GIST, the microscopic margin is negative in 70% to 95% of cases.[2] At MSKCC, 80 of 93 patients (86%) with primary disease and no metastases were able to undergo complete resection. In these 80 patients, before the advent of imatinib, the 5-year disease-specific survival rate was 54% (**Fig. 4**). Forty percent of the patients in this study had a recurrence. Other studies report 26% to 44% recurrence rates.[3-5] There are no standard protocols for postoperative follow-up after complete resections. Given that imatinib is now available for use in treating recurrences, routine axial imaging is an integral part of postoperative follow-up. Current recommendations are CT scans with intravenous contrast every 3 to 6 months for the first 5 years, and then yearly after that.[36]

The role of imatinib therapy in completely resected primary GIST is becoming clearer. The American College of Surgeons Oncology Group (ACOSOG) is leading a Phase II intergroup trial (Z9000) in combination with Novartis and the Cancer Therapy Evaluation Program. They are examining the effect of adjuvant imatinib (400 mg/day for 12 months) after complete macroscopic resection in patients with high-risk primary GIST (≥ 5 tumors, tumor size ≥ 10 cm, or intraperitoneal tumor rupture or hemorrhage). One hundred six patients accrued to this trial and were treated using imatinib (400 mg/day) for 1 year. The trial completed accrual in 2003, and 83% of patients completed the year of imatinib therapy.[37] At 4 years of median follow-up, overall survival rates were 97% at 3 years, with the conclusion that 1 year of imatinib after resection led to improved overall survival compared with historical controls.[38] A separate ACOSOG trial (Z9001) also studied the use of imatinib compared with placebo in patients with completely resected primary GIST that are at least 3 cm. The primary endpoint of the double-blind study was recurrence-free survival. The trial was halted after a median follow-up of 13 to 14 months because of the significant difference in recurrence-free survival between the study group (97%) and placebo group (83%).[39] The European organization for research and treatment of cancer (EORTC) is also conducting a study that is looking at 24 months of adjuvant imatinib compared with observation in patients at either intermediate or high risk of recurrence.

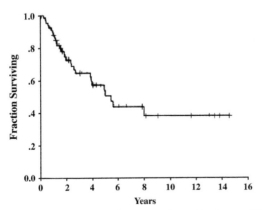

Fig. 4. Disease-specific survival after complete resection of primary GIST (n = 80). (*From* DeMatteo RP, Lewis JJ, Leung D, et al. Two hundred gastrointestinal stromal tumors: recurrence patterns and prognostic factors for survival. Ann Surg 2000;231(1):51–8; with permission.)

PRIMARY UNRESECTABLE GASTROINTESTINAL STROMAL TUMOR

When primary GIST appears to be unresectable or borderline, imatinib is the treatment of choice. A CT scan 1 month after initiation of imatinib is useful to judge tumor response and thus potential resectability. One Phase II trial by the Radiation Therapy Oncology Group (RTOG) is investigating the use of imatinib in the neoadjuvant setting when primary tumors are large and may require additional organ resection to achieve negative margins. In these trials, patients are treated with imatinib for 2 to 6 months before surgery. CT scans are used to judge the effectiveness of the imatinib, and surgical resection generally is performed within 6 to 9 months. An additional benefit may be decreased blood loss, given the hypervascularity of large GIST. One of the risks of neoadjuvant therapy is that a needle biopsy is necessary to begin treatment. Given that 15% of patients have primary resistance to imatinib, there is also a risk that the tumor will become unresectable because of the delay in surgical intervention.

RECURRENT AND METASTATIC GASTROINTESTINAL STROMAL TUMOR

Recurrent and metastatic GISTs are managed in a similar fashion. Surgery alone is limited in its value in treating recurrent GIST. Peritoneal metastases can be removed but are generally followed by another regional recurrence. In addition, only 26% of liver recurrences are resectable, and most patients have recurrence after hepatectomy.[40] The first line of treatment in patients with recurrent and metastatic disease is imatinib (**Table 3**). Initial response can be followed with CT scans or by [18]FDG-PET response. Lifelong treatment with imatinib is recommended in patients with imatinib-responsive GIST, given that it decreases the likelihood of disease progression. Approximately 45% of patients with metastatic GIST have a partial response to imatinib, whereas 30% maintain stable disease.[29,41,42] The success of imatinib is evident in that median survival was only 15 months after resection of recurrent GIST in the pre-imatinib era, whereas the median overall survival with metastatic disease is now 5 years.[29,43] The normal starting dose of imatinib is 400 mg/day. Although there is no difference in overall survival between 400 and 800 mg/day, one study does suggest there may be longer progression-free survival with twice-daily imatinib.[29]

Because of the response to imatinib in many patients with metastatic GIST, and because imatinib is not curative, there often is a role for surgery in addition to tyrosine kinase inhibition. Combining the two modalities may delay imatinib resistance and potentially be curative.[44,45] Current practice at MSKCC is to treat patients with imatinib for 3 to 6 months and then consider surgery if complete resection is suggested on imaging. Patients then are treated with postoperative imatinib to prevent recurrence. In 40 patients with metastatic GIST treated with imatinib, three subgroups were identified at the time of surgery. One group had responsive disease, another focal resistance, and the third had multifocal resistance. The median time of imatinib therapy was 7, 21, and 26 months, respectively (**Fig. 5**). Grossly negative margins were achieved in 85%, 46%, and 29% of patients, respectively. Multiple organ resections were involved in the surgery, including peritoneum (68%), stomach or intestine (48%), liver (43%), and the pancreas (13%). After a median follow-up of 15 months, there was a significant difference in progression-free survival between the groups. Although there are many potential biases confounding these results, before randomized trials can assist in providing additional data, this study does suggest that patients with imatinib-responsive disease or only focally progressive disease should be considered candidates for surgical resection.

Table 3
Trials of imatinib mesylate in metastatic gist

Trial	Phase	Year	Imatinib Mesylate Dose (n)	Follow-up	Best Response			Comments
					PR	SD	PD	
EORTC[41,52]	I	2001, 2002	400, 600, 800, or 1000 mg/d (35)	8–12 months	51%	31%	8%	TTR = 1 week MTD = 800 mg/day
U.S. Multicenter[42,43]	II	2002, 2004	400mg/d (73) 600mg/d (74)	34 months	67% 66%	16% 18%	17% 8%	No difference between groups
EORTC[29]	III	2003	400mg/d (470) 800mg/d (472)	2 years	50% 54%	32% 32%	13% 9%	32% Grade III-IV toxicity. 50% Grade III-IV toxicity. Improved PFS for 800 mg/d ($P = .03$)
Intergroup[63]	III	2003	400mg/d (350) 800mg/d (352)	12 months	49% 48%	22% 22%		36% Grade III-IV toxicity. 52% Grade III-IV toxicity. No difference in PFS

Abbreviations: PR, partial response; SD, stable disease; PD, progressive disease; TTR, time to recurrence; MTD, maximal tolerated dose; CR, complete response; PFS, progression-free survival.
From Gold JS, DeMatteo RP. Combined surgical and molecular therapy: the gastrointestinal stromal tumor model. Ann Surg 2006;244:176; with permission.

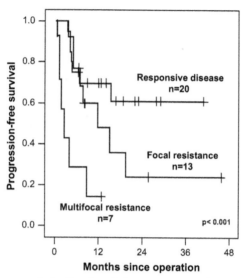

Fig. 5. Progression-free survival after imatinib treatment and metastatic GIST resection. (*From* DeMatteo RP, Maki RG, Singer S, et al. Results of tyrosine kinase inhibitor therapy followed by surgical resection for metastatic gastrointestinal stromal tumor. Ann Surg 2007;245(3):347–52; with permission.)

IMATINIB-RESISTANT GASTROINTESTINAL STROMAL TUMOR

Imatinib resistance can develop after long-term treatment. Often resistant GISTs develop a secondary *KIT* mutation at the gene that encodes parts of the kinase that are integral for imatinib binding. Approximately half of secondary mutations occur in *KIT* exon 17 and interfere with imatinib binding.[30] The other half of mutations responsible for imatinib resistance can involve activation of other kinases, increased imatinib metabolism, or, rarely, target gene amplification. Approximately 50% of GIST that progress do so in only one resistant tumor nodule that exists within or next to responding areas of metastasis. In one study, 8 of 10 such "nodules within a mass" developed a new *KIT* mutation that was not present at diagnosis.[46] In scenarios in which one nodule continues to grow, while the majority of metastatic disease responds to imatinib therapy, surgical resection of the resistant nodule should be considered. Months to years of disease control may be provided after resecting the resistant tumor and continuing imatinib therapy, especially when the primary GIST was gastric in origin.[47]

In patients who have GIST that progresses while taking imatinib at a dose of 400 mg/day, the dose can be escalated to 800 mg/day. Five percent of patients who progress at 400 mg/day will respond to the elevated dose of imatinib and achieve at least partial remission.[48] Additionally, 30% of patients will have stable disease. In patients who have imatinib-resistant GIST or who do not tolerate imatinib, sunitinib is the next line of therapy. It is a multitargeted tyrosine kinase inhibitor that has both antitumor and antiangiogenic abilities. Its mechanism involves inhibition of vascular endothelial cell growth factor receptors 1, 2, and 3; *KIT*; *PDGFRα*; *PDGFRβ*; Fms-like tyrosine kinase-3 receptor; and the ret proto-oncogene receptor. One prospective, randomized, placebo-controlled trial examined 312 patients with imatinib resistance or intolerance.[49] The investigators reported a median time to tumor progression of 6.4 weeks in the placebo group and 27.3 weeks in the sunitinib group. Fifty-eight percent of patients treated with sunitinib had stable disease compared with 48% of patients treated with placebo. The end result, even after crossover of patients from the placebo group to the treatment arm, was significantly longer overall survival in patients treated with sunitinib.

Several other treatment modalities are available, including radiation, ablation, and some novel agents. GISTs are considered radiation-resistant tumors, and there are no prospective trials of the effect of radiation therapy.[50] The only role for radiation therapy is for palliative treatment or possibly with rectal GIST. Radiofrequency ablation (RFA) is a technique that is being used more frequently with metastatic GIST in the liver. There are limited data suggesting its benefit, but based on other types of tumors in the liver, it is possible to use RFA on lesions smaller than 3 cm.[51] RFA is generally not performed with more than three to five tumors and can be used with stable or progressive disease during imatinib treatment. Hepatic artery embolization can also be useful to palliate patients with liver metastases, because the tumors often are hypervascular. In patients with diffuse hepatic metastases, half of the liver can be treated at a time. Despite its success in reducing tumor volume with metastatic GIST, there is no evidence that it improves survival.[52,53]

The results of treatment with traditional chemotherapy have not been successful.[54] Specifically, treatment with doxorubicin or gemcitabine combinations has resulted in less than a 10% response rate.[55,56] Similarly, there was no response to ifosfamide and etoposide or temozolomide in patients with metastatic GIST.[57,58] Given the failure of traditional chemotherapy agents to treat GIST, after resistance or intolerance to imatinib and sunitinib, there are several other tyrosine kinase inhibitors that are currently being studied. Vatalanib (PTK787/ZK222584) has a similar mechanism of action to sunitinib and has been shown to have an effect on imatinib-resistant GIST.[59] Dasatinib (BMS354825) is another tyrosine kinase inhibitor that may have utility in GIST with an exon 17 mutation and imatinib resistance. It also inhibits the src kinase, which is a downstream kinase that can be activated after *KIT* activation. Everolimus is another agent currently being studied. It inhibits the PI3K-Akt-mammalian target of rapamycin (mTOR) pathway that is activated by the *KIT* receptor tyrosine kinase.[60]

SUMMARY

GISTs are the most common mesenchymal tumor found in the gastrointestinal tract. The use of imatinib, and now second-generation tyrosine kinase inhibitors, for targeted therapy is a novel paradigm for treating solid tumors. Radiographic and pathologic evaluations are vital to diagnosis and prognosis of GIST. Surgical resection of primary, recurrent, and metastatic GIST, in combination with tyrosine kinase inhibition is the standard of care for treating patients with GIST. A multidisciplinary approach to GIST diagnosis and treatment is essential for successful outcomes.

REFERENCES

1. Nilsson B, Bumming P, Meis-Kindblom JM, et al. Gastrointestinal stromal tumors: the incidence, prevalence, clinical course, and prognostication in the preimatinib mesylate era – a population-based study in western Sweden. Cancer 2005; 103(4):821–9.
2. DeMatteo RP, Lewis JJ, Leung D, et al. Two hundred gastrointestinal stromal tumors: recurrence patterns and prognostic factors for survival. Ann Surg 2000; 231(1):51–8.
3. Kim TW, Lee H, Kang YK, et al. Prognostic significance of c-kit mutation in localized gastrointestinal stromal tumors. Clin Cancer Res 2004;10(9):3076–81.

4. Martin J, Poveda A, Llombart-Bosch A, et al. Deletions affecting codons 557-558 of the c-KIT gene indicate a poor prognosis in patients with completely resected gastrointestinal stromal tumors: a study by the Spanish Group for Sarcoma Research (GEIS). J Clin Oncol 2005;23(25):6190–8.

5. Wu TJ, Lee LY, Yeh CN, et al. Surgical treatment and prognostic analysis for gastrointestinal stromal tumors (GISTs) of the small intestine: before the era of imatinib mesylate. BMC Gastroenterol 2006;6:29.

6. Bumming P, Ahlman H, Andersson J, et al. Population-based study of the diagnosis and treatment of gastrointestinal stromal tumours. Br J Surg 2006;93(7): 836–43.

7. Katz SC, DeMatteo RP. Gastrointestinal stromal tumors and leiomyosarcomas. J Surg Oncol 2008;97(4):350–9.

8. Lasota J, Miettinen M. KIT and PDGFRA mutations in gastrointestinal stromal tumors (GISTs). Semin Diagn Pathol 2006;23(2):91–102.

9. Fletcher CD, Berman JJ, Corless C, et al. Diagnosis of gastrointestinal stromal tumors: a consensus approach. Hum Pathol 2002;33(5):459–65.

10. Miettinen M, Lasota J. Gastrointestinal stromal tumors: review on morphology, molecular pathology, prognosis, and differential diagnosis. Arch Pathol Lab Med 2006;130(10):1466–78.

11. Sandrasegaran K, Rajesh A, Rushing DA, et al. Gastrointestinal stromal tumors: CT and MRI findings. Eur Radiol 2005;15(7):1407–14.

12. Miettinen M, Sobin LH, Lasota J. Gastrointestinal stromal tumors of the stomach: a clinicopathologic, immunohistochemical, and molecular genetic study of 1765 cases with long-term follow-up. Am J Surg Pathol 2005;29(1):52–68.

13. Goerres GW, Stupp R, Barghouth G, et al. The value of PET, CT and in-line PET/CT in patients with gastrointestinal stromal tumours: long-term outcome of treatment with imatinib mesylate. Eur J Nucl Med Mol Imaging 2005;32(2):153–62.

14. Miettinen M, Lasota J. Gastrointestinal stromal tumors: pathology and prognosis at different sites. Semin Diagn Pathol 2006;23(2):70–83.

15. Blay P, Astudillo A, Buesa JM, et al. Protein kinase C theta is highly expressed in gastrointestinal stromal tumors but not in other mesenchymal neoplasias. Clin Cancer Res 2004;10(12 Pt 1):4089–95.

16. Ng EH, Pollock RE, Munsell MF, et al. Prognostic factors influencing survival in gastrointestinal leiomyosarcomas. Implications for surgical management and staging. Ann Surg 1992;215(1):68–77.

17. Miettinen M, Sobin LH. Gastrointestinal stromal tumors in the appendix: a clinicopathologic and immunohistochemical study of four cases. Am J Surg Pathol 2001;25(11):1433–7.

18. Singer S, Rubin BP, Lux ML, et al. Prognostic value of KIT mutation type, mitotic activity, and histologic subtype in gastrointestinal stromal tumors. J Clin Oncol 2002;20(18):3898–905.

19. Ma Y, Cunningham ME, Wang X, et al. Inhibition of spontaneous receptor phosphorylation by residues in a putative alpha-helix in the KIT intracellular juxtamembrane region. J Biol Chem 1999;274(19):13399–402.

20. Shiu MH, Farr GH, Papachristou DN, et al. Myosarcomas of the stomach: natural history, prognostic factors and management. Cancer 1982;49(1):177–87.

21. Shiu MH, Farr GH, Egeli RA, et al. Myosarcomas of the small and large intestine: a clinicopathologic study. J Surg Oncol 1983;24(1):67–72.

22. Rudolph P, Gloeckner K, Parwaresch R, et al. DNA ploidy, and biological behavior of gastrointestinal stromal tumors: a multivariate clinicopathologic study. Hum Pathol 1998;29(8):791–800.

23. Cooper PN, Quirke P, Hardy GJ, et al. A flow cytometric, clinical, and histological study of stromal neoplasms of the gastrointestinal tract. Am J Surg Pathol 1992; 16(2):163–70.

24. Gunther T, Schneider-Stock R, Hackel C, et al. Telomerase activity and expression of hTRT and hTR in gastrointestinal stromal tumors in comparison with extragastrointestinal sarcomas. Clin Cancer Res 2000;6(5):1811–8.

25. Ng EH, Pollock RE, Romsdahl MM. Prognostic implications of patterns of failure for gastrointestinal leiomyosarcomas. Cancer 1992;69(6):1334–41.

26. McGrath PC, Neifeld JP, Lawrence W Jr, et al. Gastrointestinal sarcomas. Analysis of prognostic factors. Ann Surg 1987;206(6):706–10.

27. Akwari OE, Dozois RR, Weiland LH, et al. Leiomyosarcoma of the small and large bowel. Cancer 1978;42(3):1375–84.

28. Mol CD, Dougan DR, Schneider TR, et al. Structural basis for the autoinhibition and STI-571 inhibition of c-Kit tyrosine kinase. J Biol Chem 2004;279(30): 31655–63.

29. Verweij J, Casali PG, Zalcberg J, et al. Progression-free survival in gastrointestinal stromal tumours with high-dose imatinib: randomised trial. Lancet 2004; 364(9440):1127–34.

30. Heinrich MC, Corless CL, Blanke CD, et al. Molecular correlates of imatinib resistance in gastrointestinal stromal tumors. J Clin Oncol 2006;24(29):4764–74.

31. Joensuu H, Dimitrijevic S. Tyrosine kinase inhibitor imatinib (STI571) as an anticancer agent for solid tumours. Ann Med 2001;33(7):451–5.

32. Heinrich MC, Corless CL, Demetri GD, et al. Kinase mutations and imatinib response in patients with metastatic gastrointestinal stromal tumor. J Clin Oncol 2003;21(23):4342–9.

33. Debiec-Rychter M, Sciot R, Le Cesne A, et al. KIT mutations and dose selection for imatinib in patients with advanced gastrointestinal stromal tumours. Eur J Cancer 2006;42(8):1093–103.

34. Corless CL, Schroeder A, Griffith D, et al. PDGFRA mutations in gastrointestinal stromal tumors: frequency, spectrum and in vitro sensitivity to imatinib. J Clin Oncol 2005;23(23):5357–64.

35. Blay JY, Le Cesne A, Ray-Coquard I, et al. Prospective multicentric randomized phase III study of imatinib in patients with advanced gastrointestinal stromal tumors comparing interruption versus continuation of treatment beyond 1 year: the French Sarcoma Group. J Clin Oncol 2007;25(9):1107–13.

36. Blay JY, Bonvalot S, Casali P, et al. Consensus meeting for the management of gastrointestinal stromal tumors. Report of the GIST Consensus Conference of 20-21 March 2004, under the auspices of ESMO. Ann Oncol 2005;16(4):566–78.

37. DeMatteo R, Antonescu CR, Chadaram V, et al. Adjuvant imatinib mesylate in patients with primary high risk gastrointestinal stromal tumor (GIST) following complete resection: safety results from the U.S. Intergroup Phase II trial (ACOSOG Z9000). J Clin Oncol 2005;23:9009.

38. Dematteo RP, Owzar CR, Antonescu CR, et al. Efficacy of adjuvant imatinib mesylate following complete resection of localized, primary gastrointestinal stromal tumor (GIST) at high risk of recurrence: the U.S. Intergroup phase II trial ACOSOG Z9000. [abstract]. In: American Society of Clinical Oncology 2008 Gastrointestinal Cancers Symposium; Orlando (FL): January; 2008. p. A8.

39. DeMatteo RP, Owzar CR, Maki R, et al. Adjuvant imatinib mesylate increases recurrence free survival (RFS) in patients with completely resected localized primary gastrointestinal stromal tumor (GIST): North American Intergroup phase III trial ACOSOG Z9001 [abstract]. J Clin Oncol 2007;25(Suppl 18):A10079.

40. DeMatteo RP, Shah A, Fong Y, et al. Results of hepatic resection for sarcoma metastatic to liver. Ann Surg 2001;234(4):540–7 [discussion 7–8].

41. van Oosterom AT, Judson I, Verweij J, et al. Safety and efficacy of imatinib (STI571) in metastatic gastrointestinal stromal tumours: a phase I study. Lancet 2001;358(9291):1421–3.

42. Demetri GD, von Mehren M, Blanke CD, et al. Efficacy and safety of imatinib mesylate in advanced gastrointestinal stromal tumors. N Engl J Med 2002;347(7): 472–80.

43. Blanke CD, Demetri GD, von Mehren M, et al. Long-term results from a randomized phase II trial of standard- versus higher-dose imatinib mesylate for patients with unresectable or metastatic gastrointestinal stromal tumors expressing KIT. J Clin Oncol 2008;26(4):620–5.

44. Raut CP, Posner M, Desai J, et al. Surgical management of advanced gastrointestinal stromal tumors after treatment with targeted systemic therapy using kinase inhibitors. J Clin Oncol 2006;24(15):2325–31.

45. DeMatteo RP, Maki RG, Singer S, et al. Results of tyrosine kinase inhibitor therapy followed by surgical resection for metastatic gastrointestinal stromal tumor. Ann Surg 2007;245(3):347–52.

46. Desai J, Shankar S, Heinrich MC, et al. Clonal evolution of resistance to imatinib in patients with metastatic gastrointestinal stromal tumors. Clin Cancer Res 2007; 13(18 Pt 1):5398–405.

47. Hasegawa J, Kanda T, Hirota S, et al. Surgical interventions for focal progression of advanced gastrointestinal stromal tumors during imatinib therapy. Int J Clin Oncol 2007;12(3):212–7.

48. Wen PY, Yung WK, Lamborn KR, et al. Phase I/II study of imatinib mesylate for recurrent malignant gliomas: North American Brain Tumor Consortium Study 99-08. Clin Cancer Res 2006;12(16):4899–907.

49. Demetri GD, van Oosterom AT, Garrett CR, et al. Efficacy and safety of sunitinib in patients with advanced gastrointestinal stromal tumour after failure of imatinib: a randomised controlled trial. Lancet 2006;368(9544):1329–38.

50. Von Mehren M. Imatinib-refractory gastrointestinal stromal tumors: the clinical problem and therapeutic strategies. Curr Oncol Rep 2006;8:192–7.

51. Dileo P, Randhawa E, Vansonnenberg E, et al. Safety and efficacy of percutaneous radio-frequency ablation (RFA) in patients with metastatic gastrointestinal stromal tumor (GIST) with clonal evolution of lesions refractory to imatinib mesylate. J Clin Oncol 2004;22:9024.

52. Kobayashi K, Gupta S, Trent JC, et al. Hepatic artery chemoembolization for 110 gastrointestinal stromal tumors: response, survival, and prognostic factors. Cancer 2006;107(12):2833–41.

53. Maluccio MA, Covey AM, Schubert J, et al. Treatment of metastatic sarcoma to the liver with bland embolization. Cancer 2006;107(7):1617–23.

54. Dematteo RP, Heinrich MC, El-Rifai WM, et al. Clinical management of gastrointestinal stromal tumors: before and after STI-571. Hum Pathol 2002; 33(5):466–77.

55. Edmonson JH, Marks RS, Buckner JC, et al. Contrast of response to dacarbazine, mitomycin, doxorubicin, and cisplatin (DMAP) plus GM-CSF between patients with advanced malignant gastrointestinal stromal tumors and patients with other advanced leiomyosarcomas. Cancer Invest 2002;20(5–6):605–12.

56. Von Burton G, Rankin C, Zalupski MM, et al. Phase II trial of gemcitabine as first line chemotherapy in patients with metastatic or unresectable soft tissue sarcoma. Am J Clin Oncol 2006;29(1):59–61.

57. Blair SC, Zalupski MM, Baker LH. Ifosfamide and etoposide in the treatment of advanced soft tissue sarcomas. Am J Clin Oncol 1994;17(6):480–4.
58. Trent JC, Beach J, Burgess MA, et al. A two-arm phase II study of temozolomide in patients with advanced gastrointestinal stromal tumors and other soft tissue sarcomas. Cancer 2003;98(12):2693–9.
59. Joensuu H, De Braud F, Coco P, et al. Phase II, open-label study of PTK787/ ZK222584 for the treatment of metastatic gastrointestinal stromal tumors resistant to imatinib mesylate. Ann Oncol 2008;19(1):173–7.
60. Rossi F, Ehlers I, Agosti V, et al. Oncogenic Kit signaling and therapeutic intervention in a mouse model of gastrointestinal stromal tumor. Proc Natl Acad Sci U S A 2006;103(34):12843–8.
61. Wong NA, Young R, Malcomson RD, et al. Prognostic indicators for gastrointestinal stromal tumours: a clinicopathological and immunohistochemical study of 108 resected cases of the stomach. Histopathology 2003;43(2):118–26.
62. van Oosterom AT, Judson IR, Verweij J, et al. Update of phase I study of imatinib (STI571) in advanced soft tissue sarcomas and gastrointestinal stromal tumors: a report of the EORTC Soft Tissue and Bone Sarcoma Group. Eur J Cancer 2002;38(Suppl 5):S83–7.
63. Benjamin RS, Rankin C, Fletcher C, et al. Phase III dose-randomized study of imatinib mesylate (ST1571) for GIST: Intergroup S0033 early results. Proc Am Soc Clin Oncol 2003;22:814.

Soft Tissue Sarcomas: Current Management and Future Directions

Robert J. Kenney, DO[a], Richard Cheney, MD[b], Margaret A. Stull, MD[c], William Kraybill, MD[c,d],*

KEYWORDS

- Soft tissue sarcoma • Radiation • Cancer
- Chemotherapy • Tissue sampling

Soft-tissue sarcomas (STSs) are a heterogeneous group of neoplasms arising from cells of mesenchymal origin. They are divided into tumors of adipocytic, fibroblastic, smooth muscle, skeletal muscle, vascular, osseous, fibrohistiocytic, and uncertain histogenesis.[1] Tumors are generally categorized according to the 2002 World Health Organization (WHO) classification, which is based on the tissue or cell of origin.[2] As the molecular genetics of STS becomes more clearly understood, current classifications will likely evolve into more prognostically useful groups. Tumors previously classified as malignant fibrous histiocytoma (MFH) have been reclassified into more specific entities (ie, leiomyosarcoma, dedifferentiated liposarcoma) based on their molecular genetics and cellular differentiation as determined by immunohistochemistry[3] This article discusses current epidemiology, diagnosis, and treatment of soft tissue sarcomas of the extremities, abdomen, and retroperitoneum.

EPIDEMIOLOGY

STSs account for less than 1% of all malignant neoplasms. The specific incidence patterns depend on the definition of STS used. Toro and colleagues[4] studied the epidemiology of STS from 1978 to 2001 using the Surveillance, Epidemiology, and End Results database. Rates of STS ranged from 4.5 to 6.5 cases per 100,000

[a] Department of Surgery, University of Missouri-Kansas City, 2301 Holmes, Kansas City, MO 64108, USA
[b] Department of Pathology and Laboratory Medicine, Roswell Park Cancer Institute, Elm and Carlton Streets, Buffalo, NY 14263, USA
[c] Department of Diagnostic Radiology, St. Luke's Hospital of Kansas City, 4401 Wornall Road, Kansas City, MO 64111-3220, USA
[d] Department of Surgery, University of Missouri-Kansas City, 2301 Holmes, Kansas City, MO 64108, USA
* Corresponding author. 4320 Wornall Road, Suite 240, Kansas City, MO 64111.
E-mail address: gress250@gmail.com (W. Kraybill).

Surg Clin N Am 89 (2009) 235–247
doi:10.1016/j.suc.2008.09.020
0039-6109/08/$ – see front matter © 2009 Elsevier Inc. All rights reserved.
surgical.theclinics.com

person-years. Rates were slightly higher in men than women, and highest in black women, possibly because of the inclusion of uterine leiomyosarcomas in the study. Generally, the rates of STS increase with age.

ETIOLOGY

Most STS are believed to arise spontaneously and are of an unknown cause; however, several observations have suggested specific etiologies. Rare heritable conditions are known to predispose patients to STS. Li-Fraumeni syndrome involves a cancer-pre-disposing mutation of the TP53 gene. Individuals who have this autosomal dominant condition have an increased rate of developing multiple primary malignancies, partic-ularly STS, breast cancer, leukemia, osteogenic sarcoma, melanoma, and cancers of the colon, pancreas, adrenal cortex, and brain. TP53 is a tumor suppressor gene in-volved in regulating cell cycle and apoptosis.

Retinoblastoma, the most common malignant ocular neoplasm of childhood, is caused by mutation of the tumor suppressor gene, RB1, which may be sporadic or heritable. Childhood survivors of retinoblastoma are at risk for developing an STS later in life.[5] TP53 and Rb1 gene mutations are commonly found mutated in sporadic STS. Mutation or deletion of the tumor suppressor gene, NF1, is associated with neurofibro-matosis type I, and places patients at risk for developing malignant peripheral nerve sheath tumors.

Ionizing radiation has long been known to increase the risk for STS. Tumors typically develop approximately 7 to 10 years after radiation exposure. Radiation-induced mu-tations of the TP53 gene have been shown to play an integral role in radiation-induced STS.[6] Severe, chronic lymphedema predisposes patients to developing cutaneous angiosarcoma. Stewart-Treves syndrome represents angiosarcoma arising in the set-ting of prolonged severe lymphedema from any acquired or congenital cause. It oc-curs in the upper extremity of approximately 0.07% of postmastectomy patients after axillary dissection.[7] Postlymphedema angiosarcomas are fairly aggressive tu-mors, with an average survival of 19 months.[8] Lymphedema of other sites and causes also predisposes patients to the development of STS. The only virus known to have a role in human STS is HHV-8, which plays a role in the development of Kaposi sarcoma.[3,9]

When genetic syndromes and radiation-induced tumors are excluded, patients di-agnosed with a STS have around a 16% risk for developing a second malignancy.[10] These patients probably have an unknown and complex genetic predisposition to malignancy.

Although understanding the complex molecular genetics of STS may provide more useful prognostic classifications, this knowledge will undoubtedly provide insight for more specific therapeutic options. Currently, gastrointestinal stromal tumors, are the prototype of targeted molecular therapy with imatinib targeting the c-Kit (CD 117) receptor.

STAGING AND PROGNOSIS

Staging of STS is most commonly performed using the American Joint Committee on Cancer (AJCC) system in the United States and the WHO system in the rest of the world. These systems are very similar. Unique to the staging of STS is the addition of tumor grade to the traditional TNM system. Tumor grade is one of the most impor-tant prognostic factors.[11] Grade is typically determined using either the National Can-cer Institute or the French Federation of Cancer Centers Sarcoma Group systems. Both systems are three-tiered. The French system has a slightly greater ability to predict metastases.[12] Histologic grade considers cellularity, mitotic rate, cellular pleo-morphism, and necrosis. How closely the tumor recapitulates normal tissue is also considered. STSs generally metastasize hematologically. Lymph node involvement is uncommon, and often represents aggressive disease. Nodal involvement is currently considered stage IV disease.

Limitations of traditional staging methods of determining survival have been noted. Sarcoma-specific death has been noted to be as high as 50%, but a wide variation is reported in the literature.[13] A detailed and accurate method of determining risk for sarcoma-specific death in an individual patient would be useful. The current AJCC system does not incorporate many known prognostic factors, and risk for sarcoma-specific death can vary widely among stages.

Kattan and colleagues[14] at the Memorial Sloan-Kettering Cancer Center (MSKCC) developed a nomogram to better predict risk for sarcoma-specific death (MSKCC Sarcoma Nomogram). The MSKCC nomogram considers age, histology, grade, location, depth, and size to determine the likelihood of 12-year sarcoma-specific survival. A prospective study of the validity of the nomogram proved it to have good predictive value.[15] The proposed 7th edition of the AJCC staging manual, to be published within 2 years, should provide improved prognostic information.

Management, General Considerations

Optimal patient care of STS is best provided by a multidisciplinary team (consisting of radiology, medical and surgical oncology, radiation medicine, pathology, and psycho-social experts) with experience dealing with these types of tumors. Noria and colleagues[16] found that approximately one third of patients who have excisional biopsies of an extremity sarcoma had residual disease on reexcision. A study in Florida showed that patients who had STS treated at high volume centers had improved survival and functional outcomes.[17] Multidisciplinary centers generally treat more than 50 newly diagnosed sarcomas per year, participate in sarcoma research, and have an active sarcoma patient multidisciplinary management conference.[18] Although all soft tissue masses and even soft tissue sarcomas cannot be treated at designated sarcoma centers, patients identified as having high-risk sarcomas and advanced sarcomas are best managed at these locations, with adherence to the principles of evaluating soft tissue masses as outlined here and elsewhere.[1] The coordinated use of multiple disciplines and therapeutic modalities is necessary to achieve optimal outcome in patients who have STS.

MEDICAL IMAGING

Diagnostic imaging should be performed before invasive procedures so that soft tissue edema and hemorrhage do not complicate evaluation of the lesion. Anatomic localization of the mass and the extent of regional and metastatic disease may be established through state-of the-art medical imaging techniques. Advanced imaging technology is used for monitoring response to chemotherapy, radiation treatment, and posttreatment follow-up of patients who have STS.

MRI

MRI is the most useful imaging modality for determining the extent of lesion, presurgical planning, and monitoring the disease during and after treatment. The superior soft tissue contrast resolution and multiplanar capabilities of MRI allow identification of the tumor margins and show the relationship of the tumor to muscle compartments and neurovascular and osseous structures. Different pulse sequences may assist in tissue characterization. Fat, fluid, fibrous tissue, blood, and chondroid and osteoid matrix have distinctive imaging features. Intratumoral hemorrhage has a variable appearance depending on the stage of its evolution. Hematoma must be differentiated from a hemorrhagic neoplasm and should be followed up to ensure resolution of the soft tissue mass. If the presumed hematoma does not involute or continues to enlarge, then evaluation for an underlying tumor must be instituted.[19]

Using intravenous contrast may distinguish areas of devitalized/necrotic tumor from cystic or myxomatous areas, and viable tumor must be identified to direct appropriate site of biopsy. Contrast-enhanced MRI may be used to evaluate the surgical bed in a postoperative patient who has positive tumor margins, monitor response to neoadjuvant chemotherapy and radiation therapy, and assess for tumor recurrence. Signal characteristics of the tumor will change over time and with treatment, thereby allowing differentiation of viable from nonviable tissue and scar formation from residual or recurrent tumor in many patients.[19] Posttreatment changes may mimic residual and recurrent disease on MRI. Indeterminate findings may necessitate the need for functional imaging with positron emission tomography (PET).

MRI or CT angiography has replaced conventional angiography for the evaluation of tumor vascularity. Conventional angiography is needed for presurgical embolization.

CT

Recently manufactured multidetector/multichannel CT scans can acquire high-detail, submillimeter slice–thickness images. Two-dimensional and three-dimensional reformations can be generated in any plane or obliquity and may help determine the extent of the lesion and integrity of adjacent neurovascular and osseous structures, particularly in patients who cannot undergo MRI. CT and radiographs may show lucency in fat-containing tumors and intratumoral mineralization, such as dystrophic calcification, matrix mineralization, and phleboliths, in vascular tumors (**Fig. 1**). CT can determine the integrity of the cortex of an adjacent bone. CT is commonly used for image-guided biopsy of the mass and can be correlated with MRI for tumor localization.

Chest CT is required in all patients who have STS, because they have a high incidence of lung metastases. CT scanning of the abdomen and pelvis should be performed to evaluate for lymphadenopathy or other signs of metastatic disease.

Ultrasound

Ultrasound is a useful adjunct in the evaluation of STS when performed by experienced operators and in select patients. Lesion identification using ultrasound may be limited in the detection of deep masses and in patients who have large body habitus. Ultrasound can differentiate cystic from solid components of the tumor. Tumor vascularity may be assessed with Doppler ultrasonography. Ultrasound may be used to guide biopsy and may be preferable to CT guidance, depending on the expertise of the physician performing the procedure. Postoperative fluid collections may also be evaluated with ultrasound.

POSITRON EMISSION TOMOGRAPHY

Functional imaging evaluation of tumor metabolism is performed using whole-body PET and combined PET-CT scanning. The radiopharmaceutical glucose analog, fluorodeoxyglucose (FDG), may localize abnormally increased metabolic activity in primary and recurrent STS and allows evaluation of the entire patient. High- and intermediate-grade tumors have higher glycolytic metabolic activity as opposed to

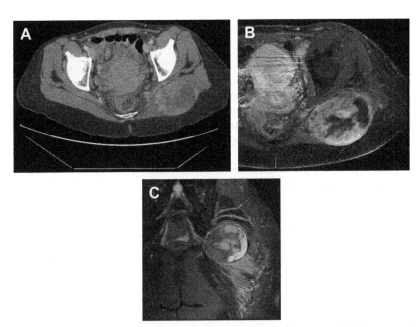

Fig. 1. Pleomorphic sarcoma in the left buttock of a 48-year-old woman. (*A*) Postcontrast CT shows lobulated areas of enhancement in the large heterogeneous mass. (*B*) The postcontrast axial fat-suppressed T1-weighted image best displays the area of tumor enhancement and the cystic/necrotic portions of the STS. (*C*) The coronal fat-suppressed T2-weighted MRI image shows the heterogeneous signal characteristics of the soft tissue sarcoma and extensive peritumoral edema.

low-grade STS or benign tumors.[20] The standardized uptake value (SUV) provides a semiquantitative measurement of glucose metabolism in a region of abnormal concentration and is typically greater than 2.0 in intermediate- and high-grade STS.[20]

PET and combined PET-CT can direct biopsy of the most biologically active area in a large STS and may show unexpected nodal and distant metastases. These techniques can be used to identify the primary tumor in patients who present with metastatic disease.

PET and combined PET-CT may be used to monitor response to chemotherapy, radiation treatment, or radiofrequency ablation, and for long-term surveillance. PET and PET-CT scanning may help differentiate posttherapeutic changes from tumor recurrence in patients who have equivocal or indeterminate MRI findings.[21] Metallic medical devices, such as orthopedic hardware, pacemakers, and dental devices, do not interfere with PET imaging.

EXTREMITY/TRUNK SOFT TISSUE SARCOMAS
Clinical Presentation

Although numerous exceptions exist, STSs of the extremities are generally painless and frequently become large before patients present. Lesions believed to be deep to fascia are suspicious for a STS and evaluated as such. Expert generally believe that superficial lesions smaller than 5 cm are unlikely to be malignant and can simply be excised. However, caution is advised, depending on the location (ie, hands, feet, face, neck) and clinical characteristics. Lesions that cannot be explained should be properly evaluated.

Tissue Sampling

Incisional or excisional biopsy has been the traditional method. Mankin and colleagues[22,23] showed the hazards of open biopsy in 1982 and again in 1992. They showed that complications from an inappropriate biopsy can have a negative impact on patient outcome, including increased use of radiation therapy and an increased rate of amputation. Core biopsy has become the preferred technique to establish diagnosis in soft tissue lesions.

Skrzynski and colleagues[24] studied cost, comparing open versus percutaneous core biopsy, and showed that the cost of an open biopsy was around seven times higher than percutaneous biopsy. Several recent studies have shown the accuracy and low morbidity than can be achieved using image-guided (CT or ultrasound) core biopsies of these tumors.[25,26] STS may be diagnosed with fine needle aspiration at institutions that have cytopathology expertise. It is advantageous for pathology to be present during the biopsy for real-time evaluation of the specimen to determine adequacy, triage tissue for special studies such as flow cytometry, or molecular diagnostics or cryopreservation. This stage is also favorable for obtaining tissue for banking and enrollment in clinical trials, if considered.[27]

Surgical Management

Principles of good management begin when patients present with a soft tissue mass. In general, if an undiagnosed mass cannot be excised with widely negative margins, it should first be imaged and then an FNA, core needle biopsy (which the authors prefer), or an open incisional biopsy performed. When performing any diagnostic procedure, one should always plan for the next operation. Incisional and needle biopsies should be performed in the plane of any planned resection with the knowledge that the biopsy scar will have to be excised during the next procedure.

Current surgical treatment emphasizes function-preserving procedures with preoperative or postoperative radiation therapy. In their classic study comparing amputation with limb-sparing surgery plus radiation, Rosenberg and colleagues[28] showed no difference in overall survival, although a small increase in local recurrence was seen in the limb-sparing group. Limb-sparing surgery entails compartmental resection or wide local excision. Compartmental resections can cause significant functional loss of the extremity; however, the approach can be modified in selected patients to allow improved function.

Standard care for surgical treatment is wide local excision that includes resection of the biopsy tract/scar with approximately 2 cm of normal tissue around the tumor. The goal of surgery is to achieve complete (R0) resection, because microscopic (R1) or grossly positive (R2) margins are associated with increased local recurrence and decreased survival.[29] Small (<5 cm) tumors, regardless of grade, may be treated with surgical excision alone if an excision margin of uninvolved tissue of larger than 1 cm can be achieved. If margins of 1 to 2 cm cannot be obtained, preoperative or postoperative radiation therapy may result in an improved local control rate and adequate function.

Proximity of the tumor to major neurovascular structures has been considered a contraindication to limb-sparing surgery, but reports have shown encouraging results for en bloc resections coupled with major vascular reconstruction in the lower extremities and retroperitoneum.[30,31] Tumors that require sacrifice of major lower extremity nerves, particularly the sciatic nerve, have traditionally been considered an indication for amputation. Studies have shown an acceptable functional outcome with resection of the sciatic, peroneal, tibial, and femoral nerves.[32,33] With appropriate reconstruction, tendon transfers, and rehabilitation, good functional outcomes have resulted. Considerable experience and judgment are required to estimate the potential for good quality of life when managing more advanced tumors. Local recurrence of STS in some patients may be treated with repeated wide local excision with no difference in survival compared with amputations.[34]

Amputation is currently reserved for treatment of primary disease or extensive local recurrence when the function of the limb would be severely impaired after tumor resection. Generally, these are large, high-grade tumors located more distal in the extremity. Increased rates of distant, usually pulmonary metastases in these patients after primary amputation is likely because of the risk factors, size, and high tumor grade.[35]

Hyperthermic isolated limb perfusion (HILP) with tumor necrosis factor and melphalan is used extensively in Europe for limb salvage in STSs of the extremities. Studies have shown response rates of approximately 75%, with long-term limb salvage rates of 80%,[36] in patients described as having advanced, frequently multicentric STSs. Radiation therapy is often given in addition to limb perfusion to increase local control.[37] Vascular insufficiency may develop as a late complication of limb perfusion and sometimes requires amputation.[38]

Patients who have a previously unplanned excision of a STS present a special circumstance for surgical management. Routine reexcision has shown residual tumor in 50% of cases.[16] Reexcision after an unplanned excision, although standard practice, is a challenging operation because the residual disease is rarely palpable to guide the surgical approach. After adequate reexcision, increased local relapse rates have been reported, whereas another series found rates similar to patients undergoing an adequate initial operation.[16,39] Higher rates of distant metastasis have been noted in groups with residual disease in the reexcision specimen.[39]

Radiation

To improve local control, radiation therapy is an effective adjuvant therapy, whether given pre- or postoperatively. Selected patients who have widely negative margins may not require radiation.[40] Extremity STS can be treated with pre- or postoperative radiation. Preoperative radiotherapy allows a decreased radiation field and radiation dose, which may diminish complications associated with radiation. Giving radiation preoperatively avoids delays in giving radiation because of postoperative wound complications. However, an increased rate of postoperative wound complications is seen in patients undergoing preoperative radiation compared with those undergoing postoperative radiation. Coordination with a reconstructive surgery team may help limit these complications, although rates of major wound complications are still significant even when sophisticated reconstruction techniques are used.[41] Postoperative radiation requires larger doses and can induce a greater long-term functional impairment. A recent randomized trial of pre- versus postoperative radiation for extremity STS showed slightly better overall survival in the preoperative group ($P<.05$), although an increased rate of wound complications was seen (35% versus 17%).[42] Surgical resection is generally performed 4 to 8 weeks after radiation therapy. Brachytherapy has resulted in reduced rates of local recurrence, especially for high-grade tumors.[43,44]

Chemotherapy

Most randomized trials assessing the role of adjuvant chemotherapy in primary STSs are small and have had varying results. A large meta-analysis performed by the

Sarcoma Meta-Analysis Collaboration, including patients who had all grades, sizes, and locations of tumors, showed a 10% decrease in overall recurrence-free survival and a 4% increase in overall survival at 10 years (not statistically significant) with adjuvant chemotherapy.[45] Criticisms of the study include concerns about inclusion of patients who had tumors in varied locations and inclusion of low-grade tumors, unlikely to metastasize, which could have overestimated the value of chemotherapy.[46] Large (>5 cm), high-grade tumors have been shown to develop distant metastasis around 35% to 60% of the time.[47] Although response to aggressive neoadjuvant and adjuvant chemotherapy has been documented using doxorubicin, ifosfamide, and dacarbazine, proof of efficacy in improving long-term survival remains controversial. This regimen and most others are extraordinarily toxic.[48] The role of neoadjuvant chemotherapy and adjuvant chemotherapy in primary STSs remains controversial. New regimens, perhaps in combination with newer targeted therapies, are greatly needed for these tumors.

Retroperitoneal/Abdominal Sarcomas

Clinical presentation
Patients who have abdominal or retroperitoneal STS generally present with sensations of fullness or obstructive symptoms of the alimentary or renal systems. Given the slow onset and vague symptoms, tumors frequently grow to an enormous size and present at an advanced stage. Patients typically present to primary care doctors with vague symptoms and findings that contribute to the delay in diagnosis of these tumors. CT scan of the abdomen and pelvis with intravenous and oral contrast should be performed for any suspicious symptoms or physical findings. In addition to STS, the differential diagnosis for a retroperitoneal mass includes germ cell tumors, lymphoma, abscess, and renal, adrenal, and neurogenic tumors, and undifferentiated carcinoma (primary or metastatic).

Tissue sampling
Image-guided core biopsy is generally efficacious, safe, and accurate. In general, retroperitoneal masses are malignant and require resection. The authors prefer to biopsy retroperitoneal masses to confirm the diagnosis before resecting the tumor. This technique may also allow placement of selected patients on specific protocols. Biopsy would be required for neoadjuvant radiation therapy. However, retroperitoneal lipomatous lesions are difficult to biopsy with core needles unless the tumor of interest contains heterogenous enhancing areas.

SURGICAL MANAGEMENT

Retroperitoneal sarcomas are treated primarily with surgical excision. If neoadjuvant radiation is a therapeutic consideration, a core needle biopsy is essential. The lesion should be resected with as wide a margin as possible, even if neoadjuvant therapy is not used. The tumors should be removed en bloc with surrounding organs as necessary.

Radiation
Retroperitoneal tumors have shown some benefits with adjuvant or neoadjuvant radiation therapy, although definitive studies are not available. The presence of the tumor can help keep abdominal viscera out of the radiation field, making preoperative therapy attractive and reducing the incidence of radiation enteritis, bowel obstruction, and other complications associated with abdominal radiation. Intraoperative radiation and brachytherapy may also be used selectively. Using preoperative therapy with either an

intraoperative boost or brachytherapy could favorably affect local recurrence and 5-year survival for intermediate- and high-grade tumors.[49]

Chemotherapy

Chemotherapy for localized retroperitoneal sarcomas is controversial, and no large controlled studies have been reported. Patients who have metastatic disease may be considered for chemotherapy, but no evidence exists of significant benefit.[50] Smaller, completely excised lesions without metastasis do not require chemotherapy. Clinical trials using chemotherapy are underway for patients who have unresectable retroperitoneal sarcomas.

SURVEILLANCE

Patients who have completed therapy and show no active disease require close observation and follow-up to monitor for recurrent or metastatic disease. For extremity/trunk STS, a recent update of the National Comprehensive Cancer Network (NCCN) recommends a history/physical and chest CT or radiograph be done every 3 to 6 months for 2 to 3 years, then every 6 months for the next 2 years and then should be done annually. Consideration should be given to imaging the primary site depending on the estimated risk for local recurrence and the primary site.[51] Routine imaging of the affected extremity is beneficial if the patient's body habitus prohibits a good physical examination.[52] Having a good baseline image of the operative site is always advantageous. In selected patients, physical examination may be adequate, but for the most part imaging at least twice a year is the prudent course. Patients who have treated retroperitoneal sarcomas and no known active disease should have abdominal and pelvic CT scans every 3 to 6 months for 2 years and then annually.[51]

METASTATIC DISEASE

STS most commonly metastasizes to the lung. Isolated pulmonary metastasis occurs in approximately 20% of patients.[53] Surgical resection (metastectomy) of these metastases is the mainstay of treatment. Resection can be performed using minimally invasive techniques, median sternotomy, unilateral posterolateral thoracotomy, staged bilateral thoracotomy, or a clamshell thoracotomy, depending on surgeon experience and the location of recurrence. Reports of 3-year survival rates after pulmonary metastectomy range from 28% to 54%.[54,55] Factors associated with a prolonged survival include complete resection of pulmonary disease and greater than 1 year disease-free before development of metastatic disease.[56] Between 40% and 80% of patients will develop recurrent disease in the lung after pulmonary resection. These patients should be considered for re-resection if complete resection of disease can be obtained.[57] If the disease cannot be completely excised, little can be gained from metastectomy unless the patient is symptomatic.

Patients who have unresectable metastatic disease have few options. Doxorubicin-based palliative chemotherapy has not been shown to increase survival, and toxic side effects of the treatments are significant.[58] Newer regimens using gemcitabine and docetaxel have shown some improvement in survival.[59] Care must be taken when selecting patients for palliative chemotherapy.

FUTURE DIRECTIONS

Sarcomas are rare (approximately 7000 cases annually in the United States) heterogeneous tumors that involve multiple specialties in patient care. Research at individual centers may be difficult. The Sarcoma Progress Review Group[18] recommended the creation of a Sarcoma Research Consortium that would guide and focus research into more fruitful directions. This group recommended that research focus on the molecular characterization of STS.

STSs have recently been molecularly categorized into two broad groups. The first group includes tumors with simple karyotypes, simple translocations, or point mutations (c-KIT in gastrointestinal stromal tumors). The second group consists of tumors with complex karyotypes and nonspecific cytogenetic aberrations (approximately two thirds of all STS).[60]

Newer molecular classification of tumors may result in a reclassification of many tumor types. Tumors previously classified as MFH have been shown to have similar gene expression patterns to liposarcomas and some leiomyosarcomas, supporting the hypothesis that MFH is a member of this group of tumors.[61] Gene microarray analysis is crucial in determining these molecular patterns. Acquisition of fresh and archival formalin-fixed, paraffin embedded tissue obtained before treatment will provide resources for correlating outcomes with molecular patterns. Future hope for patients who have STSs is that more precise molecular genetic characterization of sarcomas will lead to an enhanced array of more specific and less toxic therapeutic options than currently exists.

REFERENCES

1. Pisters P, Bramwell V, Rubin B, et al. Sarcomas of soft tissue. In: Abeloff M, Armitage J, Niederhuber J, et al, editors. Clinical Oncology. 3rd edition. Philadelphia: Elsevier Inc; 2004. p. 2573–626.
2. Fletcher C, Unni KK, Mertens F. WHO Classification of Soft Tissue Tumors. In: Fletcher C, Unni KK, Mertens F, editors. Pathology and Genetics: Tumors of Soft Tissue and Bone. World Health Organization Classification of Tumors. International Agency for Research on Cancer Press; 2002. p. 9–12.
3. Skubitz K, D'Adamo D. Sarcoma. Mayo Clin Proc 2007;82(11):1409–32.
4. Toro J, Travis L, Wu HJ, et al. Incidence patterns of soft tissue sarcomas, regardless of primary site, in the Surveillance, Epidemiology, and End Results Program, 1978–2001: an analysis of 26,758 cases. Int J Cancer 2006;119:2922–30.
5. Hawkins MM, Draper GJ, Kingston JE. Incidence of second primary tumours among childhood cancer survivors. Br J Cancer 1987;56:339–47.
6. Gonin-Laurent N, Hadj-Hamou NS, Vogt N, et al. RB1 and TP53 pathways in radiation-induced Sarcomas. Oncogene 2007;26(41):6106–12.
7. Stewart NJ, Pritchard DJ, Nascimento AG, et al. Lymphangiosarcoma following mastectomy. Clin Orthop Relat Res 1995;320:135–41.
8. Schiffman S, Berger A. Stewart-Treves syndrome. J Am Coll Surg 2007;204(2): 328.
9. Memar OM, Rady PL, Tyring SK. Human herpesvirus-8: detection of novel herpesvirus-like DNA sequences in Kaposi's sarcoma and other lesions. J Mol Med 1995;73:603–9.
10. Fernebro J, Bladstrom A, Rydholm A, et al. Increased risk of malignancies in a population-based Study of 818 soft-tissue sarcoma patients. Br J Cancer 2006;95:986–90.
11. Coindre JM. Grading of soft tissue sarcomas: review and update. Arch Pathol Lab Med 2006;130:1448–53.
12. Guillou L, Coindre JM, Bonichon F, et al. Comparative study of the National Cancer Institute and French Federation of Cancer Centers Sarcoma Group Grading

Systems in a population of 410 adult patients with soft tissue sarcoma. J Clin Oncol 1997;15:350–62.

13. Mariani L, Miceli R, Kattan M, et al. Validation and adaptation of a nomogram for predicting the survival of patients with extremity soft tissue sarcoma using a three-grade system. Cancer 2005;103(2):402–8.

14. Kattan MW, Leung DH, Brennan MF. Postoperative nomogram for 12-year sarcoma-specific death. J Clin Oncol 2002;20:791–6.

15. Eilber F, Kattan MW. Sarcoma nomogram: validation and a model to evaluate impact of therapy. J Am Coll Surg 2007;205(4S):S90–5.

16. Noria S, Davis A, Kandel R, et al. Residual disease following unplanned excision of a soft-tissue sarcoma of an extremity. J Bone Joint Surg Am 1996;78(5):650–5.

17. Gutierrez JC, Perez EA, Moffat FL, et al. Should soft tissue sarcomas be treated at high-volume centers? An analysis of 4205 Patients. Ann Surg 2007;245(6):952–8.

18. Sarcoma Progress Review Group. A roadmap for sarcoma research. US Department of Health and Human Services; 2004. Available at: http://plan2005.cancer.gov/disease.html. Accessed June 2008.

19. Ilaslan H, Sundaram M. Advances in musculoskeletal tumor imaging. Orthop Clin North Am 2006;37(3):375–91.

20. Ioannidis JPA, Lau J. ^{18}F-FDG PET for the diagnosis and grading of soft-tissue sarcoma: a meta-analysis. J Nucl Med 2003;44:717–24.

21. Bredella MA, Caputo GR, Steinbach LS. Value of FDG positron emission tomography in conjunction with MR imaging for evaluating therapy response in patients with musculoskeletal sarcomas. Am J Roentgenol 2002;179:1145–50.

22. Mankin HJ, Lange TA, Spanier SS. The hazards of biopsy in patients with malignant primary bone and soft-tissue tumors. J Bone Joint Surg Am 1982;64:1121–7.

23. Mankin HJ, Mankin CJ, Simon M. The hazards of the biopsy, revisited. For the Members of the Musculoskeletal Tumor Society. J Bone Joint Surg Am 1996; 78(5):656–63.

24. Skrzynski MC, Biermann JS, Montag A, et al. Diagnostic accuracy and charge-savings of outpatient core needle biopsy compared with open biopsy of musculoskeletal tumors. J Bone Joint Surg Am 1996;78(5):644–9.

25. Altuntas A, Flavin J, Smith P. Accuracy of computed tomography core needle biopsy of musculoskeletal tumours. ANZ J Surg. 2005;75:187–91.

26. Soudack M, Nachtigal A, Vladovski E, et al. Sonographically guided percutaneous needle biopsy of soft tissue masses with histopathologic correlation. J Ultrasound Med 2006;25:1271–7.

27. Kenney R, Cheney R, Kraybill W. Core biopsy for diagnosis and tissue procurement. J Surg Oncol 2008;97(5):374–5.

28. Rosenberg SA, Tepper J, Glatstein E, et al. The treatment of soft tissue sarcoma of the extremities: prospective randomized evaluation of 1) limb-sparing surgery plus radiation therapy compared with amputation and 2) the role of adjuvant chemotherapy. Ann Surg 1982;196:305–15.

29. Pisters PW, Leung DH, Woodruff J, et al. Analysis of prognostic factors in 1,041 patients with localized soft tissue sarcomas of the extremities. J Clin Oncol 1996;14:1679–89.

30. McKay A, Motamedi M, Temple W, et al. Vascular reconstruction with the superficial femoral vein following major oncologic resection. J Surg Oncol 2007;96:151–9.

31. Schwarzbach MH, Hormann Y, Hinz U, et al. Results of limb-sparing surgery with vascular replacement for soft tissue sarcoma in the lower extremity. J Vasc Surg 2005;42(1):88–97.

32. Shafir M, Holland J, Cohen B, et al. Radical retroperitoneal tumor surgery with resection of the psoas major muscle. Cancer 1985;56(4):929–33.

33. Brooks A, Gold J, Graham D, et al. Resection of the sciatic, peroneal, or tibial nerves: assessment of functional status. Ann Surg Oncol 2002;9(1):41–7.

34. Stojadinovic A, Jaques D, Denis H, et al. Amputation for recurrent soft tissue sarcoma of the extremity: indications and outcome. Ann Surg Oncol 2001;8(6): 509–18.

35. Ghert M, Abudu A, Driver N, et al. The indications for and the prognostic significance of amputation as the primary surgical procedure for localized soft tissue sarcoma of the extremity. Ann Surg Oncol 2005;12(1):10–7.

36. Schlag P, Tunn P. Isolated limb perfusion in advanced soft tissue sarcomas. In: Schlag P, Tunn P, editors. Regional Cancer Therapy. Totowa: Humana Press Inc.; 2007. p. 407–17.

37. Thijssens KM, van Ginkel RJ, Pras E, et al. Isolated limb perfusion with tumor necrosis factor alpha and melphalan for locally advanced soft tissue sarcoma: the value of adjuvant radiotherapy. Ann Surg Oncol 2006;13(4):518–24.

38. Hoven-Gondrie M, Thijssens KM, Van den Dungen JJ, et al. Long-term locoregional vascular morbidity after isolated limb perfusion and external-beam radiotherapy in soft tissue sarcoma of the extremity. Ann Surg Oncol 2005;12(5): 406–11.

39. Fiore M, Casali P, Rosalba M, et al. Prognostic effect of re-excision in adult soft tissue sarcoma of the extremity. Ann Surg Oncol 2006;13(1):110–7.

40. Pisters PW, Pollock RE, Lewis VO, et al. Long-term results of prospective trial of surgery alone with selective use of radiation for patients with T1 extremity and trunk soft tissue sarcomas. Ann Surg 2007;246(4):675–81.

41. Tseng JF, Ballo MT, Langstein HN, et al. The effect of preoperative radiotherapy and reconstructive surgery on wound complications after resection of extremity soft-tissue sarcomas. Ann Surg Oncol 2006;13(9):1209–15.

42. O'Sullivan B, Davis A, Turcotte R, et al. Preoperative versus postoperative radiotherapy in soft-tissue sarcoma of the limbs: a randomised trial. Lancet 2002;359: 2235–41.

43. Pisters PW, Harrison LB, Woodruff JM, et al. A prospective randomized trial of adjuvant brachytherapy in the management of low-grade soft tissue sarcomas of the extremity and superficial trunk. J Clin Oncol 1994;12:1150–5.

44. Pisters PW, Harrison LB, Leung DH, et al. Long-term results of a prospective randomized trial of adjuvant brachytherapy in soft tissue sarcoma. J Clin Oncol 1996;14(3):859–68.

45. Sarcoma Meta-analysis Collaboration. Adjuvant chemotherapy for localised resectable soft-tissue sarcoma of adults: meta-analysis of individual data. Lancet 1997;350:1647–54.

46. Bramwell V. Adjuvant chemotherapy for adult soft tissue sarcoma: is there a standard of care? J Clin Oncol 2001;19(5):1235–7.

47. Spiro I, Gebhardt M, Jennings L, et al. Prognostic factors for local control of sarcomas of the soft tissues managed by radiation and surgery. Semin Oncol 1997; 24:540–6.

48. Kraybill W, Harris J, Spiro I, et al. Phase II study of neoadjuvant chemotherapy and radiation therapy in the management of high-risk, high-grade, soft tissue sarcomas of the extremities and body wall: Radiation Therapy Oncology Group Trial 9514. J Clin Oncol 2006;24(4):619–25.

49. Pawlik T, Pisters P, Mikula L, et al. Long-term results of two prospective trials of preoperative external beam radiotherapy for localized intermediate- or high-grade retroperitoneal soft tissue sarcoma. Ann Surg Oncol 2006;13(4):508–17.

50. Woodall CE, Scoggins CR. Retroperitoneal and visceral sarcomas: issues for the general surgeon. Am Surg 2007;73:631–5.

51. Demetri GD, Heslin MJ, Pfeifer JD, et al. Practice Guidelines in oncology: soft tissue sarcoma. Available at: www.NCCN.org. Accessed November 9, 2008.

52. Whooley BP, Mooney MM, Gibbs JF, et al. Effective follow-up strategies in soft tissue sarcoma. Semin Surg Oncol 1999;17(1):83–7.

53. Gadd MA, Casper ES, Woodruff JM, et al. Development and treatment of pulmonary metastases in adult patients with extremity soft tissue sarcoma. Ann Surg 1993;218(6):705–12.

54. Jablons D, Steinberg S, Roth J, et al. Metastectomy for soft tissue sarcoma. Further evidence for efficacy and prognostic indicators. J Thorac Cardiovasc Surg 1989;97(5):695–705.

55. van Geel AN, Pastorino U, Jauch KW, et al. Surgical treatment of lung metastases: the European Organization for Research and Treatment of cancer-soft tissue and Bone Sarcoma Group Study of 255 patients. Cancer 1996;77(4):675–82.

56. Billingsley K, Burt M, Jara E, et al. Pulmonary metastases from soft tissue sarcoma: analysis of patterns of disease and postmetastasis survival. Ann Surg 1999;229(5):602–10.

57. Weiser M, Downey R, Leung D, et al. Repeat resection of pulmonary metastases in patients with soft-tissue sarcoma. J Am Coll Surg 2000;191(2):184–90.

58. Bramwell V, Anderson D, Charette M, et al. Doxorubicin-based chemotherapy for the palliative treatment of adult patients with locally advanced or metastatic soft tissue sarcoma. Cochrane Database Syst Rev 2001;4:CD003293.

59. Maki R, Wathen J, Shreyaskumar R, et al. Randomized phase II study of gemcitabine and docetaxel compared with gemcitabine alone in patients with metastatic soft tissue sarcomas: results of sarcoma alliance for research through collaboration study 002. J Clin Oncol 2007;25(19):2755–63.

60. Borden E, Baker L, Bell R, et al. Soft tissue sarcomas of adults: state of the translational science. Clin Cancer Res 2003;9:1941–56.

61. Nielsen T, West R, Linn S, et al. Molecular characterisation of soft tissue tumours: a gene expression study. Lancet 2002;359:1301–7.

The Surgical and Systemic Management of Neuroendocrine Tumors of the Pancreas

Gerard J. Abood, MD, MS[a], Aileen Go, MD[c], Deepak Malhotra, MD[c], Margo Shoup, MD, FACS[b],*

KEYWORDS

- Neuroendocrine tumor • Surgical resection
- Metastatic neuroendocrine tumor • Surgical intervention

Neuroendocrine tumors of the pancreas are rare tumors that are considered to originate from the embryonic endodermal cells that later give rise to the islet cells of Langerhans. Previous classification of this distinct type of tumor was based on its ability to take up and decarboxylate aromatic amines or their precursors, giving rise to the term APUD (amine precursor uptake and decarboxylation) cells or apudomas.[1] Currently, these tumors are designated as neuroendocrine neoplasms of the pancreas. Although similar in many aspects, neuroendocrine tumors represent a distinct group from carcinoid tumors.

The overall incidence of neuroendocrine tumors is estimated to be 1 to 1.5 per 100,000 in the general population, resulting in approximately 2500 cases per year in the United States. They account for 1% to 2% of all pancreatic neoplasms.[2] The tumors have a peak incidence at age 30 to 60 with no gender preference.[3] Neuroendocrine tumors are characterized histologically by the presence of neurosecretory granules, which demonstrate positive staining for chromogranin, synaptophysin, or Gremilius stains and neuron-specific enolase.[4] Further staining for specific hormones may allow for further tumor characterization or may confirm clinical suspicion.

Neuroendocrine tumors are classified based on their clinical presentation as functioning and nonfunctioning tumors. Functional tumors are reported to have a prevalence of 10 per million population, with an incidence of clinical significance of 3.6 to

[a] Department of General Surgery, Loyola University Medical Center, 2160 South First Avenue, Maywood, IL 60153, USA
[b] Division of Surgical Oncology, Department of General Surgery, Loyola University Medical Center, 2160 South First Avenue, Maywood, IL 60153, USA
[c] Division of Hematology and Oncology, Loyola University Medical Center, Cardinal Bernardin Cancer Center, 2160 South First Avenue, Maywood, IL 60154, USA
* Corresponding author.
E-mail address: mshoup@lumc.edu (M. Shoup).

Surg Clin N Am 89 (2009) 249–266
doi:10.1016/j.suc.2008.10.001
0039-6109/08/$ – see front matter © 2009 Elsevier Inc. All rights reserved.

surgical.theclinics.com

4 per million population per year.[5] These tumors are described as functional by virtue of the tumor's ability to secrete one or more biologically active peptides that result in systemic clinical symptoms. Nonfunctional tumors, which account for 15% to 30% of all neuroendocrine tumors, are histologically similar to functional tumors but differ in that they are not associated with clinical endocrinopathy.[6] Most nonfunctional pancreatic neuroendocrine tumors are discovered incidentally during imaging studies for other reasons, typically during evaluations for nonspecific abdominal pain or during the course of a evaluation for biliary or bowel obstruction.[7]

Because of the nonspecific and intermittent nature of their symptoms, diagnosis of neuroendocrine tumors is often delayed for months to years, even in functional tumors.[8] As such, approximately 75% of patients with neuroendocrine tumors have metastatic disease at presentation, most commonly in the liver and, infrequently, in bone.[9] Although the clinical presentation of neuroendocrine tumors is similar to that of pancreatic adenocarcinoma, the associated prognosis is different. Whereas the 5-year survival rate of pancreatic adenocarcinoma is 5% to 10% after curative resection, long-term survival is not uncommon for patients with malignant neuroendocrine tumors, particularly nonfunctioning neuroendocrine tumors.[10–12] Although pathologic features of neuroendocrine tumors are suggestive of malignancy (**Box 1**),[3] their natural history has been shown to correlate with the clinical syndrome present rather than histochemical features.[13]

Preoperative imaging and localization are recommended for individuals with suspected neuroendocrine tumors of the pancreas. With the exception of insulinomas, CT of the abdomen and pelvis and MRI of the liver and pancreas are able to detect the primary tumor and metastatic disease of the liver and lymph nodes. Because pancreatic neuroendocrine tumors express a high density of somatostatin receptor subtypes capable of binding somatostatin analogs, indium-111 somatostatin receptor scintigraphy is currently the most sensitive test for localization of most neuroendocrine tumors.[14,15] The use of positron emission tomography scanning holds significant potential for improving visualization of neuroendocrine tumors. Recent reports using 5-hydroxtryptophan labeled with ^{11}C revealed that more than 95% of neuroendocrine tumors of the pancreas were identified and anatomically localized.[16–18]

The two principal surgical strategies for neuroendocrine tumor removal are enucleation and resection. Enucleation of tumors of the pancreas without reconstruction

---

Box 1
Pathologic features of neuroendocrine tumors suggestive of malignancy[3]

Tumor size

Invasion of nearby tissue of submucosa

Evidence of angioinvasion or perineural spaces

Structural atypia with prevalence of broad, solid areas

Cellular atypia with reduced nuclear cytoplasmic ratio

More than two mitoses per 10 high power fields

Presence of necrosis

Nuclear p53 accumulation

Increased Ki-67 positive nuclei counts

Cellular dedifferentiation (loss of chromogranin A)

should be undertaken only for tumors without evidence of malignancy, if the main pancreatic duct can be preserved, and if no major pancreatic paranchymal defect will result from the enucleation. The use and necessity of intraoperative ultrasound have been demonstrated and strongly advocated in further localization of pancreatic neuroendocrine tumors at the time of operation.[19] Small tumors generally lend themselves to enucleation, as do larger tumors growing on the border of the pancreas. Resections are performed for tumors in which these criteria are not met. Segmental resections, including pancreaticoduodenectomy, central segmental resection, and distal pancreatectomy, have been described. For pancreatic head masses not amenable to enucleation, pancreaticoduodenectomy remains the preferred procedure.[20] For tumors located in the body of the pancreas, central segmental resection, instead of distal pancreatectomy, has the advantage of preserving the distal pancreas while reducing the risk of postoperative diabetes and exocrine insufficiency.[21–23] Although the fistula rate with central pancreatectomy is slightly higher compared with distal pancreatectomy, most of these fistulas have been reported to be benign and rarely require surgical intervention.[24]

The increased use of CT imaging has resulted in the location of pancreatic tumors more frequently.[25] Many of these tumors are identified in the course of evaluation for nonspecific abdominal complaints—pain typically caused by mass effect that causes biliary or bowel obstruction. Although these tumors have histologic features similar to functional neuroendocrine tumors, their inability to induce clinical endocrinopathies is likely multifactorial. Several theories as to why these tumors behave differently are invalidated. Some potential theories include the tumor's inability to actually produce hormones, inability to produce sufficient quantities, or production of inactive forms of the hormone.[26] Because of the size and presence of metastatic disease at the time of presentation, more than 50% of all nonfunctioning neuroendocrine tumors are considered malignant.[27] Although these tumors are slow growing and biologically indolent, surgical resection remains the mainstay of treatment. Most of the nonfunctional tumors are located in the head of the pancreas, which necessitates pancreaticoduodenectomy. They have a significantly better prognosis than pancreatic adenocarcinomas and can be differentiated from adenocarcinoma by their positive immunohistochemical staining for chromogranin A. Although hepatic resection for metastatic neuroendocrine tumors has been demonstrated to improve survival, other modalities, including hepatic embolization, obviate the need for aggressive hepatic resection.[28,29]

Although a significant proportion of neuroendocrine tumors is not associated with hormone overproduction, as many as half of these tumors are associated with the secretion of one or more biologically active peptides. Five phenotypically distinct clinical syndromes may develop, the two most common of which are the insulinoma syndrome[30] and gastrinoma syndrome.[31] The remaining three distinct syndromes are the vasoactive intestinal peptide tumor (VIPoma) syndrome,[32] glucogonoma syndrome,[33] and somatostatinoma syndrome.[34]

INSULINOMA

Insulinomas are the most common functional islet cell tumor. They are more common in women (2:1) and usually occur in the fifth or sixth decade of life.[35] They generally occur at a younger age in the context of multiple neuroendocrine neoplasia type 1 (MEN-1), in which patients usually present in the third decade of life. Most commonly, patients present with fatigue, weakness, tremulousness, and hunger, with the symptoms worsening with fasting.[8] Approximately 80% to 90% of insulinomas are small (< 2 cm), solitary, benign tumors equally distributed among the head, body, and tail of the pancreas, with approximately 5% to 10% occurring as multiple islet cell tumors in the setting of MEN-1.[36,37] Most benign insulinomas are between 0.5 and 2 cm in diameter. Tumors appear reddish brown in color because of increased vascularity. The diagnosis of malignancy is made at the time of surgery by the identification of either lymph node of liver metastases or recurrence after resection.[38]

Because of their small size, preoperative localization of insulinomas tends to be difficult. Noninvasive imaging modalities, such as ultrasound CT and MRI, have demonstrated a low sensitivity for localization, ranging from 7% to 46%.[38] Unlike most other pancreatic neuroendocrine tumors that express a high density of somatostatin receptor subtypes capable of binding somatostatin analogs, insulinomas do not. As such, somatostatin receptor scintingraphy has no role in preoperative localization. Recent studies using endoscopic ultrasound reported sensitivities of 75% to 86% in identifying intrapancreatic neuroendocrine tumors, but it was less reliable in identifying extrapancreatic disease.[39,40] Because neuroendocrine tumors tend to be highly vascular, angiography has been used in localization efforts. In several small studies, sensitivity rates ranged from 66% to 100% for portal venous sampling for insulin and arterial stimulation using calcium gluconate for insulin release.[41,42]

Despite preoperative testing, 20% to 60% of insulinomas remain undetected at the time of surgery. Many authorities have argued that extensive preoperative imaging is unnecessary.[43–45] When the diagnosis of insulinoma is made, operative exploration by an experienced pancreatic surgeon remains the mainstay of treatment. Studies have demonstrated that the single best modality in localizing insulinomas during surgery is intraoperative ultrasound.[19,46] Surgical exploration with exposure and palpation of the pancreas combined with the use of intraoperative ultrasound is accepted as the most cost-effective approach for primary insulinomas, even when other preoperative studies produce negative results.[44]

Although medical therapy is the initial treatment of patients diagnosed with insulinomas, surgical resection is ultimately indicated to avoid the permanent neurologic deficits that may result from prolonged hypoglycemia. Presurgical therapy frequently involves instructing the patient to eat small frequent meals; medical therapy includes prescribing diazoxide and verapamil. Although medical therapy with diazoxide and verapamil is capable of transiently reducing insulin secretion, surgical resection is the only curative intervention for insulinomas.[43,47] Before proceeding to surgery, the presence of MEN-1 should be excluded by testing for other components, including primary hyperparathyroidism and pituitary tumors.[48] Preoperative optimization involves close glucose monitoring with dextrose infusions as necessary to maintain normglycemia. Dextrose infusions are often stopped before surgical manipulation to permit intraoperative glucose monitoring as a rough indication of biochemical cure.[26]

Access to the pancreas is most typically gained through the lesser sac by traversing the gastrocolic omentum. Wide kocherization of the duodenum combined with the separation of the transverse mesocolon from the inferior border of the pancreas allows for complete mobilization of the pancreas. After complete mobilization, the entire pancreas should be visually inspected and bimanually palpated to identify the presence of tumors. Insulinomas are typically small, solitary, encapsulated, reddish-brown tumors located throughout the pancreas. Intraoperative ultrasound is critical during surgery for insulinomas because it facilitates identification and removal of these tumors. Although most insulinomas are amenable to enucleation, segmental resections also may be surgical options. In patients with MEN-1, resection rather than enucleation is normally required; however, the goal of surgery still should be to remove only tumor while preserving as much normal pancreas as possible. When multiple tumors are identified throughout the pancreas, judicious resection should be used—total pancreatectomy is not indicated for insulinomas.

Surgery in patients with malignant insulinomas may be curative, but only if all tumor can be removed completely.[36,49] Debulking also may lessen the signs and symptoms of hypoglycemia, especially in patients who do not respond well to medical therapy. Surgical resection results in a biochemical cure in more than 95% of patients.[47,50,51] When feasible, concomitant hepatic resection with curative or palliative intent has been shown to be advantageous and may offer survival advantage.[52]

GASTRINOMA

Gastrinomas, which are the second most frequent common functional islet cell tumor, classically present with fulminant peptic ulcer disease, commonly referred to as Zollinger-Ellison (ZE) syndrome. ZE syndrome is caused by excessive and unregulated secretion of the hormone gastrin, which stimulates gastric acid secretion and leads to peptic ulcer disease.[53,54] The mean age at diagnosis is 50 years, with a slight male predominance, and a male to female ratio of 2:1. Gastrinomas occur in 0.1% of all patients with peptic ulcer disease and in 2% of patients with recurrent ulcer disease.[55,56]

Approximately two thirds of gastrinomas are sporadic, whereas the familial or inherited form occurs in approximately 20% of cases.[57] The familial form is associated with MEN-1 syndrome. In the context of MEN-1–associated tumors, most functional tumors are gastrinomas.[58] Although most gastrinomas tend to be slow growing, approximately 60% are malignant. Gastrinomas associated with MEN-1 tend to be multifocal, with 50% of patients presenting with lymph node, liver, or distant metastases at the time of diagnosis.[59] Despite the presence of metastases, most gastrinomas follow a protracted and indolent course, with 10-year survival rates approaching 90% to 100%.[60–62] Individuals with gastrinomas associated with MEN-1 syndrome had a better 20-year survival rate when compared with individuals with sporadic gastrinomas.[63]

Despite the recent development and improvement of antisecretory medicines, including proton-pump inhibitors, the role of surgery remains an important adjunct in affecting the natural history of gastrinomas.[64–67] The literature supports the notion that surgical resection of gastrinomas alters the natural history by decreasing the prevalence of hepatic metastases and decreasing the requirement for medical therapy. As such, surgery should be offered to all patients with sporadic gastrinomas. ZE syndrome can be accurately diagnosed in all patients by measuring an elevated fasting serum level of gastrin and an elevated basal acid output. Patients should be off all antisecretory medications for 3 to 7 days to reduce the false-positive association. One hundred percent of patients with ZE syndrome have a fasting serum gastrin level of more than 100 pg/mL.[59] If the diagnosis remains uncertain, the results of the secretin stimulation test allow further validation, particularly in individuals who have undergone previous operations to reduce acid output. An increase of 200 pg/mL in the serum gastrin level after secretin administration is consistent with the diagnosis of ZE syndrome.

The accuracy of CT scanning depends on the size of the gasrinoma.[68] Tumors smaller than 1 cm are rarely visualized. Somatostatin receptor scintigraphy is considered the imaging test of choice for localizing primary and metastatic gastrinomas. A reported 90% of tumors can be imaged, with a specificity of nearly 100%.[69,70] As in the case of insulinomas, intraoperative ultrasound has proven use and should be the standard of therapy in localization and resection of gastrinomas.

The goals of surgery are twofold: resection of primary tumor for potential cure and prevention of malignant progression. The malignant potential of the tumor is the main determinant of long-term survival. After attempts at preoperative localization, attention can be focused primarily in the "gastrinoma triangle," which is defined as a line joining the confluence of the cystic and common bile ducts superiorly, the junction of the second and third portion of the duodenum inferiorly, and the junction of the neck and body of the pancreas medially, where 80% of gastrinomas are typically located. As in the case of insulinomas, the entire pancreas should be mobilized to allow for bimanual palpation and intraoperative ultrasound. Small, well-encapsulated tumors in the pancreas can be removed by enucleation or segmental resection. Large, unencapsulated lesions located deep within the parenchyma may require segmental resection, including Whipple or distal pancreatectomy.[26]

During surgery for gastrinoma, it is important to remember that these tumors can occur in extrapancreatic locations, particularly the duodenum. Regardless of the results of intraoperative ultrasound, a duodenotomy is indicated in all cases of gastrinoma. This procedure allows for visualization and more careful palpation of the duodenum, including the medial wall.[19] During surgery, a tumor is found in approximately 95% of patients who present with sporadic gastrinomas. In 5% to 8% of cases, the surgeon is unable to localize the gastrinoma.[61] In that situation, a highly selective vagotomy can be performed to decrease the postoperative requirement of antisecretory medications. Surgery remains the major effective treatment for metastatic gastrinoma. Distant metastatic disease becomes the most important determinant of mortality, with a 5-year survival rate of approximately 40%.[59] Aggressive surgery in appropriate patients with hepatic metastases demonstrates a survival advantage. Even if complete resection is not possible, selected patients may benefit from debulking.[71,72]

In patients with MEN-1, hyperparathyroidism is the most common abnormality. When patients with MEN-1 have pancreatic islet tumors, gastrinomas are the most common pancreatic tumor. In the case of MEN-1 with primary hyperparathyroidism and ZE syndrome, studies have shown that successful neck exploration for resection of parathyroid hyperplasia can reduce the end-organ effects of hypergastrinemia.[59] In patients with MEN-1 who have hyperparathyroidism in conjunction with ZE syndrome, neck exploration and subtotal parathyroidectomy should be performed before attempting gastrinoma resection.[48] Patients with MEN-1 typically have multiple pancreatic or duodenal neoplasms, many of which are not predictably functional.[62,73] As such, the identification of all functional tumors is imprecise, which results in a lower cure rate.

VASOACTIVE INTESTINAL PEPTIDE TUMOR

The VIPoma was first described by Verner and Morrison in 1958.[32] The mean age at diagnosis is 50 years, and there is a slight female preponderance.[74] Its typical presentation includes significant watery diarrhea, hypokalemia, and acholorhydria, which earns it the moniker WHDA syndrome. VIPomas typically induce a severe secretory diarrhea that is persistent despite abstaining from oral intake. This state ultimately leads to hypokalemia, hypochlorhydria, hypovolemia, and dehydration, with an average of 5 to 10 L of stool output per day. The diagnosis of VIPoma is made when fasting plasma levels of VIP are more than 500 pg/mL in the presence of secretory diarrhea. Approximately 85% to 90% of VIPomas arise within the pancreas, but extrapancreatic duodenal VIPomas have been described.[75] VIPomas are usually solitary tumors located in the tail of the pancreas and have an average reported size of more than 3 cm. Given the size of most VIPomas at time of presentation, preoperative localization is usually possible with CT scan, with more than 50% of reported cases having associated metastasis.[76]

Because of significant diarrhea, preoperative preparation requires aggressive correction of the resulting fluid and electrolyte abnormalities. Octreotide dramatically reduces serum VIP levels and secretory diarrhea in more than 80% of patients and greatly simplifies fluid and electrolyte resuscitation before surgery.[77–79] Bimanual palpation of the pancreas and intraoperative ultrasound are able to reliably locate most VIPomas. Most tumors are located in the tail of the pancreas, making distal pancreatectomy the more common procedure. If no tumor is found, however, examination of the retroperitoneum, including the autonomic chain and within the adrenals, is warranted.[26] Extensive and radical resection is seldom necessary because of the response of VIPomas to octreotide administration.

GLUCAGONOMA

Glucagonomas are rare tumors with a reported incidence of 0.2 cases per million per year. These tumors, which usually present during the fifth or sixth decade of life, secrete excessive amounts of glucagon, resulting in the "4-D syndrome" of glucagonomas: diabetes mellitus type 2, deep venous thrombosis, depression, and dermatitis.[80] The characteristic pruritic red rash, called necrolytic migratory erythema, can be caused by amino acid deficiency, zinc deficiency, or excess glucagons and typically involves the pretibial, perioral, and intertriginous areas. Other symptoms include weight loss, anemia, painful glossitis, and pulmonary emboli.[33]

The biochemical diagnosis of glucagonoma is made by measuring elevated plasma levels of glucagons (> 500 pg/mL) and decreased levels of amino acids. Because of tumor-induced cachexia, most patients require total parenteral nutrition. Although skin biopsies may confirm necrolytic migratory erythema, the diagnosis of necrolytic migratory erythema is suggestive but not diagnostic of glucagonoma.[81] The long-term management of patients with metastatic glucagonoma has included octreotide, which has been demonstrated to reduce circulating plasma levels of glucagons and improve the rash and malnutrition.[82]

Because diagnosis is often delayed, patients tend to present with large tumors (> 5 cm) that are easily localized with conventional imaging. Somatostatin receptor scintigraphy has been demonstrated to be useful in localization and long-term follow-up.[83,84] Unlike gastrinomas, glucagonomas are almost exclusively located in the pancreas, with the tail of the pancreas being the most common location. Distal pancreatectomy with resection of lymph nodes and liver metastases is typically the operative approach. Although surgery offers the only likelihood for cure, most tumors tend to be large (> 5–10 cm) and either locally advanced or metastatic and unresectable. Complete resection of primary tumor and metastatic disease is possible in only 30% of cases.[85]

SOMATOSTATINOMA

Somatostatinomas are rare neuroendocrine tumors that arise primarily in the pancreas and duodenum. The mean age at presentation is 51 to 53 years.[86] Although exceedingly rare, the somatostatinoma syndrome, which includes steatorrhea, cholelithiasis, diabetes mellitus type 2, and hypochloridria, is most commonly associated with pancreatic somatostatinomas. Duodenal somatostatinomas are typically associated with von Recklinghausen syndrome and the presence of psammoma bodies. Most somatostatinomas are malignant at the time of presentation; at the time of surgical exploration, more than 75% of patients have evidence of metastases, particularly in patients with tumors sizes larger than 2 cm.[87,88] Most somatostatinomas are located in the head of the pancreas. Surgical resection requires pancreaticoduodenectomy. In patients without metastatic disease, mean 5-year survival rate is 100%. Despite the high prevalence of metastatic disease, mean 5-year survival rate of patients with metastatic disease approaches 60%.[89]

METASTATIC NEUROENDOCRINE TUMORS OF THE LIVER

Unlike hepatic metastases from other primary malignancies, neuroendocrine hepatic malignancies can progress unsuspectingly until symptoms associated with pain, mass effect, or hormone overproduction occurs. Generally speaking, no prophylactic intervention, particularly chemotherapy, has been shown to improve survival after initial resection before the occurrence of hepatic metastases. In the presence of hepatic metastases, however, several treatment options have developed over time. Because of the indolent nature of the neuroendocrine tumors, asymptomatic patients can undergo serial observation with CT scans. In individuals with functional neuroendocrine tumors, hormone-related symptoms can be managed medically; however, in patients with hormonally active tumors, rapidly progressing tumors, uncontrolled pain, and mass effect, intervention is required.

When feasible, surgical resection in select patients remains the treatment option of choice for curative and palliative intent. Although hepatic resection for cure is possible in less than 10% of affected patients, it should be noted that cure is rarely—if ever—possible because most patients experience recurrence within the first 2 years after resection.[90,91] Curative surgery should be considered for patients with unilobar metastases that occupy less than 75% of the liver parenchyma; palliative resection for pain or uncontrolled hormonal symptoms can be performed if more than 90% of the tumor can be excised safely.[9,92] The literature supports the notion that patients in whom more than 75% of the liver is involved with tumor have a poor prognosis, and surgery should be avoided.[9] In the absence of curative intent, alternate therapies should be considered.

Recent reports demonstrated the use of hepatic artery embolization for metastatic disease. Selective hepatic artery embolization is based on the fact that the blood supply to the hypervascular tumors is preferentially derived from the hepatic artery, whereas normal hepatic tissue is preferentially supplied by the portal venous system. Embolization, which can be performed with gelatin foam, starch powder, or cytotoxic drugs, produces a biochemical response with or without regression of metastases.[93,94] Complications associated with embolization include pain, fever, infection, and bleeding. Recent reports suggested that hepatic artery embolization results in clinical and radiographic responses in patients with unresectable liver metastases with low associated morbidity.[95]

Other promising modalities for the management of hepatic metastatic neuroendocrine tumors include radiofrequency ablation. Recent reports of radiofrequency ablation demonstrated improved symptomatic control.[96–98] Ablation allows for treatment of smaller metastases that are deep in the liver parenchyma without the need for resection. Ablation also can be used as an adjunct to surgery, particularly in individuals with previous liver resection. More recently, institutional experience with yttrium-90 microspheres has been reported in the literature. The yttrium-90 microsphere approach is a form of targeted radiation treatment for unresectable hepatic neoplasms using selective angiography of the hepatic artery to offer a theoretic more potent dose of radiation.[99–101] Early reports suggested its potential benefit as a safe and effective palliative treatment for patients with progressive hepatic metastatic disease.

SYSTEMIC THERAPY FOR GASTROENTEROPANCREATIC NEUROENDOCRINE TUMORS

Gastroenteropancreatic neuroendocrine tumors are rare malignancies that present as a treatment challenge. They are frequently clinically silent and are diagnosed at a late stage, with symptoms related to bulky disease. Approximately 50% of pancreatic neuroendocrine tumors express at least one active hormone, including insulin, gastrin, glucagon, and VIP. Hormonal secretion can cause distinct clinical syndromes, including carcinoid syndrome. The cornerstone of therapeutic management is surgery; however, because of advanced disease, many patients are not candidates for aggressive surgical therapy. Tumor growth control and symptom management are achieved through medical approaches that include use of somatostatin analogs, chemotherapy, interferon and, more recently, targeted therapy. Most of the studies that have been published are noncomparative, mainly phase II studies, which leads to difficulty in interpreting the results.[102,103]

SOMATOSTATIN ANALOGS AND IMMUNOTHERAPY

The mainstays of treatment for functional metastatic gastroenteropancreatic neuroendocrine tumors require the control of excessive hormone activity using secretory inhibitors such as somatostatin analogs and interferon alfa. The most effective formulations of somatostatin analogs include octreotide (50 μg, 100 μg, 500 μg) or lantreotide autogel (60 mg, 90 mg, or 120 mg). The initial dosage of subcutaneous octreotide is usually 50 μg administered twice or three times daily. Upward titration is frequently required. After 2 weeks, responders may be transitioned to octreotide LAR (10 mg, 20 mg, or 30 mg) given intramuscularly at 4-week intervals. Patients should continue to receive daily octreotide injections subcutaneously for at least 2 to 3 weeks after the initial injection of octreotide LAR because of its need to reach therapeutic levels. These drugs are well tolerated and safe, with mild adverse effects, especially after sustained use. Infrequent side effects include diarrhea, abdominal pain, steatorrhea, and cholelithiasis. Treatment discontinuation related to these side effects is rare.[102–104]

Given the observed antiproliferative effects of somatostatin analogs and interferon alfa, several retrospective studies have suggested that the combination of the two may enhance such effects. A prospective, randomized, multicenter study was conducted in therapy-naïve patients with metastatic gastroenteropancreatic neuroendocrine tumors to investigate antiproliferative and symptom-controlling effects of the somatostatin analogs and interferon alfa in single agents and in combination. Eighty therapy-naïve patients with histologically verified neuroendocrine tumors were randomly treated with lantreotide, 1 mg three times a day, or interferon alfa, 5×10^6 U three times a week, or both. Within 12 months of therapy, tumor progression was observed in 14 of 25 patients (lantreotide), 15 of 27 patients (interferon alfa), and 14 of 28 patients (lantretode plus interferon alfa). There was no significant difference in the rates of partial remission, stable disease, or tumor progression among treatment groups. A symptomatic and biochemical response was studied in 29 patients who had functional neuroendocrine tumors. The frequency of tumor-related symptoms decreased under therapy in each of therapeutic group. Although a reduction of symptoms was observed in all therapeutic arms, a statistically significant reduction was noted only in the observation arm. Treatment with lantreotide was generally well tolerated, and only a few minor side effects were observed. Interferon alfa–related side effects were more common. Side effects that led to interruption of therapy were more frequent in the combination group.[104]

CYTOTOXIC CHEMOTHERAPY

Optimal treatments for metastatic carcinoid and gastroenteropancreatic neuroendocrine tumors remain undefined, and the role of chemotherapy for symptomatic patients with progressive disease is uncertain. Systemic chemotherapy using single agents has been evaluated in metastatic carcinoid, with variable rates of tumor response. Single agents used include streptozocin (STZ), fluorouracil (FU), doxorubicin (DOX), and chlorozotocin and dacarbazine (DTIC), but they usually produce low response rates. Earlier studies tried to use a combination of STZ and FU compared with STZ and cyclophosphamide. The response rates were 33% in the STZ/FU arm compared with 26% in the STZ/cyclophosphamide arm with no difference in survival. A more recent Eastern Cooperative Oncology Group study (ECOG 1281) compared FU/STZ to FU/DOX in the treatment of selected patients with metastatic carcinoid. Two hundred forty-nine patients were randomized to either FU/DOX or FU/STZ. There were no differences between the two groups in terms of response rates (15.9% versus 16%) and progression-free survival (4.5 versus 5.3 months). There was a significant advantage in terms of median survival; patients in the FU/STZ arm had a median survival of 24.3 months, whereas patients in the FU/DOX arm had median survival of 15.7 months ($P = .0267$). In this trial, however, 34.8% of the patients developed significant renal toxicity. This and other toxicities, combined with the modest efficacy, precluded the common use of STZ-based chemotherapy as first line in this disease.[105,106]

Several studies seem to indicate a more robust response to chemotherapy in pancreatic neuroendocrine tumors. One hundred five patients with advanced islet cell carcinoma were randomly assigned to receive treatments with STZ/FU, STZ/DOX, or chlorozotocin. STX/DOX was found to be superior to STZ/FU in terms of rate of tumor regression (69% versus 45%), time to progression (20 versus 6.9 mo), and survival (2.2 versus 1.4 years). A retrospective analysis of 84 patients with metastatic pancreatic neuroendocrine tumors who received a three-drug regimen of STZ, FU, and DOX showed an overall response rate of 39% and a median survival duration of 37 months. While this combination demonstrated clinical response, the results were less dramatic than previous combination studies.[107,108]

DTIC is an alternative to STZ-based therapy in gastroenteropancreatic neuroendocrine tumors. An ECOG (E6282) phase II study of DTIC in patients with pancreatic neuroendocrine tumors who had no prior chemotherapy showed an overall response rate of 33% in 42 patients who had measurable disease, with a median overall survival of 19.3 months. In the earlier ECOG 1281 study, after receiving STZ-based therapy, patients were allowed to cross over to single-agent DTIC treatment after disease. The response rate of DTIC was 8.2%, with a median survival of 11.9 months.[105,109,110] Temozolamide is another cytotoxic alkylating agent that was developed as an oral alternative to DTIC. In a phase II study, 29 patients with pancreatic neuroendocrine tumors, pheochromocytomas, and carcinoid tumors were treated with a combination of temozolomide, 150 mg/m^2, for 7 days every other week and thalidomide, 50 to 400 mg, daily. The objective biochemical response rate was 40% and the radiologic response rate was 25%. The median duration of response was 13.5 months, with a 1-year survival rate of 79% and a 2-year survival rate of 61%. Grades 3 to 4 toxicity included lymphopenia in 69% of the patients; 10% of the patients developed opportunistic infections.[111] It is recommended that patients receive prophylaxis with trimethoprim-sulfamethoxazole while on therapy.

NEW DRUGS AND TARGETED THERAPY

Advanced neuroendocrine tumors lack an accepted standard treatment. Recent studies in neuroendocrine tumors showed potential molecular targets, including epidermal growth factor receptor, vascular endothelial growth factor and its receptor, or insulin-like growth factor receptor, phosphoinositide-3-kinase, RAC-alpha serine/threonine-protein kinase, and mammalian target of rapamycin. Early clinical trials are assessing new drugs that target some of these molecules.[102,112]

Neuroendocrine tumors are highly vascular, which led to the initial interest in angiogenesis inhibition as a treatment modality in this disease. The overexpression of vascular endothelial growth factor, together with vascular epidermal growth factor receptor subtypes, has been observed in carcinoid and pancreatic endocrine tumors, which suggests that autocrine activation of the vascular endothelial growth factor pathway may promote tumor growth. The vascular endothelial growth factor monoclonal antibody bevacizumab (Avastin, Roche, Basilea, Switzerland) has been reported in neuroendocrine tumors. A small phase II trial with 44 patients who had advanced carcinoid tumors and were taking stable doses of octreotide were randomized to either bevacizumab, 15 mg/kg, every 3 weeks or weekly pegylated interferon alfa-2b. Bevacizumab was found to be superior to pegylated interferon alfa-2b in terms of progression-free survival after 18 weeks of monotherapy. The progression-free survival rates after 18 weeks of monotherapy were 95% in bevacizumab versus 67% in the pegylated interferon alfa-2b arm. A phase III trial by SWOG (S0158) is currently ongoing in which patients with advanced poor prognosis carcinoid tumor under stable doses of depot octreotide will be randomized to receive either subcutaneous interferon or bevacizumab. The treatment is generally well tolerated, although there is an increased risk of hypertension and thromboembolic arterial and bleeding events.[113]

Sunitinib maleate (SU-11248, Sutent; Pfizer, New York, NY) is a selective inhibitor of tyrosine kinases, such as vascular epidermal growth factor receptor-1 to -3, platelet derived growth factor receptor (PDGFR), FMS-like tyrosine kinase 3 (FLT), c-Kit, and RET. Antitumor activity is caused by the inhibition of angiogenesis and its antiproliferative effects.[113] A large phase II multicenter study was conducted to assess the safety and efficacy of sunitinib in patients with advanced neuroendocrine tumors. Repeated 6-week treatment cycles of sunitinib were administered at an oral dose of 50 mg once daily for 4 weeks, followed by 2 weeks off the medication. One hundred seven patients (carcinoid tumors, $n = 41$; pancreatic neuroendocrine tumors, $n = 66$) received sunitinib in this study. The overall objective response rate in patients with pancreatic neuroendocrine tumors was 16.7%, and 68% had stable disease. Among patients with carcinoid tumor, objective response rate was 2.4%, and 83% had stable disease. Median time to tumor progression was 7.7 months in patients with pancreatic neuroendocrine tumor and 10.2 months in patients with carcinoid tumor. The one-year survival rate was 81.1% in patients with pancreatic neuroendocrine tumor and 83.4% in patients with carcinoid tumor.[114]

Sorafenib (BAY 43-9006, Nexavar; Bayer Pharmaceuticals Corporation, West Haven, Connecticut) is an oral multitargeted agent with potent activities against Raf-Kinase and vascular epidermal growth factor receptor-2 that also results in growth inhibition of the tumor via inhibition of angiogenesis and interference with cellular proliferation.[12] A multicenter phase II study led by the Mayo Clinic is evaluating the efficacy of sorafenib in metastatic neuroendocrine tumors. Preliminary results were presented at a meeting for the American Society of Clinical Oncologists 2007. Sorafenib, 400 mg orally, twice a day had a modest activity in metastatic neuroendocrine tumors—10% partial response in carcinoid and pancreatic neuroendocrine tumors. For patients who could be evaluated, the 6-month progression-free survival rate was 40% (8/20) in patients with carcinoid tumors and 60.8% (14/23) in patients with pancreatic neuroendocrine tumors.[115]

The mammalian target of rapamycin is a serine threonine kinase that participates in the regulation of apoptosis, proliferation, and cell growth through modulation of cell cycle progression. Sirolimus (rapamycin) and its derivatives are immunosuppressive macrolides that block mammalian target of rapamycin and yield antiproliferative activity in various malignancies. Two rapamycin derivatives have been evaluated in neuroendocrine tumors: temsirolimus and everolimus.[113] Temsirolimus (CCI-779; Wyeth, Philadelphia, Pennsylvania) is a mammalian target of rapamycin inhibitor that downregulates cascades activated by the loss of the tumor suppressor PTEN. Thirty-seven patients with advanced, progressed neuroendocrine tumors were treated with weekly doses of temsirolimus, 25 mg, intravenously. The results from this multicenter study, led by the Princess Margaret Consortium II in Canada, showed that among the 15 patients who were evaluable for response thus far, 10 achieved prolonged stable disease (range: 3–11 cycles), including 1 patient with a 24% tumor shrinkage by response evaluation criteria in solid tumors (RECIST) criteria after 4 cycles and 2 patients who experienced significant clinical benefit and are on cycles 9 and 11.[116] Everolimus (RAD001; Novartis) at 5 mg orally was combined with depot octreotide in a phase II study that examined effective systemic therapies for low-grade neuroendocrine tumors. By RECIST criteria, 17% patients had partial response, 75% had stable disease, and 8% had progressive disease. The progression-free survival rate at 24 weeks was 86%, and the median duration of progression-free survival was 59 weeks. The median progression-free survival duration for patients with progressive disease at enrollment was 38 weeks. The treatment was well tolerated.[117]

On the basis of these encouraging results, the RADIANT (RAD001 in advanced neuroendocrine tumors trials) trials are under development. RADIANT-1, which is closed to accrual, is an open-label, single-arm, phase II study of evrolimus in patients with advanced pancreatic neuroendocrine tumors who failed previous cytotoxic chemotherapy. Two phase III placebo-controlled randomized trials in patients receiving depot octreotide are currently open for accrual: RADIANT-2 in patients with advanced carcinoid tumors and RADIANT-3 in patients with advanced pancreatic islet cell tumors.

The emerging knowledge of the molecular biology of neuroendocrine tumors has facilitated the development of new targeted therapies. Several early phase II data involving antiangiogenic agents and mammalian target of rapamycin inhibitors seem promising, yet caution must be applied when interpreting disease stabilization because many of these trials did not require patients to have progressive disease or provide a precise extent of disease progression as an inclusion criteria. More studies to confirm safety, efficacy, and tolerability of said drugs are needed. The combination of classical cytotoxic chemotherapy with some of the novel agents is also warranted.[113]

SUMMARY

Neuroendocrine tumors of the pancreas comprise a class of rare tumors that can be associated with symptoms of hormone overproduction. While complete surgical resection offers the only hope for cure, understanding the basic biology of the tumors has advanced the medical management in metastatic disease. Surgical resection of hepatic metastases offers survival advantage and should be performed when feasible. Currently, hepatic artery embolization is the preferred mode of palliation for pain and hormonal symptoms. Further experience with ablation therapies, including cryoablation, radiofrequency ablation and yttrium-90 microspheres, will be necessary to demonstrate both safety and efficacy.

REFERENCES

1. Kloppel G, Heitz PU. Classification of normal and neoplastic neuroendocrine cells. Ann N Y Acad Sci 1994;733:19–23.

2. Delcore R, Friesen SR. Gastrointestinal neuroendocrine tumors. J Am Coll Surg 1994;178(2):187–211.
3. Rindi G, Capella C, Solcia E. Introduction to a revised clinicopathological classification of neuroendocrine tumors of the gastroenteropancreatic tract. Q J Nucl Med 2000;44(1):13–21.
4. Nash SV, Said JW. Gastroenteropancreatic neuroendocrine tumors: a histochemical and immunohistochemical study of epithelial (keratin proteins, carcinoembryonic antigen) and neuroendocrine (neuron-specific enolase, bombesin and chromogranin) markers in foregut, midgut, and hindgut tumors. Am J Clin Pathol 1986;86(4):415–22.
5. Metz DC, Jensen RT. Gastrointestinal neuroendocrine tumors: pancreatic endocrine tumors. Gastroenterology 2008;135:1469–92.
6. Cheslyn-Curtis S, Sitaram V, Williamson RC. Management of non-functioning neuroendocrine tumours of the pancreas. Br J Surg 1993;80(5):625–7.
7. Oberg K, Eriksson B. Endocrine tumours of the pancreas. Best Pract Res Clin Gastroenterol 2005;19(5):753–81.
8. Grama D, Eriksson B, Martensson H, et al. Clinical characteristics, treatment and survival in patients with pancreatic tumors causing hormonal syndromes. World J Surg 1992;16(4):632–9.
9. Chamberlain RS, Canes D, Brown KT, et al. Hepatic neuroendocrine metastases: does intervention alter outcomes? J Am Coll Surg 2000;190(4):432–45.
10. Eriguchi N, Aoyagi S, Imayama H, et al. Endocrine tumor of the pancreas: an evaluation of eighteen patients who underwent resection followed by long-term survival. Kurume Med J 1999;46(2):105–10.
11. Madura JA, Cummings OW, Wiebke EA, et al. Nonfunctioning islet cell tumors of the pancreas: a difficult diagnosis but one worth the effort. Am Surg 1997;63(7): 573–7 [discussion: 577–8].
12. Tsiotos GG, Farnell MB, Sarr MG. Are the results of pancreatectomy for pancreatic cancer improving? World J Surg 1999;23(9):913–9.
13. Wick MR, Graeme-Cook FM. Pancreatic neuroendocrine neoplasms: a current summary of diagnostic, prognostic, and differential diagnostic information. Am J Clin Pathol 2001;115(Suppl):S28–45.
14. Rappeport ED, Hansen CP, Kjaer A, et al. Multidetector computed tomography and neuroendocrine pancreaticoduodenal tumors. Acta Radiol 2006;47(3): 248–56.
15. Virgolini I, Traub-Weidinger T, Decristoforo C. Nuclear medicine in the detection and management of pancreatic islet-cell tumours. Best Pract Res Clin Endocrinol Metab 2005;19(2):213–27.
16. Eriksson B, Orlefors H, Oberg K, et al. Developments in PET for the detection of endocrine tumours. Best Pract Res Clin Endocrinol Metab 2005;19(2):311–24.
17. Orlefors H, Sundin A, Garske U, et al. Whole-body (11)C-5-hydroxytryptophan positron emission tomography as a universal imaging technique for neuroendocrine tumors: comparison with somatostatin receptor scintigraphy and computed tomography. J Clin Endocrinol Metab 2005;90(6):3392–400.
18. Sundin A, Eriksson B, Bergstrom M, et al. PET in the diagnosis of neuroendocrine tumors. Ann N Y Acad Sci 2004;1014:246–57.
19. Norton JA. Intra-operative procedures to localize endocrine tumours of the pancreas and duodenum. Ital J Gastroenterol Hepatol 1999;31(Suppl 2):S195–7.
20. Solorzano CC, Lee JE, Pisters PW, et al. Nonfunctioning islet cell carcinoma of the pancreas: survival results in a contemporary series of 163 patients. Surgery 2001;130(6):1078–85.

21. Christein JD, Kim AW, Golshan MA, et al. Central pancreatectomy for the resection of benign or low malignant potential neoplasms. World J Surg 2003;27(5): 595–8.

22. Iacono C, Bortolasi L, Serio G. Indications and technique of central pancreatectomy: early and late results. Langenbecks Arch Surg 2005;390(3):266–71.

23. Yamaguchi K, Yokohata K, Ohkido M, et al. Which is less invasive, distal pancreatectomy or segmental resection? Int Surg 2000;85(4):297–302.

24. Balzano G, Zerbi A, Veronesi P, et al. Surgical treatment of benign and borderline neoplasms of the pancreatic body. Dig Surg 2003;20(6):506–10.

25. O'Grady HL, Conlon KC. Pancreatic neuroendocrine tumours. Eur J Surg Oncol 2008;34(3):324–32.

26. Azimuddin K, Chamberlain RS. The surgical management of pancreatic neuroendocrine tumors. Surg Clin North Am 2001;81(3):511–25.

27. Eckhauser FE, Cheung PS, Vinik AI, et al. Nonfunctioning malignant neuroendocrine tumors of the pancreas. Surgery 1986;100(6):978–88.

28. Gupta S, Johnson MM, Murthy R, et al. Hepatic arterial embolization and chemoembolization for the treatment of patients with metastatic neuroendocrine tumors: variables affecting response rates and survival. Cancer 2005;104(8): 1590–602.

29. Madoff DC, Gupta S, Ahrar K, et al. Update on the management of neuroendocrine hepatic metastases. J Vasc Interv Radiol 2006;17(8):1235–49 [quiz 1250].

30. Burgos L, Burgos ME [Pancreatic neuroendocrine tumors]. Rev Med Chil 2004; 132(5):627–34 [Spanish].

31. Tamburrano G, Paoloni A, Pietrobono D, et al. Pancreatic endocrine tumours. Ital J Gastroenterol Hepatol 1999;31(Suppl 2):S104–7.

32. Verner JV, Morrison AB. Islet cell tumor and a syndrome of refractory watery diarrhea and hypokalemia. Am J Med 1958;25(3):374–80.

33. Stacpoole PW. The glucagonoma syndrome: clinical features, diagnosis, and treatment. Endocr Rev 1981;2(3):347–61.

34. Ganda OP, Weir GC, Soeldner JS, et al. "Somatostatinoma:" a somatostatin-containing tumor of the endocrine pancreas. N Engl J Med 1977;296(17): 963–7.

35. Perry RR, Vinik AI. Endocrine tumors of the gastrointestinal tract. Annu Rev Med 1996;47:57–68.

36. Park BJ, Alexander HR, Libutti SK, et al. Operative management of islet-cell tumors arising in the head of the pancreas. Surgery 1998;124(6):1056–61 [discussion: 1061–2].

37. Sheppard BC, Norton JA, Doppman JL, et al. Management of islet cell tumors in patients with multiple endocrine neoplasia: a prospective study. Surgery 1989; 106(6):1108–17 [discussion: 1117–8].

38. Machado MC, da Cunha JE, Jukemura J, et al. Insulinoma: diagnostic strategies and surgical treatment. A 22-year experience. Hepatogastroenterology 2001; 48(39):854–8.

39. Ardengh JC, Rosenbaum P, Ganc AJ, et al. Role of EUS in the preoperative localization of insulinomas compared with spiral CT. Gastrointest Endosc 2000; 51(5):552–5.

40. Ardengh JC, Valiati LH, Geocze S [Identification of insulinomas by endoscopic ultrasonography]. Rev Assoc Med Bras 2004;50(2):167–71 [Portuguese].

41. Aoki T, Sakon M, Ohzato H, et al. Evaluation of preoperative and intraoperative arterial stimulation and venous sampling for diagnosis and surgical resection of insulinoma. Surgery 1999;126(5):968–73.

42. Doppman JL, Chang R, Fraker DL, et al. Localization of insulinomas to regions of the pancreas by intra-arterial stimulation with calcium. Ann Intern Med 1995; 123(4):269–73.
43. Boukhman MP, Karam JH, Shaver J, et al. Insulinoma: experience from 1950 to 1995. West J Med 1998;169(2):98–104.
44. Hashimoto LA, Walsh RM. Preoperative localization of insulinomas is not necessary. J Am Coll Surg 1999;189(4):368–73.
45. Lo CY, Lam KY, Kung AW, et al. Pancreatic insulinomas: a 15-year experience. Arch Surg 1997;132(8):926–30.
46. Hiramoto JS, Feldstein VA, LaBerge JM, et al. Intraoperative ultrasound and preoperative localization detects all occult insulinomas. Arch Surg 2001;136(9): 1020–5 [discussion: 1025–6].
47. Doherty GM, Doppman JL, Shawker TH, et al. Results of a prospective strategy to diagnose, localize, and resect insulinomas. Surgery 1991;110(6):989–96 [discussion: 996–7].
48. Norton JA, Cornelius MJ, Doppman JL, et al. Effect of parathyroidectomy in patients with hyperparathyroidism, Zollinger-Ellison syndrome, and multiple endocrine neoplasia type I: a prospective study. Surgery 1987;102(6):958–66.
49. Fraker DL, Norton JA. The role of surgery in the management of islet cell tumors. Gastroenterol Clin North Am 1989;18(4):805–30.
50. D'Herbomez M, Pattou F, Nocaudie M, et al [Usefulness and limits of intraoperative hormone measurements in surgery of endocrine duodeno-pancreatic tumors: experience of 72 cases]. Ann Biol Clin (Paris) 1999;57(2):185–90 [French].
51. Machado MC, Jukemura J, da Cunha JE, et al [Surgical treatment of insulinoma: study of 59 cases]. Rev Assoc Med Bras 1998;44(2):159–66 [Portuguese].
52. Yedibela S, Reck T, Hohenberger W [Resection of liver metastases: goal, timing and results]. Ther Umsch 2001;58(12):713–7 [German].
53. Isenberg JI, Walsh JH, Grossman MI. Zollinger-Ellison syndrome. Gastroenterology 1973;65(1):140–65.
54. Zollinger RM, Ellison EH. Primary peptic ulcerations of the jejunum associated with islet cell tumors of the pancreas. Ann Surg 1955;142(4):709–23 [discussion: 724–8].
55. Modlin IM, Jaffe BM, Sank A, et al. The early diagnosis of gastrinoma. Ann Surg 1982;196(5):512–7.
56. Perry RR, Vinik AI. Clinical review 72: diagnosis and management of functioning islet cell tumors. J Clin Endocrinol Metab 1995;80(8):2273–8.
57. Meko JB, Norton JA. Management of patients with Zollinger-Ellison syndrome. Annu Rev Med 1995;46:395–411.
58. Veldhuis JD, Norton JA, Wells SA Jr, et al. Surgical versus medical management of multiple endocrine neoplasia (MEN) type I. J Clin Endocrinol Metab 1997; 82(2):357–64.
59. Norton JA. Gastrinoma: advances in localization and treatment. Surg Oncol Clin N Am 1998;7(4):845–61.
60. Alexander HR, Bartlett DL, Venzon DJ, et al. Analysis of factors associated with long-term (five or more years) cure in patients undergoing operation for Zollinger-Ellison syndrome. Surgery 1998;124(6):1160–6.
61. Norton JA, Doppman JL, Jensen RT. Curative resection in Zollinger-Ellison syndrome: results of a 10-year prospective study. Ann Surg 1992;215(1):8–18.
62. Wu PC, Alexander HR, Bartlett DL, et al. A prospective analysis of the frequency, location, and curability of ectopic (nonpancreaticoduodenal, nonnodal) gastrinoma. Surgery 1997;122(6):1176–82.

63. Weber HC, Venzon DJ, Lin JT, et al. Determinants of metastatic rate and survival in patients with Zollinger-Ellison syndrome: a prospective long-term study. Gastroenterology 1995;108(6):1637–49.

64. Jensen RT. Gastrointestinal endocrine tumours: gastrinoma. Baillieres Clin Gastroenterol 1996;10(4):603–43.

65. Li ML, Norton JA. Gastrinoma. Curr Treat Options Oncol 2001;2(4):337–46.

66. Miller TA. Zollinger-Ellison syndrome: surgery should still play an important role in its management. Gastroenterology 1995;108(5):1600–2.

67. Norton JA, Fraker DL, Alexander HR, et al. Surgery increases survival in patients with gastrinoma. Ann Surg 2006;244(3):410–9.

68. Wank SA, Doppman JL, Miller DL, et al. Prospective study of the ability of computed axial tomography to localize gastrinomas in patients with Zollinger-Ellison syndrome. Gastroenterology 1987;92(4):905–12.

69. Gibril F, Reynolds JC, Chen CC, et al. Specificity of somatostatin receptor scintigraphy: a prospective study and effects of false-positive localizations on management in patients with gastrinomas. J Nucl Med 1999;40(4):539–53.

70. Gibril F, Reynolds JC, Lubensky IA, et al. Ability of somatostatin receptor scintigraphy to identify patients with gastric carcinoids: a prospective study. J Nucl Med 2000;41(10):1646–56.

71. Gomez D, Malik HZ, Al-Mukthar A, et al. Hepatic resection for metastatic gastrointestinal and pancreatic neuroendocrine tumours: outcome and prognostic predictors. HPB (Oxford) 2007;9(5):345–51.

72. McEntee GP, Nagorney DM, Kvols LK, et al. Cytoreductive hepatic surgery for neuroendocrine tumors. Surgery 1990;108(6):1091–6.

73. MacFarlane MP, Fraker DL, Alexander HR, et al. Prospective study of surgical resection of duodenal and pancreatic gastrinomas in multiple endocrine neoplasia type 1. Surgery 1995;118(6):973–9 [discussion: 979–80].

74. Mekhjian HS, O'Dorisio TM. VIPoma syndrome. Semin Oncol 1987;14(3):282–91.

75. Long RG, Bryant MG, Mitchell SJ, et al. Clinicopathological study of pancreatic and ganglioneuroblastoma tumours secreting vasoactive intestinal polypeptide (VIPomas). Br Med J (Clin Res Ed) 1981;282(6278):1767–71.

76. Capella C, Polak JM, Buffa R, et al. Morphologic patterns and diagnostic criteria of VIP-producing endocrine tumors: a histologic, histochemical, ultrastructural, and biochemical study of 32 cases. Cancer 1983;52(10):1860–74.

77. Arnold R, Frank M, Kajdan U. Management of gastroenteropancreatic endocrine tumors: the place of somatostatin analogues. Digestion 1994;55(Suppl 3): 107–13.

78. Nikou GC, Toubanakis C, Nikolaou P, et al. VIPomas: an update in diagnosis and management in a series of 11 patients. Hepatogastroenterology 2005;52(64): 1259–65.

79. Schoevaerdts D, Favet L, Zekry D, et al. Vipoma: effective treatment with octreotide in the oldest old. J Am Geriatr Soc 2001;49(4):496–7.

80. Norton JA. Neuroendocrine tumors of the pancreas and duodenum. Curr Probl Surg 1994;31(2):77–156.

81. Boden G. Glucagonomas and insulinomas. Gastroenterol Clin North Am 1989; 18(4):831–45.

82. Maton PN. Use of octreotide acetate for control of symptoms in patients with islet cell tumors. World J Surg 1993;17(4):504–10.

83. Krausz Y, Bar-Ziv J, de Jong RB, et al. Somatostatin-receptor scintigraphy in the management of gastroenteropancreatic tumors. Am J Gastroenterol 1998;93(1): 66–70.

84. Lipp RW, Schnedl WJ, Stauber R, et al. Scintigraphic long-term follow-up of a patient with metastatic glucagonoma. Am J Gastroenterol 2000;95(7):1818–20.
85. Higgins GA, Recant L, Fischman AB. The glucagonoma syndrome: surgically curable diabetes. Am J Surg 1979;137(1):142–8.
86. Vinik AI, Strodel WE, Eckhauser FE, et al. PPomas, neurotensinomas. Semin Oncol 1987;14(3):263–81.
87. Konomi K, Chijiiwa K, Katsuta T, et al. Pancreatic somatostatinoma: a case report and review of the literature. J Surg Oncol 1990;43(4):259–65.
88. Tanaka S, Yamasaki S, Matsushita H, et al. Duodenal somatostatinoma: a case report and review of 31 cases with special reference to the relationship between tumor size and metastasis. Pathol Int 2000;50(2):146–52.
89. Soga J, Yakuwa Y. Somatostatinoma/inhibitory syndrome: a statistical evaluation of 173 reported cases as compared to other pancreatic endocrinomas. J Exp Clin Cancer Res 1999;18(1):13–22.
90. Moertel CG. Karnofsky memorial lecture: an odyssey in the land of small tumors. J Clin Oncol 1987;5(10):1502–22.
91. Sarmiento JM, Heywood G, Rubin J, et al. Surgical treatment of neuroendocrine metastases to the liver: a plea for resection to increase survival. J Am Coll Surg 2003;197(1):29–37.
92. Norton JA, Kivlen M, Li M, et al. Morbidity and mortality of aggressive resection in patients with advanced neuroendocrine tumors. Arch Surg 2003;138(8): 859–66.
93. Marlink RG, Lokich JJ, Robins JR, et al. Hepatic arterial embolization for metastatic hormone-secreting tumors: technique, effectiveness, and complications. Cancer 1990;65(10):2227–32.
94. Perry LJ, Stuart K, Stokes KR, et al. Hepatic arterial chemoembolization for metastatic neuroendocrine tumors. Surgery 1994;116(6):1111–6 [discussion: 1116–7].
95. Strosberg JR, Choi J, Cantor AB, et al. Selective hepatic artery embolization for treatment of patients with metastatic carcinoid and pancreatic endocrine tumors. Cancer Control 2006;13(1):72–8.
96. Cozzi PJ, Englund R, Morris DL. Cryotherapy treatment of patients with hepatic metastases from neuroendocrine tumors. Cancer 1995;76(3):501–9.
97. Mazzaglia PJ, Berber E, Milas M, et al. Laparoscopic radiofrequency ablation of neuroendocrine liver metastases: a 10-year experience evaluating predictors of survival. Surgery 2007;142(1):10–9.
98. Seifert JK, Cozzi PJ, Morris DL. Cryotherapy for neuroendocrine liver metastases. Semin Surg Oncol 1998;14(2):175–83.
99. Cosin O, Bilbao JI, Alvarez S, et al. Right gastric artery embolization prior to treatment with yttrium-90 microspheres. Cardiovasc Intervent Radiol 2007; 30(1):98–103.
100. McStay MK, Maudgil D, Williams M, et al. Large-volume liver metastases from neuroendocrine tumors: hepatic intraarterial 90Y-DOTA-lanreotide as effective palliative therapy. Radiology 2005;237(2):718–26.
101. Murthy R, Kamat P, Nunez R, et al. Yttrium-90 microsphere radioembolotherapy of hepatic metastatic neuroendocrine carcinomas after hepatic arterial embolization. J Vasc Interv Radiol 2008;19(1):145–51.
102. Delaunoit T, Hobday T, Neczyporenko F, et al. Medical management of pancreatic neuroendocrine tumors. Am J Gastroenterol 2008;103:475–83.
103. Modlin IM, Oberg K, Chung DC, et al. Gastropancreatic neuroendocrine tumours. Lancet Oncol 2008;9:61–72.

104. Faiss S, Ulrich-Frank P, Wiedenmann B, et al. Prospective, randomized, multi-center trial on the antiproliferative effect of lantreotide, interferon alfa, and their combination for therapy of metastatic neuroendocrine gastropancreatic tumors: the International Lantreotide and Interferon alfa study group. J Clin Oncol 2003; 21(14):2689–96.

105. Sun W, Lipsitz S, Haller D, et al. Phase II/III study of doxorubicin with fluorouracil compared with streptozocin with fluorouracil or dacarbazine in the treatment of advanced carcinoid tumors: ECOG Study E1281. J Clin Oncol 2005;23(22): 4897–904.

106. Moertel CG, Hanley JA. Combination chemotherapy trials in metastatic carcinoid tumor and the malignant carcinoid syndrome. Cancer Clin Trials 1979;2: 327–34.

107. Moertel C, Lefkopoulo M, Lipsitz S, et al. Streptozocin–doxorubicin, stretpozocin–fluorouracil, or chlorozotocin in the treatment of advanced islet-cell carcinoma. N Engl J Med 1992;326:519–23.

108. Kouvaraki M, Ajani J, Yao J, et al. Fluorouracil, doxorubicin, and streptozocin in the treatment of patients with locally advanced and metastatic pancreatic endocrine carcinomas. J Clin Oncol 2004;22:4762–71.

109. Ramanathan RK, Cnaan A, Haller DG, et al. Phase II trial of dacarbazine (DTIC) in advanced pancreatic islet cell carcinoma: study of the Eastern Cooperative Oncology Group-E6282. Ann Oncol 2001;12:1139–43.

110. Bukowski R, Johnson K, Costanzi J, et al. A phase II trial of combination chemotherapy in patients with metastatic carcinoid tumors. Cancer 1987;60:2891–5.

111. Kulke MH, Stuart K, Enzinger PC, et al. Phase II study of temozolomide and thalidomide in patients with metastatic neuroendocrine tumors. J Clin Oncol 2006; 24:401–6.

112. Nakakura EK, Bergsland EK. Islet cell carcinoma: neuroendocrine tumors of the pancreas and periampullary region. Hematol Oncol Clin North Am 2007;21: 457–73.

113. Duran I, Salazar R, Casanovas O, et al. New drug development in digestive neuroendocrine tumors. Ann Oncol 2007;18:1307–13.

114. Kulke M, Lenz HJ, Meropol NJ, et al. Activity of sunitinib in patients with advanced neuroendocrine tumors. J Clin Oncol 2008;26(20):3403–10.

115. Hobday DJ, Rubin J, Holen K, et al. MC044h, a phase 2 trial of sorafenib in patients with metastatic neuroendocrine tumors: a phase 2 consortium study. ASCO Annual Meeting Proceedings, June 2007; Chicago, IL. J Clin Oncol 2007;vol 25(No 18S) [abstract 4504].

116. Duran I, Le L, Saltman D, et al. A phase II trial of temsirolimus in metastatic neuroendocrine tumors. ASCO Annual Meeting Proceedings, June 2007; Chicago, IL. J Clin Oncol 2005;vol 23(No 16S) [abstract 3096].

117. Yao JC, Phan AT, Chang DZ, et al. Phase II study of RAD001 (everolimus) and depot octreotide (Sandostatin LAR) in patients with advanced low grade neuroendocrine carcinoma. ASCO Annual Meeting Proceedings, June 2007; Chicago, IL. J Clin Oncol 2006;vol. 24 [abstract 4042].

Multidisciplinary Treatment of Primary Melanoma

Katharine Yao, MD[a],*, Glen Balch, MD[a], David J. Winchester, MD[b]

KEYWORDS

- Melanoma • Sentinel node • Immunotherapy • Interferon
- Melanoma vaccine • Thin melanomas • Breslow thickness

The incidence of melanoma is increasing faster than all cancers except lung cancer. It accounts for the sixth highest number of newly diagnosed cancer cases and is the sixth most common cancer among men and seventh most common among women.[1] With increasing public awareness, the number of melanoma cases will likely continue to rise and most general surgeons will encounter these cases in their daily practice. Fortunately, 80% of melanomas present in an early stage and are easily treated with surgery alone, indeed the 5- and 10-year survival rates are 91% and 89% respectively; overall, localized melanomas have a 99% 5-year survival rate.[1] On the other hand, the 5-year survival rates for regional and distant disease are 65% and 15% respectively.[1] As with many cancers, melanoma is best approached in a multidisciplinary fashion. The main disciplines that participate in the care of most melanoma patients are dermatology, pathology, surgical oncology, and medical oncology. Rarely, radiation oncology will be involved. With the limited effectiveness of adjuvant treatment for melanoma, it is essential that patients also have access to ongoing clinical immunotherapy trials. In this article, we present the standard management of melanoma from the perspective of each discipline and discuss outcome studies supporting these practice guidelines.

DERMATOLOGIC APPROACH FOR MELANOMA

Dermatologists mainly play a role in the prevention and detection of melanoma. Most melanomas are diagnosed in a dermatologist's office and dermatologists are often the

Financial Disclosure: The authors have no financial relationships to disclose.
[a] Department of Surgery, Northwestern University Feinberg School of Medicine, NorthShore University HealthSystem, Evanston Hospital-Walgreen Bldg Suite 2507, 2650 Ridge Ave, Evanston, IL 60201, USA
[b] Division of Surgical Oncology and General Surgery, Department of Surgery, Northwestern University Feinberg School of Medicine, NorthShore University HealthSystem, Evanston Hospital-Walgreen Bldg Suite 2507, 2650 Ridge Ave, Evanston, IL 60201, USA
* Corresponding author.
E-mail address: kyao@northshore.org (K. Yao).

doctors who initiate and coordinate the patient's treatment process. Additionally, dermatologists are properly equipped to perform a skin biopsy to get the most accurate microstaging information on a melanoma. Because as many as 5% of patients with newly diagnosed melanomas will have another skin cancer detected, it is essential all melanoma patients undergo a thorough skin examination by a dermatologist. Dermatologists often identify patients at increased risk for melanoma such as those with family history of melanoma, previous skin cancers, multiple nevi, dysplastic nevi, immunosuppressed, type I skin, blue eyes, red hair, and freckling. They screen patients for melanoma using dermoscopy and whole body photography. Dermoscopy is widely used in Europe and one study showed that the diagnostic accuracy for melanoma diagnosis was significantly higher using dermoscopy.[2] Often dermatologists will widely excise in situ or thin melanomas if a sentinel lymphadenectomy is not indicated. Last, all melanoma patients need lifelong dermatologic screening. Dermatologists also advise patients on how to prevent future melanomas by pursuing proper sun protection and how to perform proper self-examination. In two studies, patients detected their own melanomas 40% to 57% of the time;[3,4] thus, self-examination is important in this group of patients.

SURGICAL THERAPY FOR MELANOMA

Most newly diagnosed melanoma patients are referred by a dermatologist directly to a surgeon. Surgical excision is usually the first step in treatment of melanoma followed by possibly adjuvant systemic therapy or enrollment onto a clinical trial.

Surgical Excision

Surgical management of early-stage melanomas is guided mainly by the Breslow thickness of the lesion (**Table 1**). The Breslow thickness dictates the excision margin and the necessity for sentinel lymphadenectomy. There have been five randomized trials in both Europe and the United States examining the amount of excision margin needed for certain thickness of melanoma. The first of these trials, conducted by the World Health Organization (WHO)[5] showed that 1-cm versus 3-cm margins were equivalent in terms of recurrence and survival and that a 1-cm margin for melanomas less than 2.0-mm thick was feasible and safe. In contrast, the other two trials looked at 2 cm versus 5 cm for less than 2.0-mm thick melanomas and concluded that 2 cm was just as safe as 5 cm.[6,7] The last two trials examined thicker melanomas, 1- to 4-mm thick and more than 2.0-mm thick. The Intergroup Melanoma Trial showed that a 2-cm margin was equivalent to 4 cm in terms of locoregional recurrence and overall survival.[8] In the fifth trial, from the United Kingdom,[9] a significantly worse local recurrence and disease-free survival rate was seen in the 1-cm versus the 3-cm arm for

Table 1		
Breslow thickness dictates margin excision and sentinel lymphadenectomy		
Breslow Thickness	**Recommended Excision Margin**	**Sentinel Lymphadenectomy**
<1.0 mm	1.0 cm	Not recommended[a]
1.0–2.0 mm	1.0–2.0 cm	Recommended
2.0–4.0 mm	2.0 cm	Recommended
>4.0 mm	2.0 cm	Recommended

[a] Sentinel lymphadenectomy may be performed with some thin melanomas depending on histopathologic characteristics.

melanomas more than 2.0-mm thick but no overall survival difference was seen. The investigators concluded that a 1-cm margin was not safe for melanomas more than 2.0-mm thick because of the increased risk of locoregional recurrence and possibly increased mortality risk.

Based on the results of these trials, a 1-cm margin is recommended for melanomas less than 1.0-mm thick, 1 to 2 cm for 1.0- to 2.0-mm thick melanomas, and 2 cm for melanomas more than 2.0-mm thick (**Table 2**). A 0.5-cm margin is recommended for melanoma in situ lesions.

Wide excisions should be performed with an elliptic incision with a length-to-width ratio of approximately 3:1. The excision is carried down to the muscle fascia and closure accomplished with an advancement flap. For those lesions not amenable to an elliptic incision, a rotational flap or split thickness graft can be used. The skin graft donor site should be outside any potential areas of locoregional recurrence.

Sentinel Lymphadenectomy

The need for sentinel lymphadenectomy is also dictated by the Breslow thickness. As the Breslow thickness increases, the rate of sentinel node tumor positivity increases (**Table 3**).[10] For those melanomas that are less than 1.0-mm thick, sentinel lymphade-nectomy is not routinely recommended unless more suspicious features are seen on histologic review of the biopsy such as ulceration, high mitotic count, Clark level IV or greater, vertical growth phase, or regression. Nonetheless, sentinel lymphadenectomy in thin melanomas is controversial and there are no phase III randomized studies supporting any treatment recommendation for these thin melanomas. Several single-center retrospective studies have examined histopathologic factors that would predict sentinel node positivity in thin melanomas and one study found that the sentinel node status was significant for disease and overall survival in a group of 631 patients with thin melanomas[11–20] (**Box 1**). The incidence of sentinel node

Table 2					
Randomized trials involving excision margins					
Trial	No. Patients	Year	Breslow Thickness	Margins of Excision	Significant Sifference in Local Recurrence/ Survival?
World Health Organization-10[5]	612	1988	<2.0 mm	1 versus 3 cm	No
French Group of Research[7]	337	2004	<2.1 mm	2 versus 5 cm	No
Swedish Melanoma Group[6]	989	2000	0.8–2.0 mm	2 versus 5 cm	No
United States Intergroup Trial[8]	740	2001	1.0–4.0 mm	2 versus 4 cm	No
United Kingdom[9]	900	2004	>2.0 mm	1 versus 3 cm	Yes; increased regional recurrence in 1-cm arm, no difference in survival

Table 3
Breslow thickness and sentinel node tumor positivity[10]

Breslow Thickness	Tumor Positive Sentinel Node Rate
<0.76 mm	Minimal
0.76–1.00 mm	5%–6%
1.1–1.5 mm	7%–8%
1.5–4.0 mm	18%–19%
>4.0 mm	29%–34%

Data from Gershenwald JE, Thompson W, Mansfield PF, et al. Multi-institutional melanoma lymphatic mapping experience: the prognostic value of sentinel lymph node status in 612 stage I or II melanoma patients. J Clin Oncol 1999;17:976–83.

positivity in these studies ranged from 3.6% to 6.5% demonstrating at least some need for sentinel lymphadenectomy in this group of patients.

For melanomas 1.0-mm thick or more, a sentinel lymphadenectomy is routinely recommended unless the patient has palpable adenopathy. Those with palpable adenopathy will proceed directly to complete lymph node dissection. Sentinel lymphadenectomy for melanoma has been validated at several centers and has become standard of care. In 2006, Morton and colleagues[21] published the results of the Multicenter Selective Lymphadenectomy Trial (MSLT I) and showed that immediate lymphadenectomy for patients with nodal metastases prolonged survival. There were 1269 patients with 1.2- to 3.5-mm thick melanomas randomized to wide excision alone versus wide excision and sentinel lymphadenectomy. Those in the wide excision alone arm underwent a delayed lymph node dissection when nodal metastases were clinically apparent. There was a significant difference in the 5-year disease-free survival rate (78% for wide excision/sentinel lymphadenectomy versus 73% for wide excision alone) but no difference in melanoma-specific or overall survival. However, in a subset analysis of patients with nodal metastases in both arms, the 5-year survival rate was significantly higher among those who underwent sentinel lymphadenectomy and then immediate lymph node dissection versus those who had a wide excision only and then delayed lymph node dissection (72% versus 52%

Box 1
Sentinel lymphadenectomy in thin melanomas[11–20]

Histopathologic Factors to Consider for Sentinel Lymphadenectomy for Thin Melanomas

Breslow thickness (>0.75-mm thick)

Clark Level of Invasion

Mitotic index

Vertical growth phase

Male gender

Ulceration of the primary

Young age

Regression

Discordancy between clinical findings and biopsy findings

respectively). Furthermore, there were more tumor-positive lymph nodes in the delayed dissection group versus the sentinel lymphadenectomy group (3.3 versus 1.4). These findings support a role for early lymph node dissection as opposed to waiting until nodal metastases become clinically apparent. At least two other elective lymph node dissection trials, both based in Europe, have demonstrated similar results; that is, higher 5-year survival rates for those who underwent immediate lymph node dissection versus delayed dissection.[22–24] Although no overall survival benefit was seen in this trial, this trial clearly confirms that sentinel node biopsy is the standard of care for staging the lymph nodes for patients with intermediate-thickness melanomas. It also affirms that the status of the sentinel node is still the most important prognostic factor for intermediate-thickness melanomas. Sentinel lymphadenectomy in melanoma patients participating in MSLT I detected cancer 16 months earlier than the observation arm.

Nonetheless, only 15% to 20% of sentinel node–positive patients will have additional nodal metastases on complete lymph node dissection, which means 80% of patients are undergoing an unnecessary lymph node dissection. Based on these data, Morton and colleagues[21] have launched MSLT II (Multicenter Selective Lymphadenectomy Trial II), a trial where positive sentinel node patients are randomized to complete lymph node dissection versus observation with nodal ultrasound. Ultrasound is more commonly used in Europe[24,25] as a means to identify nodal metastases. Several studies in Europe have been conducted and show it has a low sensitivity for small micrometastases in the sentinel node. This trial will hopefully establish that group of sentinel node–positive patients who would most likely benefit from a complete lymph node dissection.

Sentinel lymphadenectomy is also recommended for patients with thick melanomas (>4.0-mm thick), although these patients were not included in MSLT I and there have been no randomized trials in patients with thick melanomas. Several studies on sentinel lymphadenectomy in patients with thick melanomas show sentinel node tumor positive rates of 32% to 44%[26–30] and also consistently show that the sentinel node status is predictive for either survival or recurrence, thus arguing for the routine use of sentinel lymphadenectomy in thick melanomas.

The incidence of nodal recurrence is low after a negative sentinel lymphadenectomy, less than 5%.[10] Some studies have suggested that there is an increased rate of in-transit metastases after sentinel lymphadenectomy because of altered lymphatic pathways from the sentinel lymphadenectomy, but several large follow-up studies from well-known melanoma centers have clearly shown no increase in in-transit metastases after sentinel lymphadenectomy.[31,32] One study showed a 4.9% incidence of in-transit disease in a group of wide-excision alone patients versus a 4.5% incidence in wide excision plus sentinel lymphadenectomy patients.[33] These findings have been corroborated by the MSLT I trial as well.[20]

RADIATION THERAPY FOR MELANOMA

Because the risk of locoregional recurrence in melanoma patients with positive lymph nodes can be 30%,[34–37] several centers have conducted trials using adjuvant radiation for patients with positive lymph nodes in the inguinal, neck, and other locations.[38–45] Prospective studies of adjuvant radiation have shown improved regional control for the radiation arm but not always improved overall survival. The highest rates for locoregional control are seen in the head and neck melanomas and the lowest rates for ilioinguinal disease. Unfortunately, the main complication from radiation is lymphedema, which is not usually seen in the head and neck region but is definitely more common in the ilioinguinal region with rates up to 30% to 40%.[43,44]

Nonetheless, adjuvant radiation may be indicated for patients who are at high risk for recurrence, such as those with close margins at the primary lesion, locoregional recurrent disease, or multiple positive lymph nodes especially if extracapsular extension is present. Some of the larger cancer centers have been administering hypofractionated regimens to decrease the duration of the treatments so that patients can receive their systemic treatment in a timely fashion.[44,45] Concurrent radiation and systemic treatment appears to incur an unacceptable amount of toxicity but large studies on these regimens are lacking.

SYSTEMIC THERAPY FOR MELANOMA
Chemotherapy/Biochemotherapy

Unfortunately, multiple randomized trials of chemotherapy (dacarbazine, carmustine) for Stage II to III melanomas have not shown any survival benefit. The largest trial of adjuvant chemotherapy was reported in 1982 by Veronesi and colleagues[46] in which 761 patients were randomized to dacarbazine, bacilli Calmette-Guerin (BCG), dacarbazine + BCG, or observation after complete surgical resection. No survival benefit was seen at 3 years but patients were followed for only a mean of 41 months. In 1981, Hill and colleagues[47] compared dacarbazine to observation but no survival benefit was seen for dacarbazine. Poor trial design and low numbers of patients have contributed to these disappointing results of past chemotherapy trials, but resistance of melanoma to standard chemotherapy regimens may also be playing a role.

Biologic agents combined with chemotherapy agents have been studied for both Stage III and IV disease but again no definitive survival benefit has been demonstrated. A Southwestern Oncology Group (S0008) trial is comparing three cycles of biochemotherapy with 1 year of high-dose interferon in very high risk stage III patients but no data have been published to date.[48] Given the poor results presented for Stage IV patients, investigators are skeptical that results will be that much different for Stage III patients.

Vaccines

There have been at least eight randomized trials using different vaccine formulations for Stage IIB to IV patients but none have shown a definitive overall survival benefit (**Table 4**). Some trials did show small survival benefits for certain subgroups of patients though; in a SWOG trial studying Melacine, there was a significant 5-year relapse-free survival for patients positive for HLA-A2 and HLA-C3 compared with the control group (77% versus 64% respectively).[49,50] Unfortunately, there has been no follow-up trial specifically looking at HLA-A2– and HLA-C3–positive patients. Two trials conducted recently by Morton and colleagues[51,52] examined an allogeneic whole-cell vaccine (CancerVax) plus BCG versus BCG alone for both Stage III and IV patients. Previous studies from this group showed survival benefits for CancerVax over historical controls but results presented from the two trials showed that the CancerVax arms had worse outcomes then the control arms.[53] A trial involving immunization with ganglioside (GM2) showed that those patients who manifested GM2-specific antibodies had a survival advantage compared with a BCG-alone arm.[54] The European Organization for Research and Treatment of Cancer (EORTC) then conducted a phase III trial of GM2 but the interim analysis actually showed a worse outcome for those on the GM2 arm and thus the trial was stopped.

Nonetheless, much has been learned from these vaccine trials and the biology of the T-cell response. Investigators will need to find ways to more reliably measure T-cell

| Table 4 |||||
| Prospective randomized vaccine trials |||||
Trial	Year	Vaccine Type	Stage of Patients	DFS	OS
Livingston et al[54]	1994	GM2/BCG versus BCG	III	0.09	0.22
Wallack et al[79]	1998	Whole cell versus control	III	0.61	0.79
Mitchell et al[80]	1997	Melacine versus DCC/TAM	IV	NA	0.16
Kirkwood et al[58]	2001	GMK versus INFα2b	IIB/III	0.0015	0.009
Sondak et al[49]	2002	Melacine versus observation	IIB	0.51	NA
Hersey et al[81]	2002	Melanoma cell lysate versus observation	IIB/III	0.27	0.11
Morton et al[51]	2006	Allogeneic whole cell vaccine/ BCG versus placebo/BCG	III	0.047	0.040
Morton et al[52]	2006	Allogeneic whole cell vaccine/ BCG versus placebo/BCG	IV	0.418	0.245
Schadendorf et al[82]	2006	Peptide-pulsed dendritic cells versus DTIC	IV	NA	0.48

Abbreviations: BCG, bacilli Calmette-Guerin; DCC/TAM, dacarbazine, carmustine, cisplatin/tamoxifen; DFS, disease-free survival; DTIC, dacarbazine; GMK, GM2 keyhole limpet hemocyanin-QS-21; INFα, interferon alpha; NA, not available; OS, overall survival.

responses and how to correlate these T-cell responses with clinical responses. Moreover, investigators are learning how tumors evade the immune system and how to manipulate this response to their advantage. They are focusing on cytotoxic T cells and how to enhance antigen presentation with dendritic cells and to block down-regulation of T cells using monoclonal antibodies that block cytotoxic T lymphocyte–associated antigen 4 (anti-CTLA-4). Phase I and II trials using these approaches have shown promising results and phase III trials are ongoing.[55]

Interferon Alpha

There have been three Eastern Cooperative Oncology Group (ECOG) randomized trials of high-dose interferon for 1 year compared with other treatment regimens for patients with positive nodes or melanomas more than 4.0-mm thick with only one trial demonstrating a clear survival benefit (**Table 5**). High-dose interferon involves 1 month of intravenous therapy, Monday through Friday, followed by subcutaneous injections three times a week for 11 months. The first interferon trial, ECOG 1684, studied 1 year of high-dose interferon compared with observation and initially showed an overall survival benefit, but with 12-year follow-up the overall survival benefit disappeared although the disease-free survival benefit persisted.[56] This trial led to the US Food and Drug Administration (FDA) approval of interferon in 1996 for high-risk melanoma patients. The second interferon trial, ECOG 1690, compared high-dose interferon to low-dose interferon to no treatment. There was no overall survival benefit for any of the groups.[57] In the third interferon trial, ECOG 1694, high-dose interferon was compared with a GM2 vaccine for high-risk melanoma patients.[58] The trial was stopped early because of a significant disease-free and overall survival benefit for the high-dose interferon arm. Unfortunately, there was no observation arm in this trial so it is impossible to know if the vaccine was equivalent to observation or better and whether interferon was really conferring a better survival than just observation alone. Survival curves were the same for interferon in this trial compared with the previous two interferon trials, suggesting that the GM2 vaccine arm was probably equivalent to no therapy. Nonetheless, the use of interferon is controversial, namely because

Table 5
Interferon trials

Trial	No. Patients	Dose/Duration	DFS Benefit	OS Benefit
ECOG 1684[56]	287	1-y high-dose versus observation	Yes	No
ECOG 1690[57]	642	High-dose versus low-dose versus observation	Yes	No
ECOG 1694[58]	880	High-dose versus GM2 vaccine	Yes	Yes
EORTC 18,952[62]	1388	25-month versus 13-month versus observation	No	No
EORTC 18,991[63]	1256	5 y pegylated IFN versus observation	Yes	No
Creagan et al[60]	262	High dose for 3 mo versus observation	Yes, only for Stage II patients[a]	No
Cascinelli et al[59]	444	Low dose for 3 y versus observation	No	No
French Cooperative Group[61]	499	Lose dose for 18 mo versus observation	Yes, relapse-free survival benefit	No

Abbreviations: DFS, disease-free survival; ECOG, Eastern Cooperative Oncology Group; EORTC, European Organization for Research and Treatment of Cancer; IFN, interferon; OS, overall survival.
[a] This effect was seen only on an adjusted analysis.

the small survival (if any) benefit may not justify the toxicity of the treatment. In these trials, anywhere from 20% to 50% of patients underwent dose reductions of interferon because of side effects and the treatment is expensive.[56–58] For these reasons, there have been several trials examining shortened courses of high-dose interferon (3 months) or low doses of interferon for a 3-year period or 18-month period.[59–61] Unfortunately, none showed a survival benefit. One study that examined high-dose interferon for 3 months and found a disease-free survival benefit for Stage II patients only.[60] EORTC 18,952 looked at intermediate doses of interferon for Stage IIB to III disease but no statistically significant difference in survival was seen, and it was difficult to tell if these differences in survival were because of the duration of therapy or the dose of interferon.[62] A recently published EORTC 18,991 trial compared 5 years of pegylated interferon α-2b to observation: the recurrence-free survival was 45.6% in the interferon group compared with 38.9% in the observation arm.[63] There was no difference in overall survival. Pegylated interferon allows patients to undergo prolonged weekly injections with the potential to improve the toxicity of interferon. When the subgroup of patients with microscopic tumor involvement was studied, a distant metastasis-free survival benefit was seen. Interferon may have a more important survival benefit in those with microscopic disease as opposed to those with palpable adenopathy. These findings demonstrate the wide variation in prognosis for those patients with nodal micrometastases versus macrometastases and the importance of sentinel node microstaging for these patients.

LIMB PERFUSION/INFUSION

Limb perfusion/infusion strategies for advanced locoregional disease include hyperthermic isolated limb perfusion, hyperthermic isolated limb infusion, radiation therapy, or a combination of these treatments. These modalities do not improve overall survival but may extend disease-free survival. Klopp was the first to recognize the value of intra-arterial chemotherapy.[64] Creech advanced this concept further using an extracorporeal circuit to isolate the affected limb during the treatment.[65] Hyperthermia was added in 1969 based upon the observation of synergistic activity of heat and alkylating agents.[66] Subsequent reports of limb perfusion have described response rates as high as 90% as well as a high percentage of complete responses in patients with extensive, unresectable disease using Melphalan.[67–69] Randomized studies have not demonstrated any additional benefit of tumor necrosis factor in addition to Melphalan.[70] Although effective, the limb perfusion approach is complex and expensive, requiring an extensive dissection and mobilization of inflow and outflow blood vessels and branches, a continuous monitoring system to detect a systemic leak of the perfusate with nuclear medicine, and a perfusionist to assist in the delivery of an oxygenated hyperthemic circuit. Recognizing the potential for localized toxicity, this treatment offers patients an excellent option for treatment that would otherwise be limited to amputation.

A simpler, less extensive modification of this technique, hyperthermic isolated limb infusion (ILI) was developed by John Thompson and colleagues from the Sydney Melanoma Unit.[71] This does not involve any dissection but depends upon the use of percutaneous catheters and pneumatic tourniquets to isolate the affected limb. Due to consistently low leak rates, this does not require monitoring. ILI uses a hyperthermic infusate consisting of Dactinomycin and Melphalan and occurs over a shorter time course without oxygenation. Although the hospital stay is significantly shorter, the toxicity and response rates are similar to isolated limb perfusion.[72] Regional chemotherapy may be redelivered, depending upon the initial response. These techniques

---

Box 2
Summary points

- The incidence of melanoma is increasing

- Survival rates for early-stage melanoma are 90% at 5 years; for regional and distant disease they are 65% and 15% respectively

- Melanoma patients need lifelong screening; >40% of the time patients will detect their own melanomas on follow-up

- Excision margins for melanomas <1.0-mm thick should be 1 cm, for melanomas 1.0- to 2.0-mm thick 1 to 2 cm, and for melanomas >2.0-mm thick a 2-cm margin is needed

- Sentinel lymphadenectomy is recommended for all melanomas >1.0-mm thick and even for melanomas >4.0-mm thick. Select cases of thin (<1.0-mm thick) melanomas may also be candidates for sentinel lymphadenectomy

- The results of a randomized sentinel lymphadenectomy trial reported in 2006 showed that sentinel lymphadenectomy and immediate lymphadenectomy had a survival benefit over delayed lymph node dissection

- Radiation therapy may be indicated for some high-risk melanomas and results are especially favorable in the head and neck region

- Chemotherapy and biochemotherapy regimens for melanoma have not shown promising results, only high-dose interferon has shown a disease-free survival benefit; overall survival benefit from interferon is controversial

- There have been several randomized vaccine trials but none have shown a definitive overall survival benefit; only subsets of patients have had survival benefits

may help limit the morbidity of locally advanced disease and have the potential to contribute to disease-free survival.

FOLLOW-UP CARE

The risk for a second primary melanoma ranges from 0.2% to 8.6%[73,74] and all melanoma patients need lifelong dermatologic screening at least annually. Because 76% to 94% of recurrences are detected by either physical examination or complete history, it is imperative that patients have proper follow-up care.[75–77] The National Comprehensive Cancer Network (NCCN) recommends that in situ melanoma patients have an annual skin examination for life, and history and physical every 3 to 12 months for 5 years and then annually.[78] All other melanoma patients need an annual skin examination for life, and history and physical examination every 3 to 6 months for 2 years, then every 3 to 12 months for 2 years, then annually as indicated. CT scans should be considered to screen Stage IIB and higher patients (**Box 2**).

ACKNOWLEDGMENTS

We thank Debbie Affinati for her assistance in the preparation of this article.

REFERENCES

1. Cancer Facts and Figures. Available at: http://www.cancer.org. 2007; Accessed November 4, 2008.
2. Kittler H, Pehamberger H, Wolff K, et al. Diagnostic accuracy of dermoscopy. Lancet Oncol 2002;3:159–65.
3. Brady MS, Oliveria SA, Christos PJ, et al. Patterns of detection in patients with cutaneous melanoma. Cancer 2000;89:342–7.
4. Carli P, DeGiorgi V, Palli D, et al. Dermatologist detection and skin self-examination are associated with thinner melanomas: results from a survey of the Italian Multidisciplinary Group on Melanoma. Arch Dermatol 2003;139:607–12.
5. Veronesi U, Cascinelli N, Adamus J, et al. Thin stage I primary cutaneous malignant melanoma. Comparison of excision with margins of 1 or 3 cm. N Engl J Med 1988;318:1159–62.
6. Cohn-Cedermark G, Lars ER, Andersson R, et al. Long term results of a randomized study by the Swedish melanoma study group on 2-cm versus 5-cm resection margins for patients with cutaneous melanoma with a tumor thickness of 0.8–2.0mm. Cancer 2000;89(7):1495–501.
7. Khayat D, Rixe O, Martin G. Surgical margins in cutaneous melanoma (2 cm versus 5 cm for lesions measuring less then 2.1-mm thick). Long-term results of a large European multicentric phase III study. Cancer 2003;97(8):1941–6.
8. Balch CM, Urist MM, Karakousis CP, et al. Efficacy of 2-cm surgical margins for intermediate-thickness melanomas (1 to 4 MM). Results of a multi-institutional randomized surgical trial. Ann Surg 1993;218(3):262–9.
9. Thomas JM, Newton-Bishop J, A'Hern R, et al. Excision margins in high-risk malignant melanoma. N Engl J Med 2004;350(8):757–66.
10. Gershenwald JE, Thompson W, Mansfield PF, et al. Multi-institutional melanoma lymphatic mapping experience: the prognostic value of sentinel lymph node status in 612 stage I or II melanoma patients. J Clin Oncol 1999;17:976–83.
11. Bleicher RJ, Essner R, Foshag LJ, et al. Role of sentinel lymphadenectomy in thin invasive cutaneous melanoma. J Clin Oncol 2003;21(7):1326–31.

12. Jacobs IA, Chang CK, DasGupta TK, et al. Role of sentinel lymph node biopsy in patients with thin (<1mm) melanoma. Ann Surg Oncol 2003;10(5): 558–61.

13. Karakousis GC, Gimotty PA, Botbyl JD, et al. Predictors of regional nodal disease in patients with thin melanomas. Ann Surg Oncol 2006;13(4):533–41.

14. Karakousis GC, Gimotty PA, Czerniecki BJ, et al. Regional nodal metastatic disease is the strongest predictor of survival in patients with thin vertical growth phase melanomas: a case for SLN staging biopsy in these patients. Ann Surg Oncol 2007;14(5):1596–603.

15. Morris KT, Busam KJ, Bero S, et al. Primary cutaneous melanoma with regression does not require threshold for sentinel lymph node biopsy. Ann Surg Oncol 2008; 15(1):316–22.

16. Ranieri JM, Wagner JD, Wenck S, et al. The prognostic importance of sentinel lymph node biopsy in thin melanoma. Ann Surg Oncol 2006;13(7):927–32.

17. Sondak VK, Taylor JM, Sabel MS, et al. Mitotic rate and younger age are predictors of sentinel lymph node positivity: lessons learned from the generation of a probabilistic model. Ann Surg Oncol 2004;11(3):233–5.

18. Stitzenberg KB, Groben PA, Stern SL, et al. Indications for lymphatic mapping and sentinel lymphadenectomy in patients with thin melanoma (Breslow thickness < or =1.0mm). Ann Surg Oncol 2004;11(10):900–6.

19. Wong SL, Brady MS, Busam KJ, et al. Results of sentinel lymph node biopsy in patients with thin melanoma. Ann Surg Oncol 2006;13(3):302–9.

20. Wright BE, Scheri RP, Ye X, et al. Importance of sentinel lymph node biopsy in patients with thin melanoma. Arch Surg 2008;143(9):892–9.

21. Morton DL, Thompson JF, Cochran AJ, et al. Sentinel-node biopsy or nodal observation in melanoma. N Engl J Med 2006;355:1307–17.

22. Cascinelli N, Morabito A, Santinami M, et al. Immediate or delayed dissection of regional nodes in patients with melanoma of the trunk: a randomized trial. WHO Melanoma Programme. Lancet 1998;351:793–6.

23. Kretschmer L, Hilgers R, Mohrle M, et al. Patients with lymphatic metastasis of cutaneous malignant melanoma benefit from sentinel lymphonodectomy and early excision of their nodal disease. Eur J Cancer 2004;40:212–8.

24. Voit CA, van Akkooi ACJ, Schaefer-Hesterberg G, et al. Reduction of need for operative sentinel node procedure in melanoma patients: fifty percent identification rate of sentinel node positivity by ultrasound (US)-guided fine needle aspiration cytology (FNAC) in 400 consecutive patients (abstract 3BA). Eur J Cancer Suppl 2007;5(6):11.

25. Voit C, Kron M, Schafer G, et al. Ultrasound-guided fine needle aspiration cytology prior to sentinel lymph node biopsy in melanoma patients. Ann Surg Oncol 2006;12:1682–9.

26. Carlson GW, Murray DR, Hestley A, et al. Sentinel lymph node mapping for thick (≥4mm) melanoma: should we be doing it? Ann Surg Oncol 2003;10(4):408–15.

27. Cecchi R, Buralli L, Innocenti S, et al. Sentinel lymph node biopsy in patients with thick (= 4 mm) melanoma: a single-centre experience. J Eur Acad Dermatol Venereol 2007;21(6):758–61.

28. Essner R, Chung MH, Bleicher R, et al. Prognostic implications of thick (>4-mm) melanoma in the era of intraoperative lymphatic mapping and sentinel lymphadenectomy. Ann Surg Oncol. 2002;9(8):754–61.

29. Gershenwald JE, Mansfield PF, Lee JE, et al. Role for lymphatic mapping and sentinel lymph node biopsy in patients with thick (>4 mm) primary melanoma. Ann Surg Oncol 2000;7(2):160–5.

30. Jacobs IA, Chang CK, Salti GI, et al. Role of sentinel lymph node biopsy in patients with thick (>4 mm) primary melanoma. Am Surg 2004;70(1):59–62.

31. Kretschmer L, Beckmann I, Thoms KM, et al. Sentinel lymphonodectomy does not increase the right of loco-regional cutaneous metastases of malignant melanomas. Eur J Cancer 2005;41:531–8.

32. van Poll D, Thompson JF, Colman MH, et al. A sentinel node biopsy does not increase the incidence of in-transit metastasis in patients with primary cutaneous melanoma. Ann Surg Oncol 2005;12(8):597–608.

33. Pawlik TM, Ross MI, Thompson JF, et al. The risk of intransit melanoma metastasis depends on tumor biology and not the surgical approach to regional lymph nodes. J Clin Oncol 2005;23:4588–90.

34. Pathak I, Gilbert R, Yoo J, et al. Outcome of neck dissection for node-positive melanoma. J Otolaryngol 2002;31:147–9.

35. Meyer T, Merkel S, Gohl J, et al. Lymph node dissection for clinically evident lymph node metastases of malignant melanoma. Eur J Surg Oncol 2002;28:424–30.

36. Hughes TM, A'Hern RP, Thomas JM. Prognosis and surgical management of patients with palpable inguinal lymph node metastases from melanoma. Br J Surg 2000;87:892–901.

37. Kretschmer L, Neumann C, Preusser KP, et al. Superficial inguinal and radical ilioinguinal lymph node dissection in patients with palpable melanoma metastases to the groin—an analysis of survival and local recurrence. Acta Oncol 2001;40:72–8.

38. Shen P, Wanek LA, Morton DL. Is adjuvant radiotherapy necessary after positive lymph node dissection in head and neck melanomas? Ann Surg Oncol 2000;7: 554–9.

39. Lee RJ, Gibbs JF, Proulx GM, et al. Nodal basin recurrence following lymph node dissection for melanoma: implications for adjuvant radiotherapy. Int J Radiat Oncol Biol Phys 2000;46:467–74.

40. O'Brien CJ, Coates AS, Petersen-Schaefer K, et al. Experience with 998 cutaneous melanomas of the head and neck over 30 years. Am J Surg 1991;162: 310–4.

41. Calabro A, Singletary SE, Balch CM. Patterns of relapse in 1001 consecutive patients with melanoma nodal metastases. Arch Surg 1989;124:1051–5.

42. Mendenhall WM, Amdur RJ, Grobmyer SR, et al. Adjuvant radiotherapy for cutaneous melanoma. Cancer 2008;112:1189–96.

43. Burmeister BH, Mark SB, Burmeister E, et al. A prospective phase II study of adjuvant postoperative radiation therapy following nodal surgery in malignant melanoma-Trans Tasman Radiation Oncology Group (TROG) Study 96.06. Radiother Oncol 2006;81:136–42.

44. Ballo MT, Zagars GK, Gershenwald JE, et al. A critical assessment of adjuvant radiotherapy for inguinal lymph node metastases from melanoma. Ann Surg Oncol 2004;11:1079–84.

45. Stevens G, Thompson JF, Firth I, et al. Locally advanced melanoma: results of postoperative hypofractionated radiation therapy. Cancer 2000;88:88–94.

46. Veronesi U, Adamus J, Aubert C, et al. A randomized trial of adjuvant chemotherapy and immunotherapy in cutaneous melanoma. N Engl J Med 1982;307:913–6.

47. Hill GJ 2nd, Moss SE, Golomb FM, et al. DTIC and combination therapy for melanoma III. DTIC (NSC 45388) Surgical Adjuvant Study COG PROTOCOL 7040. Cancer 1981;47:2556–62.

48. Atkins MB, Lee S, Flaherty LE, et al. A prospective randomized phase III trial of concurrent biochemotherapy (BCT) with cisplatin, vinblastine, dacarbazine

(CVD), IL-2 and interferon alpha-2b (INF) versus CVD alone in patients with metastatic melanoma (E3695): an ECOG coordinated intergroup trial. Proc Am Soc Clin Oncol 2003;22:2847.

49. Sondak VK, Liu PY, Tuthill RJ, et al. Adjuvant immunotherapy of resected, intermediate thickness, node-negative melanoma with an allogeneic tumor vaccine: overall results of a randomized trial of the Southwest Oncology Group. J Clin Oncol 2002;20:2058–66.

50. Sosman JA, Unger JM, Liu PY, et al. Southwest Oncology Group. Adjuvant immunotherapy of resected, intermediate-thickness, node negative melanoma with an allogenic tumor vaccine: impact of HLA class I antigen expression on outcome. J Clin Oncol 2002;20(8):2067–75.

51. Morton DL, Hsueh EC, Essner R, et al. Prolonged survival of patients receiving active immunotherapy with canvaxin therapeutic polyvalent vaccine after complete resection of melanoma metastatic to regional lymph nodes. Ann Surg 2002;235:438–49.

52. Morton DL, Mozzillo N, Thompson JF, et al. An international randomized, double-blind, phase 3 study of the specific active immunotherapy agent, Onamelatucel-L (Canvaxin™), compared to placebo as a post-surgical adjuvant in AJCC stage IV melanoma. Ann Surg Oncol 2006;13:5.

53. Hsueh EC, Essner R, Foshag LJ, et al. Prolonged survival after complete resection of disseminated melanoma and active immunotherapy with a therapeutic cancer vaccine. J Clin Oncol 2002;20(23):4549–54.

54. Livingston PO, Wong GYC, Adluri S, et al. Improved survival in stage III melanoma patients with GM2 antibodies: a randomized trial of adjuvant vaccination with GM2 ganglioside. J Clin Oncol 1994;12:1036–44.

55. Kirkwood JM, Tarhini AA, Panelli MC, et al. Next generation of immunotherapy for melanoma. J Clin Oncol 2008;26:3445–55.

56. Kirkwood JM, Strawderman MH, Ernstoff MS, et al. Interferon alfa-2b adjuvant therapy of high-risk resected cutaneous melanoma: The Eastern Cooperative oncology Group Trial EST 1684. J Clin Oncol 1996;14:7–17.

57. Kirkwood JM, Ibrahim JG, Sondak VK, et al. High and low-dose interferon alfa-2b in high-risk melanoma: first analysis of intergroup trial E1690/S9111/C9190. J Clin Oncol 2000;19:2444–58.

58. Kirkwood JM, Ibrahim JG, Sosman JA, et al. High-dose interferon alfa-2b significantly prolongs relapse-free and overall survival compared with the GM2-KLH/QS-21 vaccine in patients with resected stage IIB-III melanoma: results of intergroup trial E1694/S9512/C509801. J Clin Oncol 2001;19:2370–80.

59. Cascinelli N, Belli B, MacKie R, et al. Effect of long-term adjuvant therapy with interferon alpha-2a in patients with regional node metastases from cutaneous melanoma: a randomized trial. Lancet 2001;358:866–9.

60. Creagan ET, Dalton RJ, Ahmann DL, et al. Randomized, surgical adjuvant clinical trail of recombinant interferon alfa-2a in selected patients with malignant melanoma. J Clin Oncol 1995;13(11):2776–83.

61. Grob JJ, Dreno B, de la Salmoniere P, et al. Randomised trial of interferon α-2a as adjuvant therapy in resected primary melanoma thicker than 1.5 mm without clinically detectable node metastases. French Cooperative Group on Melanoma. Lancet 1998;351:1905–10.

62. Eggermont AMM, Suciu S, MacKie R, et al. Post-surgery adjuvant therapy with intermediate doses of interferon alfa 2b versus observation in patients with stage IIb/III melanoma (EORTC 18952): randomized controlled trial. Lancet 2005;366: 1189–96.

63. Eggermont AMM, Suciu S, Santinami M, et al. Adjuvant therapy with pegylated interferon alfa-2b versus observation alone in resected stage III melanoma: final results of EORTC 18991, a randomized phase III trial. Lancet 2008;372:117–26.
64. Klopp CT, Alford TC, Bateman J, et al. Fractionated intra-arterial cancer chemotherapy with a methylbisamine hydrochloride. Preliminary report. Ann Surg 1950; 132:811.
65. Creech OJ Jr, Krementz ET, Ryan RF, et al. Chemotherapy of cancer. Regional perfusion using an extracorporeal circuit. Ann Surg 1958;148:616.
66. Stehlin SJ Jr. Hyperthermic perfusion with chemotherapy for cancers of the extremitites. Surg Gynecol Obstet 1969;129:305–8.
67. Storm FK, Morton DL. Value of therapeutic hyperthermic limb perfusion in advanced recurrent melanoma of the lower extremity. Am J Surg 1985;150:32–5.
68. Minor DR, Allen RE, Alberts D, et al. A clinical and pharmacokinetic study of isolated limb perfusion with heat and melphalan for melanoma. Cancer 1985;55: 2638–44.
69. Skene AI, Bulman AS, Williams TR, et al. Hyperthermic isolated perfusion with melphalan in the treatment of advanced malignant melanoma of the lower limb. Br J Surg 1990;77:765–7.
70. Cornett WR, McCall LM, Petersen RP, et al. Randomized multicenter trial of hyperthermic isolated limb perfusion with melphalan alone compared with melphalan plus tumor necrosis factor: American College Surgeons Oncology Group Trial Z0020. Journal of Clinical Oncology 2006;24(25):4196–201.
71. Thompson JF, Kam PC, Waugh RC, et al. Isolated limb infusion with cytotoxic agents: a simple alternative to isolated limb perfusion. Semin Surg Oncol 1998; 14:238–47.
72. Lindnér P, Doubrovsky A, Kam PCA, et al. Prognostic Factors After Isolated Limb Infusion With Cytotoxic Agents for Melanoma. Annals of Surgical Oncology 2002; 9(2):127–36.
73. Goggins WB, Tsao H. A population-based analysis of risk factors for a second primary cutaneous melanoma among melanoma survivors. Cancer 2003;97:639–43.
74. Ferrone CR, Ben Porat L, Panageas KS, et al. Clinicopathological features of and risk factors for multiple primary melanomas. JAMA 2005;294:1647–54.
75. Mooney MM, Kulas M, McKinley B, et al. Impact on survival by method of recurrence detection in stage I and II cutaneous melanoma. Ann Surg Oncol 1998;5: 54–63.
76. Poo-Hwu JJ, Ariyan S, Lamb L, et al. Follow-up recommendations for patients with American Joint Committee on Cancer Stages I-III malignant melanoma. Cancer 1999;86:2252–8.
77. Weiss M, Loprinzi CL, Creagan ET, et al. Utility of follow up tests for detecting recurrent disease in patients with malignant melanomas. JAMA 1995;274:1703–5.
78. National Comprehensive Cancer Network. Available at: http://www.nccn.org. 2007; Accessed November 4, 2008.
79. Wallack MK, Sivanandham M, Balch CM, et al. Surgical adjuvant active specific immunotherapy for patients with stage III melanoma: the final analysis of data from a phase III, randomized, double blind, multicenter vaccinia melanoma oncolysate trial. J Am Coll Surg 1998;187:69–79.
80. Mitchell MS, Von Eschen KB. Phase III trial of Melacine melanoma vaccine versus combination chemotherapy in the treatment of stage IV melanoma. Proc Am Soc Clin Oncol 1997;16:494a.

81. Hersey P, Coates AS, McCarthy WH, et al. Adjuvant immunotherapy of patients with high-risk melanoma using vaccinia viral lysats of melanoma: results of a randomized trial. J Clin Oncol 2002;20:4181–90.
82. Schadendorf D, Ugurel S, Schuler-Thurner B, et al. DC study group of the De-COG Dacarbazin (DTIC) versus vaccination with autologous peptide-pulsed dendritic cells (DC) in first-line treatment of patients with metastatic melanoma: a randomized phase III trial of the DC study group of the DeCOG. Ann Oncol 2006;17:563–70.

Index

Note: Page numbers of article titles are in **boldface** type.

Surg Clin N Am 89 (2009) 283–294
doi:10.1016/S0039-6109(09)00010-3
0039-6109/09/$ – see front matter © 2009 Elsevier Inc. All rights reserved.

surgical.theclinics.com

Moving?

Make sure your subscription moves with you!

To notify us of your new address, find your **Clinics Account Number** (located on your mailing label above your name), and contact customer service at:

E-mail: elspcs@elsevier.com

800-654-2452 (subscribers in the U.S. & Canada)
314-453-7041 (subscribers outside of the U.S. & Canada)

Fax number: 314-523-5170

Elsevier Periodicals Customer Service
11830 Westline Industrial Drive
St. Louis, MO 63146

*To ensure uninterrupted delivery of your subscription, please notify us at least 4 weeks in advance of move.

Printed and bound by CPI Group (UK) Ltd, Croydon, CR0 4YY

03/10/2024

01040453-0010